The Role of Epiglottis in Obstructive Sleep Apnea

Springer Nature More Media App

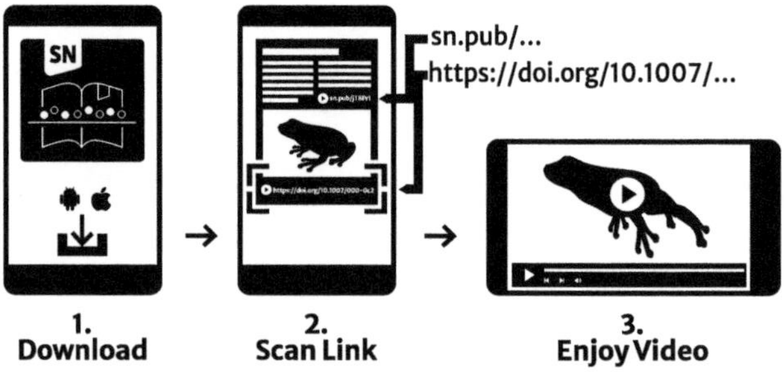

Support: customerservice@springernature.com

Matej Delakorda • Nico de Vries
Editors

The Role of Epiglottis in Obstructive Sleep Apnea

Springer

Editors
Matej Delakorda
General Hospital Celje
Celje, Slovenia

Nico de Vries
Jan Tooropstraat
Onze Lieve Vrouwe Gasthuis
Amsterdam, The Netherlands

ISBN 978-3-031-34991-1 ISBN 978-3-031-34992-8 (eBook)
https://doi.org/10.1007/978-3-031-34992-8

This Springer imprint is published by the registered company Springer Nature Switzerland AG
The registered company address is: Gewerbestrasse 11, 6330 Cham, Switzerland

Paper in this product is recyclable.

To my parents for teaching me how
To my wife for showing me why
To my children for making it worth it
—Matej Delakorda, Celje

This book is dedicated to my wife Judith and
our wonderful kids David, Lisa, and Maurits.
—Nico de Vries, Amsterdam

Foreword

Dear Colleague,

Thanks for choosing this book and for reading this foreword. I'll try to explain why in my opinion you have made a good decision to study this book. As an expert in sleep medicine and sleep surgery you are aware that the epiglottis has become an area of interest in this field. Many years ago, we used to focus in particular on the nose, the palate, the tongue, and the facial bone framework, while the epiglottis as a source of obstruction was mostly neglected. There might be several reasons for this: in the first place, the epiglottis is not visualized by standard physical examination, as performed by pulmonologists and neurologists; it is mostly diagnosed by drug-induced sleep endoscopy. Secondly, it was until recently regarded as a rare phenomenon. In the last place, most OSA care givers would reason that epiglottis collapse, if present anyhow, would be effectively treated by CPAP. This probably explains both the apathy in the sleep community regarding the epiglottis and the relatively low number of papers on this topic in the sleep surgery literature. This book however indicates that epiglottis collapse is not rare at all, it discusses different ways to diagnose it, and that epiglottis collapse in fact might be a reason for CPAP failure. The increasing amount of worldwide clinical data seems to disclose an underevaluated problem, and epiglottis collapse might very well be much more prevalent than we used to think. Moreover, the pathophysiology of epiglottis instability and collapse, primary or secondary, may explain many challenging and not well-understood situations (e.g., unexpected and unexplained CPAP failures, residual OSA after upper airway surgery, etc.) in the daily practice. This book is intended as another contribution in helping you to build a better understanding of the role of the epiglottis in upper airway collapse during sleep. Most of the available basic and advanced data is organized in a logical sequence, giving you the possibility to get into the problem in a very smooth and comprehensive way. After a general introductory overview of the problem about definition, epidemiology, pathogenesis, and outcome definitions, several main sections are expanded. A first section is devoted to the proper identification of epiglottis dysfunction during sleep. Clinical and endoscopical information is discussed within a wide range of additional options (sleep studies, DISE, imaging and manometry) in order to build up a sound diagnostic approach workup. Some situations that deserve special attention are described in detail for their relative more complex profile: epiglottis collapse in childhood (laryngomalacia), the role of obesity in epiglottis collapse, and the role of the nose as related to hypopharyngeal obstructions. The last couple of chapters are intended to highlight the great variety of treatment options, conservative and surgical, in a comprehensive, detailed and critical way. CPAP therapy, myofunctional therapy, oral appliances, and positional therapy are described in the nonsurgical section. All the state-of-the-art updated surgical techniques are a matter of discussion in a special section. Last but not least, the long experience and competence of all authors in the field of sleep disorders makes this book a real treasure of knowledge and an useful compass in the still dark sea of epiglottis collapse in OSA. Enjoy the lecture.

Department of Otolaryngology and Head-Neck Surgery
Morgagni-Pierantoni Hospital,
Forlì, Italy
Claudio Vicini

Contents

Contributors

Ghizlane Aarab, DDS, PhD Department of Orofacial Pain and Dysfunction, Academic Center for Dentistry Amsterdam (ACTA), University of Amsterdam and Vrije Universiteit Amsterdam, Amsterdam, The Netherlands

Mohamed Abdelwahab, MD, PhD Sleep Surgery Division, Department of Otolaryngology Head and Neck Surgery, Medical University of South Carolina, Charleston, SC, USA

Rakha Abdelwahab, MD, PhD Department of Otolaryngology, Head and Neck Surgery, School of Medicine, Mansoura University, Mansoura, Egypt

Vikas Agrawal, MD, MBBS, MS, DORL, FCPS Speciality ENT Hospital, Mumbai, Maharashtra, India

Muhammad Firas Alhammad, MBBCH Department of Anaesthesia, ICU and Perioperative Medicine, Hamad Medical Corporation, Doha, Qatar

Marco Barbieri, MD ENT Dept. IRCCS Ospedale Policlinico San Martino, Genoa, Italy

Department of Surgical Sciences and Integrated Diagnostics (DISC), University of Genoa, Genoa, Italy

Robson Capasso, MD, FAASM Division of Sleep Surgery, Department of Otolaryngology-Head & Neck Surgery, Stanford University Medical Center, Stanford, CA, USA

A. Simon Carney, BSc, MB ChB, FRCS, FRACS, DM College of Medicine and Public Health, Flinders University, Adelaide, Australia

Adelaide Institute for Sleep Health, Flinders University, Adelaide, Australia

Joana Vaz de Castro, MD, Phd ISAMB, Medicine of University of Lisbon, Lisbon, Portugal

Centro de Electroencefalografia e Neurofisiologia Clínica (CENC), Lisbon, Portugal

Comprehensive Health Research Centre - CHRC, Lisbon, Portugal

Peter G. Catcheside, PhD, BSc(Hons), CRFS College of Medicine and Public Health, Flinders University, Adelaide, Australia

Adelaide Institute for Sleep Health, Flinders University, Adelaide, Australia

Peter A. Cistulli, MD, PhD, MBA, FRACP Centre for Sleep Health and Research, Royal North Shore Hospital, Sydney, NSW, Australia

Charles Perkins Centre, The University of Sydney, Sydney, NSW, Australia

Abdulrahman Dardeer, FCAI, MCAI, ABHS-AIC Department of Anaesthesia, ICU and Perioperative Medicine, Hamad Medical Corporation, Doha, Qatar

Matej Delakorda, MD, PhD General Hospital Celje, Celje, Slovenia

Danny J. Eckert, PhD College of Medicine and Public Health, Flinders University, Adelaide, Australia

Adelaide Institute for Sleep Health, Flinders University, Adelaide, Australia

Marco Fragale, MD Department of Medical and Surgical Sciences and Advanced Technologies "GF Ingrassia", ENT Section, University of Catania, Catania, Italy

Michael Friedman, MD, FACS Division of Sleep Surgery, Department of Otolaryngology-Head and Neck Surgery, Rush University Medical Center, Chicago, IL, USA

Department of Otolaryngology, Advanced Center for Specialty Care, Advocate Illinois Masonic Medical Center, Chicago, IL, USA

Clemens Heiser, MD, PhD, MHBA Department of Otorhinolaryngology, Head and Neck Surgery, Klinikum Rechts der Isar, Technical University of Munich, Munich, Germany

Translational Neurosciences, University of Antwerp, Antwerp, Belgium

Simon D. Herkenrath, MD Department of Pneumology at the Protestant Hospital Bergisch Gladbach, Solingen, Germany

Antonius A. J. Hilgevoord, MD, PhD Department of Clinical Neurophysiology, OLVG, Amsterdam, The Netherlands

Jean-Pierre T.F. Ho, MD, DDS Department of Oral and Maxillofacial Surgery, Amsterdam UMC and Academic Centre for Dentistry Amsterdam (ACTA), University of Amsterdam, Amsterdam, The Netherlands

Department of Oral and Maxillofacial Surgery, Northwest Clinics, Alkmaar, The Netherlands

Zhengfei Huang, DMD, MSc Department of Clinical Neurophysiology, OLVG, Amsterdam, The Netherlands

Stacey L. Ishman, MD, MPH Division of Pediatric Otolaryngology-Head and Neck Surgery, Cincinnati Children's Hospital Medical Center, Cincinnati, OH, USA

Srinivas Kishore, MD, MBBS, MS AIG Hospitals, Hyderabad, Telangana, India

Bhik T. Kotecha, MBBCh, MPhil, FRCS, DLO Nuffield Health Brentwood, Essex, UK

Vijaya Krishnan, MD, MBBS, DNB, DLO, MNAMS Department of Snoring & Sleep Disorders, Madras ENT Research Foundation, Chennai, Tamil Nadu, India

Jan de Lange, MD, DDS, PhD Department of Oral and Maxillofacial Surgery, Amsterdam UMC and Academic Centre for Dentistry Amsterdam (ACTA), University of Amsterdam, Amsterdam, The Netherlands

Mickey Leentjens, MD Department of Otorhinolaryngology, OLVG, Location West, Amsterdam, The Netherlands

Federico Leone, MD Unit of Otorhinolaryngology – Head and Neck Surgery – Snoring and OSA Research Centre, Humanitas San Pio X, Milan, Italy

Hsin-Ching Lin, MD, FACS Department of Otolaryngology, Kaohsiung Chang Gung Memorial Hospital, Kaohsiung, Taiwan

Sleep Center, Robotic Surgery Center, Center for Quality Management, Kaohsiung Chang Gung Memorial Hospital, Kaohsiung, Taiwan

College of Medicine, Chang Gung University, Taoyuan and Kaohsiung, Taiwan

Department of Business Management and Institute of Biomedical Science, Institute of Healthcare Management, National Sun Yat-sen University, Kaohsiung, Taiwan

Russell Chung-Wei Lin, MD Department of Otolaryngology, Kaohsiung Chang Gung Memorial Hospital, Kaohsiung, Taiwan

Marina Carrasco-Llatas, MD, PhD, AP Department of Otorhinolaringology, Hospital Universitario Dr. Peset, Valencia, Spain

Department of Otorhinolaryngology, IMED Hospital, Valencia, Spain

Frank Lobbezoo, DDS, PhD Department of Orofacial Pain and Dysfunction, Academic Center for Dentistry Amsterdam (ACTA), University of Amsterdam and Vrije Universiteit Amsterdam, Amsterdam, The Netherlands

Blaz Maver, MD General Hospital Celje, Celje, Slovenia

Davide Mocellin, MD IRCCS Ospedale Policlinico San Martino, Genoa, Italy

ENT Dept., Ospedale S.Paolo, Savona, Italy

Filippo Montevecchi, MD Forlì Private Hospitals, Forlì, Italy

Carlos O'Connor Reina, MD, PhD Head of Otorhinolaryngology Department in Hospital Quironsalud, Marbella, Spain

Eli Van de Perck, MD, PhD Department of Otolaryngology – Head and Neck Surgery, Antwerp University Hospital, Edegem, Belgium

Christel A. L. de Raaff, MD, PhD Department of Albert Schweitzer Hospital, Dordrecht, The Netherlands

Winfried J. Randerath, MD, FCCP, FATS, FAASM Internal Medicine, Cardiology and Sleep Medicine, Bethanien Hospitzal, Clinic of Pneumology and Allergology, Center for Sleep Medicine and Respiratory Care, Institute of Pneumology at the University of Cologne, Solingen, Germany

Internal Medicine, Pneumology, Allergology, Sleep Medicine, Palliative Medicine, Bethanien Hospital Clinic of Pneumology and Allergology, Center for Sleep Medicine and Respiratory Care, Institute of Pneumology at the University of Cologne, Valencia, Spain

Madeline J. L. Ravesloot, MD, PhD, MSc Department of Otorhinolaryngology, OLVG, location West, Amsterdam, The Netherlands

Fabrizio Salamanca, MD Unit of Otorhinolaryngology – Head and Neck Surgery – Snoring and OSA Research Centre, Humanitas San Pio X, Milan, Italy

Department of Biomedical Sciences, Humanitas University, Milan, Italy

Nabil A. Shallik, MD, MSc Department of Anaesthesia, ICU and Perioperative Medicine, Hamad Medical Corporation, Doha, Qatar

Department of Clinical Anesthesiology, Weill Cornell Medical College in Qatar, Al Rayyan, Qatar

Department of Clinical Anesthesiology, Qatar University, Doha, Qatar

Ashley L. Soaper, MD Division of Pediatric Otolaryngology-Head and Neck Surgery, Cincinnati Children's Hospital Medical Center, Cincinnati, OH, USA

Olivier M. Vanderveken, MD, PhD Department of Otolaryngology—Head and Neck Surgery, Antwerp University Hospital, Edegem, Belgium

Faculty of Medicine and Health Sciences, University of Antwerp, Wilrijk, Belgium

Johan Verbraecken, MD, PhD Department of Pulmonary Medicine and Multidisciplinary Sleep Disorders Center, Antwerp University Hospital, Edegem, Belgium

University of Antwerp, Antwerp, Belgium

Thomas Verse, MD, PhD Department for Otorhinolaryngology, Head and Neck Surgery, Asklepios Klinikum Hamburg, Asklepios Campus, Hamburg, Germany

Claudio Vicini, MD Department of Otolaryngology and Head-Neck Surgery, Morgagni-Pierantoni Hospital, Forlì, Italy

Patty E. Vonk, MD, PhD Department of Otorhinolaryngology, Academic Medical Center Amsterdam, Amsterdam, The Netherlands

Nico de Vries, MD, PhD Jan Tooropstraat, Onze Lieve Vrouwe Gasthuis, Amsterdam, The Netherlands

Cynthia S. Wang, MD Division of Pediatric Otolaryngology-Head and Neck Surgery, Cincinnati Children's Hospital Medical Center, Cincinnati, OH, USA

Markus Wirth, MD Department of Otolaryngology Head and Neck Surgery, Technical University Munich, Munich, Germany

Department of Orofacial Pain and Dysfunction, Academic Center for Dentistry Amsterdam (ACTA), University of Amsterdam and Vrije Universiteit Amsterdam, Amsterdam, The Netherlands

Department of Otorhinolaryngology–Head and Neck Surgery, OLVG, Amsterdam, The Netherlands

Ning Zhou, MSc Department of Oral and Maxillofacial Surgery, Amsterdam UMC and Academic Centre for Dentistry Amsterdam (ACTA), University of Amsterdam, Amsterdam, The Netherlands

Department of Orofacial Pain and Dysfunction, Academic Center for Dentistry Amsterdam (ACTA), University of Amsterdam and Vrije Universiteit Amsterdam, Amsterdam, The Netherlands

List of Videos

Part I

Introduction to OSA

OSA Epidemiology

1

Hsin-Ching Lin, Russell Chung-Wei Lin, and Michael Friedman

1.1 Introduction

Obstructive sleep apnea (OSA) is characterized by repetitive obstruction(s) of the upper airway and arousal. OSA often results in episodic hypoxemia and abnormal activation of the nocturnal sympathetic nervous system during sleep. Untreated OSA is strongly associated with poor quality of life in nighttime and daytime as well as an increase in cardio- and cerebro-vascular disorders [1–3].

The nighttime symptoms of OSA, such as habitual snoring, witnessed sleep apneas, choking/gasping, restless sleep, frequent arousals, bruxism, night sweats, gastroesophageal reflux, and frequent nocturia, are commonly reported by the

H.-C. Lin (✉)
Department of Otolaryngology, Kaohsiung Chang Gung Memorial Hospital, Kaohsiung, Taiwan

Sleep Center, Robotic Surgery Center, Center for Quality Management, Kaohsiung Chang Gung Memorial Hospital, Kaohsiung, Taiwan

College of Medicine, Chang Gung University, Taoyuan and Kaohsiung, Taiwan

Department of Business Management and Institute of Biomedical Science, Institute of Healthcare Management, National Sun Yat-sen University, Kaohsiung, Taiwan
e-mail: hclin@adm.cgmh.org.tw

R. C.-W. Lin
Department of Otolaryngology, Kaohsiung Chang Gung Memorial Hospital, Kaohsiung, Taiwan

M. Friedman
Division of Sleep Surgery, Department of Otolaryngology-Head and Neck Surgery, Rush University Medical Center, Chicago, IL, USA

Department of Otolaryngology, Advanced Center for Specialty Care, Advocate Illinois Masonic Medical Center, Chicago, IL, USA

M. Delakorda, N. de Vries (eds.), *The Role of Epiglottis in Obstructive Sleep Apnea*, https://doi.org/10.1007/978-3-031-34992-8_1

patients and their bed-partners when they visit the sleep-related clinic. The daytime symptoms of OSA, which may not be recognized by the patients themselves as OSA-induced problems, include excessive daytime sleepiness (EDS)/hypersomnolence, morning headache, neurocognitive impairment, vigilance, motor coordination, mood and personality changes, depression, anxiety, irritability, sexual dysfunction, and so on.

Common risk factors for OSA include obesity (the most important risk factor), upper airway abnormalities, male gender, menopause, and age [4, 5]. Numerous characteristic findings of physical signs from the nasal cavity, pharyngeal space, and craniofacial structure could be significantly associated with upper airway obstruction in suspected OSA patients. Some of them require complex measurements with flexible fiberoptic observations or radiographs, whereas other measures will change in response to maneuvers, such as using a flexible nasopharyngoscopy with the Müller maneuver. These signs of OSA are obesity, increased neck circumference, retrognathia (a.k.a. mandibular retroposition), nasal valves narrowing, deviation of the septum, turbinate hypertrophy, adenoid hypertrophy, short lingual frenulum, macroglossia (often associated with lateral lingual scalloping by adjacent teeth), tonsil hypertrophy, redundant peripharyngeal tissue and soft palate, high arched palate, elongated uvula, higher Friedman tongue position (intraoral tongue position relative to the palatal degree of exposure) [6], prominent lateral pharyngeal walls, floppy epiglottis, etc..

Although the understanding of OSA's entirety and its impact on healthcare still continues to evolve and remain challenging, it is clear that OSA is an important cause of morbidity and mortality. Intermittent hypoxemia (IH) of OSA is now being recognized as a potentially major factor contributing to the pathogenesis of OSA-related comorbidities [7]. IH can promote oxidative stress by increased production of reactive oxygen species and angiogenesis, increased sympathetic activation with blood pressure elevation, and systemic and vascular inflammation with endothelial dysfunction. Data from observational studies in large population groups support the role of hypoxia in the pathogenesis of OSA comorbidity as well.

OSA is well recognized as an independent risk factor for cardiometabolic comorbidities, such as hypertension, coronary heart disease, arrhythmia, stroke, and metabolic disorders (e.g., diabetes and dyslipidemia). Traditionally, patients suffering from more severe OSA, longer time of sleep apneas/hypopneas, frequent nocturnal hypoxemia, and worse sleep quality are more likely to develop cardiometabolic comorbidities and neurocognitive decline [8]. The neurobehavioural morbidities of daytime sleepiness and impaired cognitive function may contribute to motor vehicle and job-related accidents [9, 10].

In addition, OSA significantly increases the risk of stroke or death from any cause; in an observational cohort study with 1022 community-based patients, moderate to severe sleep apnea is independently associated with a significantly increased risk of all-cause mortality [11].

OSA patients also commonly contend with comorbid psychiatric conditions, including depression, insomnia, and anxiety. The most common mood disorder associated with OSA is depression. Comprehensive reviews report increased rates of depression of 20–63% in patients with OSA based on a variety of screening questionnaires to determine diagnosis [11]. Dysfunctional sleep in OSA facilitates the development of insomnia by repeated awakenings during sleep. Insomnia causes sleep fragmentations that may then negatively impact the muscle tone of the upper airway, which will induce further airway collapse and vice versa [12].

As sleep surgeons/otolaryngologists, we have the responsibility to screen patients for both symptoms and signs of OSA and the possibility of OSA-related comorbidities. As experts in the upper airway, we could often view an airway clearly and identify the possible collapsed/obstructed lesion site(s) of OSA patients via scopic and imaging assistance. We all know that the most important factor for the success of OSA treatment, especially in OSA surgery, is patient selection, which includes the subjective patient's perception and exception, as well as upper airway lesion site(s) identification and treatment per adequate tools and procedures. OSA treatments over the hypopharyngeal region are usually challenging for the majority of sleep physicians. Additionally, the literature data on the obstructive site(s) that may influence procedure selection and treatment outcome are relatively limited. This chapter presents an overview of the role of the epiglottis in OSA, especially in epidemiology.

1.2 Brief Diagnostic Tools and Methods for Epiglottis Collapse

Looseness and instability of the epiglottis are commonly and well discussed in the pediatric literature as one of the possible causes of congenital laryngomalacia; however, the adult form is rarely described [12]. As we know, a variety of methods can be used to assess the anatomical locations of upper airway obstruction, but none can be considered a standard diagnostic method. In the literature, study tools for examining the epiglottis in patients with snoring with/without OSA include awake flexible nasoendoscopy, drug-induced sleep endoscopy (DISE), imaging and cephalometric study, snoring sound analysis, and so on. The majority of physicians are familiar with the scopic and imaging studies.

Fujita [13], Moore [14], and Friedman [6] proposed clinical systems for the classification of upper airway collapse, respectively. These classifications had some roles in predicting OSA surgical outcomes and are helpful in selecting the OSA patients who could benefit from a multilevel surgery of the upper airway. However, these common clinical evaluation methods are still limited in the awake state as well as subjectively mentioned the epiglottis status. In 1991, Croft and Pringle [15] described sleep nasendoscopy, a more realistic 3-D method for evaluating the upper airway under pharmacologically induced sleep. Currently, this technique is well known as drug-induced sleep endoscopy (DISE). Although DISE has been commonly used, the laxity of the epiglottis in OSA has been found to occur more frequently than previously described in the literature (see Chap. 8) [16, 17]. However, there is currently a lack of good evidence about the relationship between epiglottis collapse and OSA severity, knowledge regarding the role of the epiglottis in adult

OSA and snoring patients, and the most suitable diagnostic tools and treatment procedures for the epiglottis are still limited.

1.3 Prevalence of Epiglottis Collapse

In 1998, epiglottis collapse during sleep was first reported in adult OSA patients by Catalfumo et al. [18]. They evaluated 104 patients with persistent OSA after undergoing uvulopalatopharyngoplasty (UPPP) with awake flexible fibroscopy and found that 11.5% of the patients had an abnormal position of the epiglottis because it was retrodisplaced against the posterior pharyngeal wall at the level of the hypopharynx during inspiration.

In 2000, Golz et al. [19] found that 27 out of 187 patients examined by fiberoptic nasopharyngolaryngoscopy during night sleep were found to have narrowing to various degrees of the laryngeal inlet due to an abnormal epiglottis or its abnormal backward displacement against the posterior pharyngeal wall.

In 2011, Ravesloot et al. [20] reported the DISE findings on 100 consecutive OSA patients and found that 12% and 16% of the patients had partial and complete antero-posterior (AP) collapse, respectively. There were 2% and 8% of their patients with partial and complete lateral collapse, respectively.

In 2012, Koutsourelakis et al. [21] evaluated OSA patients by using DISE before the surgery and found that 27 (55.1%) and 7 (14.3%) of their 49 patients had complete and partial epiglottic AP collapse, respectively.

In 2013, Lin et al. [22] evaluated the efficacy of tongue base resection via transoral robotic surgery (TORS) in 12 OSA patients. Before the procedure, they performed DISE and found that 31% of their patients had obvious epiglottic AP collapse.

In 2013, Cavaliere et al. [16] compared the degrees and patterns of airway obstruction in awake endoscopy vs. DISE in 66 patients with OSA. They found that 22.7% (15/66) of patients had epiglottis collapse that was not identified during the awake status. In their results, nine (13.6%) of their 66 patients had AP collapse and 9.1% (6/66) had lateral collapse.

In 2014, Fernandez-Julian et al. [23] compared surgical decisions in 162 patients based on DISE vs. awake clinical evaluations (Friedman staging system, lateral cephalometry, and the Müller maneuver). The authors found that during DISE, the epiglottis was overall involved and contributed to upper airway obstruction in 36.4% ($n = 59$) of patients. The detection of epiglottis collapse by clinical examination, lateral cephalometry, and Müller maneuver was 24%, 25%, and 28%, respectively.

In 2014, Zhang et al. [24] evaluated the associations between the findings of DISE and upper airway computed tomography (UACT) in 62 male patients with OSA. Their results were that 9.7% ($n = 6$) had epiglottis collapse in DISE, but that none of the UACT measurements significantly differed between subjects with and without epiglottis collapse.

In 2014, Dedhia et al. [25] systematically reviewed 17 articles supporting the role of the larynx in adult OSA. Their results showed that primary epiglottic obstruction in the hypopharynx represents 15% of 515 patients with OSA unable to tolerate continuous positive airway pressure therapy (CPAP). In the enrolled patients, OSA was associated with neuromuscular disorders, anatomic abnormalities, head and neck cancer, and so on.

In 2015, Lan et al. [26] studied 64 OSA patients by DISE. They noted that 12.5% and 26.6% of the patients, respectively, had partial and complete AP epiglottis collapse by correlating DISE findings with BMI and PSG variables. Among them, there was no case having partial lateral epiglottis collapse; however, 3.1% of the patients had a complete lateral collapse.

In 2015, Kent et al. [27] studied OSA patients who were CPAP intolerant or had incomplete responses to oral appliances. They found that 31.4% (11/35) of the 35 studied patients had epiglottis collapse.

In 2015, Woodson conducted a study of 117 DISE investigations to identify the characteristics of the luminal airway by using visible landmarks identifiable on flexible endoscopy. He reported that 16% of patients had isolated obstruction caused by a ptotic epiglottis [17].

In 2016, Torre et al. [28] conducted a systematic review of epiglottis collapse in adult OSA. Year ranges for each of the databases were from the first year of each database through March 5, 2015. Their data suggest that the prevalence of epiglottis collapse in OSA is higher than previously described. The epiglottis has been implicated in 12% of cases of snoring. The prevalence of epiglottis collapse in OSA was wide ranging with prevalence, 9.7–73.5%.

In 2017, Genta et al. [29] conducted a study with 31 OSA patients with a pediatric endoscope and simultaneous nasal flow and pharyngeal pressure recordings during natural sleep. They noted that the epiglottis was a cause of pharyngeal obstruction in nine patients (29%), and the epiglottis was strongly associated with a severe degree of negative effort dependence (defined as the percent reduction in inspiratory flow from peak to plateau) and abrupt discontinuities in inspiratory flow. They also found that collapse at the epiglottis was typically intermittent of nature and often co-occurred with collapse at other upper airway levels.

In 2017, Azarbarzin et al. [30] demonstrated an alternative diagnostic tool that could identify epiglottic collapse with the airflow signal measured during a sleep study because diagnosing epiglottic collapse usually requires relatively invasive studies (imaging, endoscopy, or DISE). They studied 23 OSA patients who underwent natural sleep endoscopy. 1232 breaths were scored as epiglottic/nonepiglottic collapse. Several flow characteristics were determined from the flow signal (recorded simultaneously with endoscopy) and used to build a predictive model to distinguish epiglottic from non-epiglottic collapse. They found that epiglottic collapse was characterized by a rapid fall(s) in the inspiratory flow, more variable inspiratory and expiratory flows, and reduced tidal volume. Their cross-validated accuracy was 84%. Predictive features obtained from pneumotachograph flow and nasal pressure were strongly correlated. In their study, 244 (19.8%) of 1232 breaths in 23 OSA patients were classified as epiglottic collapse.

In 2021, Yui et al. [31] conducted a prospective, controlled clinical trial to identify possible characteristics related to low compliance with CPAP therapy due to respiratory complaints. With DISE, they noted that 61% of patients in group 1 ($n = 13$, patients trying to use CPAP for more than 12 months, but with difficulty in compliance due to respiratory symptoms) presented with partial or complete epiglottis collapse, while no patient in group 2 ($n = 6$, patients adapted to CPAP therapy without any complaint regarding the therapy for more than 12 months) presented obstruction at the epiglottis level.

In 2021, Kim et al. [32] performed an age-sex matched case-control study to analyze patients with epiglottic collapse, especially their clinical characteristics related to OSA and phenotype labeling using DISE. A total number of 522 patients underwent PSG and DISE during the 4 years' study period, 122 (23.4%) patients had epiglottic collapse. Among these 122 patients with epiglottic collapse, 106 (20.3%) patients showed epiglottic AP collapse, and 16 (3.1%) patients showed epiglottic lateral collapse. Additionally, their results showed that the body mass index was significantly lower in the group of patients with epiglottic collapse (Epi group). However, the AHI was lower in the Epi group, and the lowest oxygen saturation was significantly higher in the Epi group. The phenotype labeling on DISE showed that the prevalence of tongue-base collapse was higher in the Epi group as well as multilevel obstruction of the upper airway.

In 2021, Van den Bossche et al. [33] performed a systematic review on the role of natural sleep endoscopy in OSA patients after searching Medline, Web of Science, and the Cochrane Library up to January 31, 2021. Their results revealed an epiglottic collapse in 22.4% of patients (range: 11.5–29.0%, seven studies encompassing 143 patients) [29, 30, 34–38].

In 2021, Op de Beeck et al. [39] assessed the feasibility of concomitant flow shape analysis flow measurements during DISE by using a pneumotachograph to preliminarily assess correlations between negative effort dependence and upper airway collapse sites during DISE. Epiglottic collapse produced a sudden drop (i.e., discontinuity) in inspiratory airflow (associated with high negative effort dependence). Epiglottic collapse was found in 7 (46.7%) of 15 patients.

Literature on the prevalence of epiglottis collapse in patients with OSA is summarized in Table 1.1.

In addition to original cohort studies, there were several case reports that described OSA secondary to a floppy epiglottis, which could cause airway obstruction by collapsing into the laryngeal inlet during the inspiration even in the awake state [40–44].

Table 1.1 Summary of literature on the prevalence of epiglottis collapse in patients with OSA. *OSA* obstructive sleep apnea, *DISE* drug-induced sleep endoscopy

Author, Year	*N*	% of Epiglottis Collapse	Evaluation Tool(s)
Catalfumo et al. [18] 1998	104	11.5%	Awake flexible fibroscopy
Golz et al. [19] 2000	187	14.4%	Fiberoptic nasopharyngolaryngoscopy during night sleep
Ravesloot et al. [20] 2011	100	38%	DISE
Koutsourelakis et al. [21] 2012	49	69.4%	DISE
Lin et al. [22] 2013	12	31%	DISE
Cavaliere et al. [16] 2013	66	22.7%	Awake endoscopy and DISE
Fernandez-Julian et al. [23] 2014	162	36%, 24%, 25%, and 28% with DISE, clinical examination, lateral cephalometry, and Müller maneuver, respectively	DISE and awake clinical evaluations
Zhang et al. [24] 2014	62	9.7%	DISE
Dedhia et al. [25] 2014	515	15%	Systematically reviewed 17 articles
Lan et al. [26] 2015	64	39.1%	DISE
Kent et al. [27] 2015	35	31.4%	DISE
Woodson [17], 2015	117	16%	DISE
Torre, et al. [28] 2016	888	9.7% ~ 73.5%.	Systematic review of 38 studies
Genta, et al. [29] 2017	31	29%	Nasal flow and pharyngeal pressure recordings during natural sleep
Azarbarzin et al. [30] 2017	23	19.8%	Airflow signal measured during a sleep study
Yui, et al. [31] 2021	19	61%	DISE
Kim et al. [32] 2021	522	23.4%	DISE
Van den Bossche et al. [33] 2021	143	22.4%	DISE
OP de Beeck et al. [39] 2021	15	46.7%	DISE

1.4 Summary

Increasing studies have been reported over the past several decades focusing on the role of the epiglottis in OSA. Although the study findings are limited, they clearly show evidence of the epiglottis contributing to the pathophysiology of OSA. All sleep physicians, especially sleep surgeons, should better understand and characterize this involute relationship and then may explore more adequate diagnosis and treatment strategies.Competing Interests/Financial Disclosure**Dr. Hsin-Ching Lin** received research grants from *Intuitive Surgical Inc., Sunnyvale, CA, USA*. However, *Intuitive Surgical Inc.* had no role in the design or conduct of this chapter.

References

1. Marin JM, Agusti A, Villar I, et al. Association between treated and untreated obstructive sleep apnea and risk of hypertension. JAMA. 2012;307:2169–76.
2. Shahar E, Whitney CW, Redline S, et al. Sleep-disordered breathing and cardiovascular disease: cross-sectional results of the sleep heart health study. Am J Respir Crit Care Med. 2001;163:19–25.
3. Yaggi HK, Concato J, Kernan WN, et al. Obstructive sleep apnea as a risk factor for stroke and death. N Engl J Med. 2005;353:2034–41.
4. Young T, Palta M, Dempsey J, et al. The occurrence of sleep-disordered breathing among middle-aged adults. N Engl J Med. 1993;328:1230–5.
5. Young T, Finn L, Austin D, et al. Menopausal status and sleep-disordered breathing in the Wisconsin sleep cohort study. Am J Respir Crit Care Med. 2003;167:1181–5.
6. Friedman M, Ibrahim H, Bass L. Clinical staging for sleep disordered breathing. Otolaryngol Head Neck Surg. 2002;127:13–21.
7. Dewan NA, Nieto FJ, Somers VK. Intermittent hypoxemia and OSA: implications for comorbidities. Chest. 2015;147:266–74.
8. André S, Andreozzi F, Van Overstraeten C, et al. Cardiometabolic comorbidities in obstructive sleep apnea patients are related to disease severity, nocturnal hypoxemia, and decreased sleep quality. Respir Res. 2020;21:35.
9. George CF, Nickerson PW, Hanly PJ, et al. Sleep apnea patients have more automobile accidents. Lancet. 1987;2:447.
10. Young T, Peppard PE, Gottlieb DJ. Epidemiology of obstructive sleep apnea: a population health perspective. Am J Respir Crit Care Med. 2002;165:1217–39.
11. Dhanda Patil R, Sarber KM. Sleep Apnea treatment considerations in patients with comorbidities. Otolaryngol Clin North Am. 2020;53:339–49.
12. Hey SY, Oozeer NB, Robertson S, et al. Adult-onset laryngomalacia: case reports and review of management. Eur Arch Otorhinolaryngol. 2014;271:3127–32.
13. Fujita S. Surgical treatment of obstructive sleep apnea: UPP and lingualplasty (laser midline glossectomy). In: Guilleminault C, Partinen M, editors. Obstructive sleep Apnea syndrome: clinical research and treatment. New York, NY: Raven Press; 1990. p. 129–51.
14. Moore KE, Phillips C. A practical method for describing patterns of tongue-base narrowing (modification of Fujita) in awake adult patients with obstructive sleep apnea. J Oral Maxillofac Surg. 2002;60:252–60.
15. Croft CB, Pringle M. Sleep nasendoscopy: a technique of assessment in snoring and obstructive sleep apnea. Clin Otolaryngol. 1991;16:504–9.
16. Cavaliere M, Russo F, Iemma M. Awake versus drug-induced sleep endoscopy: evaluation of airway obstruction in obstructive sleep apnea/hypopnoea syndrome. Laryngoscope. 2013;123:2315–8.
17. Woodson BT. A method to describe the pharyngeal airway. Laryngoscope. 2015;125:1233–8.
18. Catalfumo FJ, Golz A, Westerman ST, et al. The epiglottis and obstructive sleep apnoea syndrome. J Laryngol Otol. 1998;112:940–3.
19. Golz A, Goldenberg D, Westerman ST, et al. Laser partial epiglottidectomy as a treatment for obstructive sleep apnea and laryngomalacia. Ann Otol Rhinol Laryngol. 2000;109(12 Pt 1):1140–5.
20. Ravesloot MJ, de Vries N. One hundred consecutive patients undergoing drug-induced sleep endoscopy: results and evaluation. Laryngoscope. 2011;121:2710–6.
21. Koutsourelakis I, Safiruddin F, Ravesloot M, et al. Surgery for obstructive sleep apnea: sleep endoscopy determinants of outcome. Laryngoscope. 2012;122:2587–91.
22. Lin HS, Rowley JA, Badr MS, et al. Transoral robotic surgery for treatment of obstructive sleep apnea-hypopnea syndrome. Laryngoscope. 2013;123:1811–6.

23. Fernandez-Julian E, Garcia-Perez MA, Garcia-Callejo J, et al. Surgical planning after sleep versus awake techniques in patients with obstructive sleep apnea. Laryngoscope. 2014;124:1970–4.
24. Zhang P, Ye J, Pan C, et al. Comparison of drug-induced sleep endoscopy and upper airway computed tomography in obstructive sleep apnea patients. Eur Arch Otorhinolaryngol. 2014;271:2751–6.
25. Dedhia RC, Rosen CA, Soose RJ. What is the role of the larynx in adult obstructive sleep apnea? Laryngoscope. 2014;124:1029–34.
26. Lan MC, Liu SY, Lan MY, et al. Lateral pharyngeal wall collapse associated with hypoxemia in obstructive sleep apnea. Laryngoscope. 2015;125:2408–12.
27. Kent DT, Rogers R, Soose RJ. Drug-induced sedation endoscopy in the evaluation of OSA patients with incomplete oral appliance therapy response. Otolaryngol Head Neck Surg. 2015;153:302–7.
28. Torre C, Camacho M, Liu SY, et al. Epiglottis collapse in adult obstructive sleep apnea: a systematic review. Laryngoscope. 2016;126:515–23.
29. Genta PR, Sands SA, Butler JP, et al. Airflow shape is associated with the pharyngeal structure causing OSA. Chest. 2017;152:537–46.
30. Azarbarzin A, Marques M, Sands SA, et al. Predicting epiglottic collapse in patients with obstructive sleep apnoea. Eur Respir J. 2017;50:1700345.
31. Yui MS, Tominaga Q, Lopes BCP, et al. Can drug-induced sleep endoscopy (DISE) predict compliance with positive airway pressure therapy? A pilot study. Sleep Breath. 2022;26:109–16.
32. Kim HY, Sung CM, Jang HB, l. Patients with epiglottic collapse showed less severe obstructive sleep apnea and good response to treatment other than continuous positive airway pressure: a case-control study of 224 patients. J Clin Sleep Med. 2021;17:413–9.
33. Van den Bossche K, Van de Perck E, Kazemeini E, et al. Natural sleep endoscopy in obstructive sleep apnea: a systematic review. Sleep Med Rev. 2021;60:101534. https://doi.org/10.1016/j.smrv.2021.101534; Online ahead of print.
34. Marques M, Genta PR, Azarbarzin A, et al. Retropalatal and retroglossal airway compliance in patients with obstructive sleep apnea. Respir Physiol Neurobiol. 2018;258:98–103.
35. Marques M, Genta PR, Sands SA, et al. Effect of sleeping position on upper airway patency in obstructive sleep apnea is determined by the pharyngeal structure causing collapse. Sleep. 2017;40:zsx005. https://doi.org/10.1093/sleep/zsx005.
36. Ordones AB, Grad GF, Cahali MB, et al. Comparison of upper airway obstruction during zolpidem-induced sleep and propofol-induced sleep in patients with obstructive sleep apnea: a pilot study. J Clin Sleep Med. 2020;16:725–32.
37. Azarbarzin A, Sands SA, Marques M, et al. Palatal prolapse as a signature of expiratory flow limitation and inspiratory palatal collapse in patients with obstructive sleep apnoea. Eur Respir J. 2018;51:1701419. https://doi.org/10.1183/13993003.01419-2017.
38. Park D, Kim JS, Heo SJ. Obstruction patterns during drug-induced sleep endoscopy vs natural sleep endoscopy in patients with obstructive sleep apnea. JAMA Otolaryngol Head Neck Surg. 2019;145:730–4.
39. Op de Beeck S, Van de Perck E, Vena D, et al. Flow-identified site of collapse during drug-induced sleep endoscopy: feasibility and preliminary results. Chest. 2021;159:828–32.
40. Maurer JT, Stuck BA, Hein G, et al. Videoendoscopic assessment of uncommon sites of upper airway obstruction during sleep. Sleep Breath. 2000;4:131–6.
41. Chetty KG, Kadifa F, Berry RB, et al. Acquired laryngomalacia as a cause of obstructive sleep apnea. Chest. 1994;106:1898–9.
42. Andersen AP, Alving J, Lildholdt T, et al. Obstructive sleep apnea initiated by a lax epiglottis. A contraindication for continuous positive airway pressure. Chest. 1987;91:621–3.
43. Enoz M. UPPP failure due to lingual tonsils and epiglottal laxity. Sleep Med. 2006;7:660–1.
44. Woodson BT, Fujita S. Clinical experience with lingualplasty as part of the treatment of severe obstructive sleep apnea. Otolaryngol Head Neck Surg. 1992;107:40–8.

OSA Pathogenesis 2

A. Simon Carney, Peter G. Catcheside, and Danny J. Eckert

2.1 Patient Phenotyping/Endotyping

Obstructive sleep apnea (OSA) is a complex disorder for which a "one size fits all" treatment approach fails to successfully treat many patients [1, 2]. Evidence-based research now supports the hypothesis that there are at least four main traits ("endotypes" or "phenotypes") that contribute to an individual's propensity for, and the severity of, airway collapse during sleep [3] (Fig. 2.1). Whilst a narrow and/or collapsible airway remains the major factor for the majority of patients, other non-anatomical factors, such as poor airway dilator muscle activity, unstable central respiratory control ("high loop gain"), and a low respiratory arousal threshold can all play an important causal role in OSA [1]. Identification of the presence and magnitude of these non-anatomical factors is thus important to help determine which patients are likely to do well with upper airway surgery and, more importantly, to identify patients more likely to get a poor result and for whom other treatment modalities are likely to be more preferable [1].

2.1.1 Deficient Upper Airway Anatomy

There is no doubt that a narrow and/or collapsible upper airway is a key factor in the etiology of OSA for most patients [1]. Several established interventions including CPAP, dental appliances, and multi-level sleep surgery are all specifically directed

A. S. Carney (✉) · P. G. Catcheside · D. J. Eckert
College of Medicine and Public Health, Flinders University, Adelaide, Australia

Adelaide Institute for Sleep Health, Flinders University, Adelaide, Australia

M. Delakorda, N. de Vries (eds.), *The Role of Epiglottis in Obstructive Sleep Apnea*, https://doi.org/10.1007/978-3-031-34992-8_2

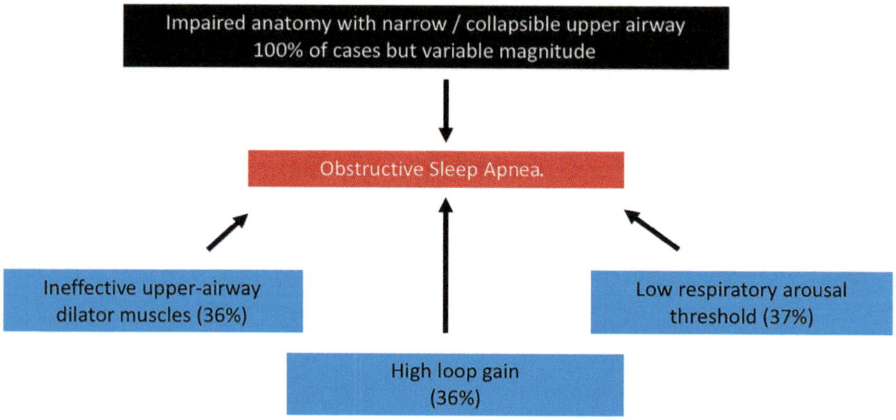

Fig. 2.1 Schematic diagram of the four main endotypes/phenotypes contributing to OSA

at resolving this problem [4]. Obesity causes increased fat deposition in the neck, pharyngeal muscles, the tongue, and abdomen, all of which may influence sleep via airway crowding, increased tissue mass, and reduced caudal tracheal traction effects. There is also evidence that the stiffness of the tongue, and potentially other airway structures, is reduced in patients with OSA [5].

Upper airway examination techniques such as Müller's maneuvre and Woodson's hypotonic method are now commonly used to help identify the site and degree of collapsibility in the awake patient [4], but they have their limitations and physicians are constantly in search of other techniques that may be more representative of the sites and degree of collapse during sleep.

The passive critical closing pressure (Pcrit) of the airway is defined as the pressure necessary to achieve total airway collapse during sleep and can be measured by the following technique. Wearing a modified CPAP device that can deliver both positive and negative pressures, the patient breathes with a fully patent airway (often requiring some degree of positive pressure) and relatively low breathing drive (and thus largely passive upper airway muscle activity). The pressure is then suddenly lowered with brief pressure drops that last at least 5 breaths. This protocol is ideally performed during non-REM sleep and is best used to induce different severities of partial airway collapse and airflow limitation, using variable positive and negative pressures as necessary. Repeated measurements can be obtained over the night, allowing a plot of average peak inspiratory flow vs. end-expiratory mask pressure. Extrapolation of the pressure versus flow relationship is performed to the point where it crosses the *x*-axis (i.e., with zero flow). This point identifies the Pcrit. Patients without OSA (or very mild airway collapse) usually show Pcrit below −2.0 cmH_2O. Moderately collapsible airways are defined as having a Pcrit at or close to atmospheric pressure (Pcrit between −2.0 and + 2.0 cmH_2O). Severely collapsible airways have a Pcrit above 2.0 cmH_2O, requiring more substantial pressure to maintain airway patency [6] (Fig. 2.2).

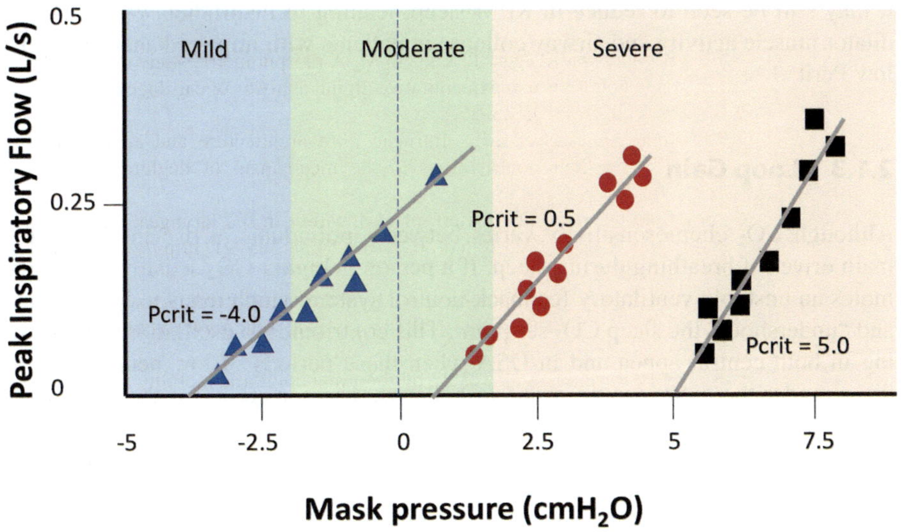

Fig. 2.2 Measurement of Pcrit. This figure shows three examples of Pcrit where multiple reductions in pressure were obtained. The point at which the regression line crosses the x-axis is used to define Pcrit

2.1.2 Muscle Responsiveness

The pharyngeal airway consists of several overlapping and inter-connected muscles. Control of this complex tube relies on coordinated neuromuscular activation via centrally controlled mechanisms to maintain airway patency [1]. Surrounding tissues can be affected by gravity and dynamic negative pressures act on the intraluminal airway throughout each breathing cycle. The two key muscular dilator muscles, genioglossus and tensor veli palatini, are activated via central neural control and reflex loops in response to respiration and, more importantly, changing airway pressure and collapse during sleep. In a normal airway, when sleep commences, genioglossus activity abruptly decreases with the loss of wake-related central control inputs, then throughout N2 to slow wave sleep there is a compensatory increase often to above wake levels [1]. Tonic muscles, such as tensor palatini, behave very differently and typically show an abrupt decrease in activity at sleep onset and throughout all phases of sleep. All skeletal muscles show quite profound hypotonia in REM sleep, explaining why OSA is typically most severe during this sleep phase. When CO_2 rises and O_2 reduces secondary to airway obstruction, we then see chemo-reflex augmentation of the drive to breathing and upper airway dilatory muscles. This, along with airway pressure changes, contributes to increased dilator muscle activity termed "muscle responsiveness," which varies across individuals. In over 33% of patient with OSA, genioglossus muscle responsiveness is low or absent. If muscle responsiveness is preserved during non-REM sleep (which protects the airway in patients with anatomical compromise and Pcrit < -5 cmH_2O), it may still be seen to reduce in REM sleep, leading to insufficient upper airway dilator muscle activity and airway collapse in patients with impaired anatomy and a low Pcrit.

2.1.3 Loop Gain

Although CO_2 chemosensitivity varies between individuals, a rise in CO_2 is the main driver of breathing during sleep. If a person is highly CO_2 sensitive, this promotes an unstable ventilatory feedback-control system which tends to “overshoot” and “undershoot” the sleep CO_2 set-point. This contributes to oscillations in breathing in both central apnea and in OSA when these periods of low neuromuscular drive render the airway more prone to collapse. The sensitivity of the ventilatory control system is described by the concept of “loop gain” which is the ratio of the magnitude of the bodies response to a ventilatory disturbance relative to the actual disturbance itself. Patients with high loop gain have large changes in breathing in response to relatively small changes in CO_2. Figure 2.3a) demonstrates the concept of high loop gain. A significant proportion of patients with OSA patients demonstrate high loop gain (33% in one particular study where loop gain was defined as 5 L/min increase to a normal 1 L/min stimulus) [1].

When patients who underwent multilevel upper airway surgery for OSA were investigated retrospectively, those with a lower loop gain achieved better outcomes from surgery than those with higher loop gain [7]. Whilst this does not necessarily

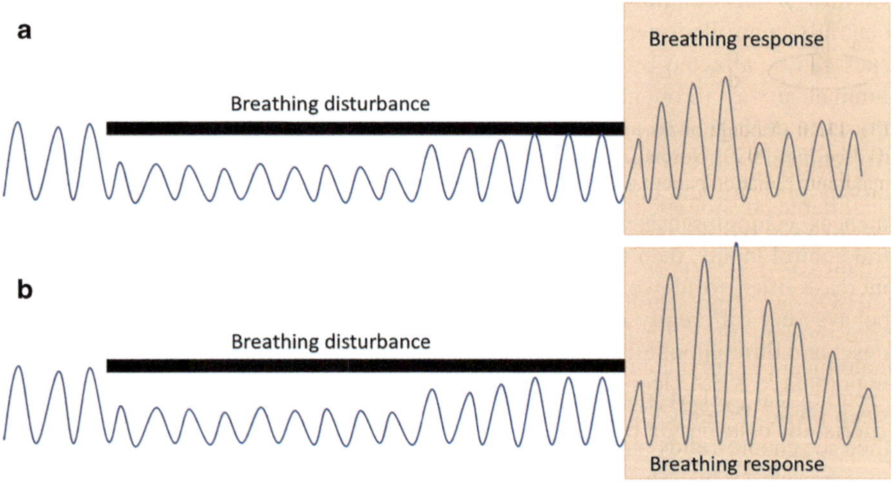

Fig. 2.3 Schematic representation of low (**a**) versus high (**b**) loop gain. After normal breathing, a reduction in CPAP occurs, creating a breathing disturbance. When breathing is restored, in (**a**), a slight increase occurs before settling back to steady state within a few breaths. In (**b**), breathing peaks of much higher magnitude are seen, taking longer to settle back to steady state normal breathing

mean that the patients with higher loop gain should be denied surgical intervention, loop gain is now established as one of several parameters that may be useful to consider in a multidisciplinary setting to help differentiate patients who are more likely to gain benefit from surgery [8]. This approach is critical to allow for better informed patient discussions, consent, and optimized patient outcomes.

2.1.4 Respiratory Arousal Threshold

It was long been presumed that cortical arousals were required to restore airflow after an obstructive event in patients with OSA. However, around 20% of such events in adults terminate without arousal [1]. This is higher in children (50%) and even more so in infants (>90%). In contrast, 20% of arousals only occur after airway patency is restored and airflow resumes, further establishing the independent nature of arousal and airflow recovery in a significant number of cases. The degree of inspiratory effort associated with respiratory-related arousal is termed the "respiratory arousal threshold." Between 30 and 50% of patients show arousal in response to quite small changes in negative intra-thoracic pressure (i.e., a low respiratory arousal threshold). This percentage is even higher in non-obese patients. In slow wave and deep sleep, the respiratory arousal threshold becomes elevated (harder to wake), which likely promotes raised inspiratory and upper airway dilator muscle activity. The majority of patients with OSA can usually achieve a proportion of deep sleep during which there are much fewer respiratory events [9]. However, in those patients with a low respiratory arousal threshold, frequent arousals can delay and even prevent progression to the deeper and more stable stages of sleep [1].

2.2 PALM Scale for Patient Phenotyping

The PALM (Pcrit, arousal threshold, loop gain, and muscle responsiveness) scale was developed to classify patients into groups aimed at directing targeted therapy to identifiable physiological deficits [1]. The various groups are identified according to the levels of Pcrit. PALM 1 (Pcrit > +2.0 cmH_2O) patients have severe anatomical collapse, PALM 2 (Pcrit −2.0 - +2.0 cmH_2O), moderate, and PALM 3 (Pcrit < −2.0 cmH_2O) only demonstrate minor anatomical problems. As PALM 2 is by far the largest group, this is further subdivided into PALM 2a with NO evidence of a non-anatomical phenotype and PALM 2b where patients have one or more of the other physiological ("ALM") features. In one study of 54 patients assessed using PALM criteria, the distribution of patients was as shown in Fig. 2.4.

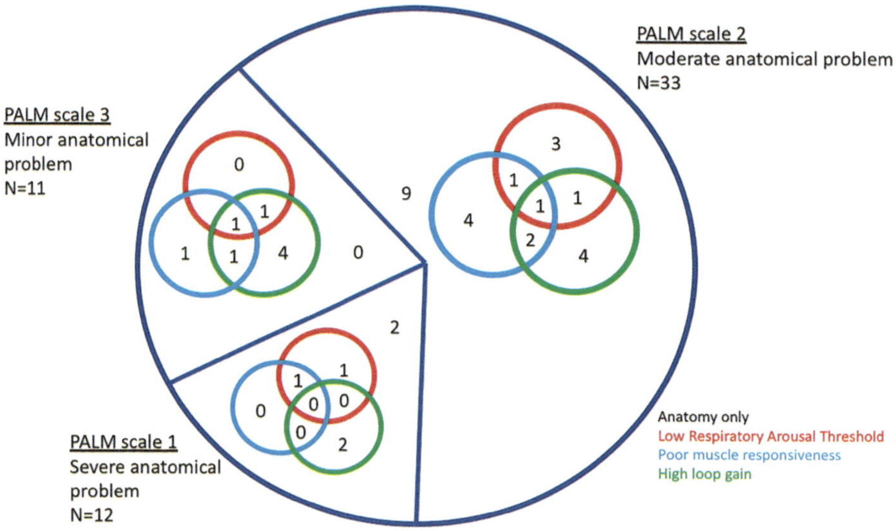

Fig. 2.4 A Venn diagram showing the overlap of the various OSA phenotypes in a study of 54 patients categorised into PALM scale

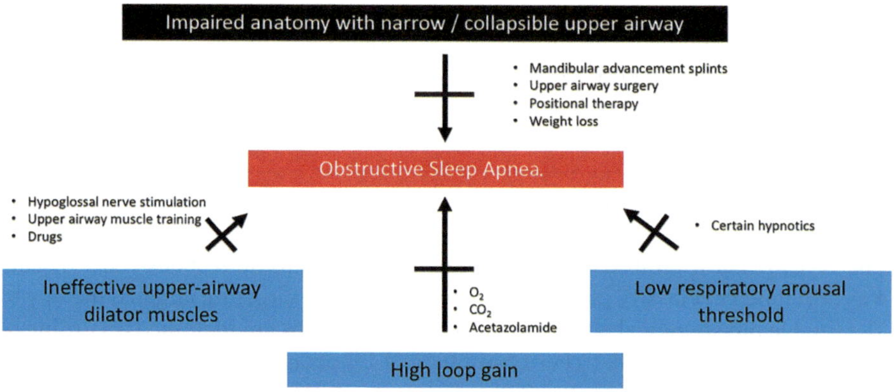

Fig. 2.5 Treatment methods applicable to OSA phenotypes

2.3 Phenotyping/Endotyping Conclusions

Patient phenotyping/endotyping is an exciting area for future research. It clearly identifies the need for multi-disciplinary input in order to identify patients most suitable for upper airway surgery [4] (or other alternative OSA treatments) when CPAP fails or is not tolerated (Fig. 2.5).

2.4 Analysis of Airflow Shape

Patients with OSA usually have narrowing or collapse in one or more anatomical areas [4]. During airway collapse, in natural sleep, the pattern of airflow reduction can be observed by using simultaneous nasal and pharyngeal pressure catheter recordings. In a study from Harvard Medical School researchers [10], 31 people with OSA were studied using airflow and pharyngeal pressure measurements and simultaneous nasendoscopic video. Amongst the group, it was possible to identify different patterns of inspiratory flow and negative effort dependence (reduced airflow despite increased respiratory effort), depending on the location of the predominant area of collapse. Different tracings occurred when collapse was in the retrolingual segment (flattened airflow pattern), the retropalatal segment (palatal movement associated with moderate negative effort dependence), or associated with lateral wall collapse. Very clear identification of epiglottic collapse was also possible [10]. With epiglottic collapse, a sudden obstruction of the airway (with a characteristic cessation of airflow) was observed (Figs. 2.6 and 2.7). Whilst these airflow

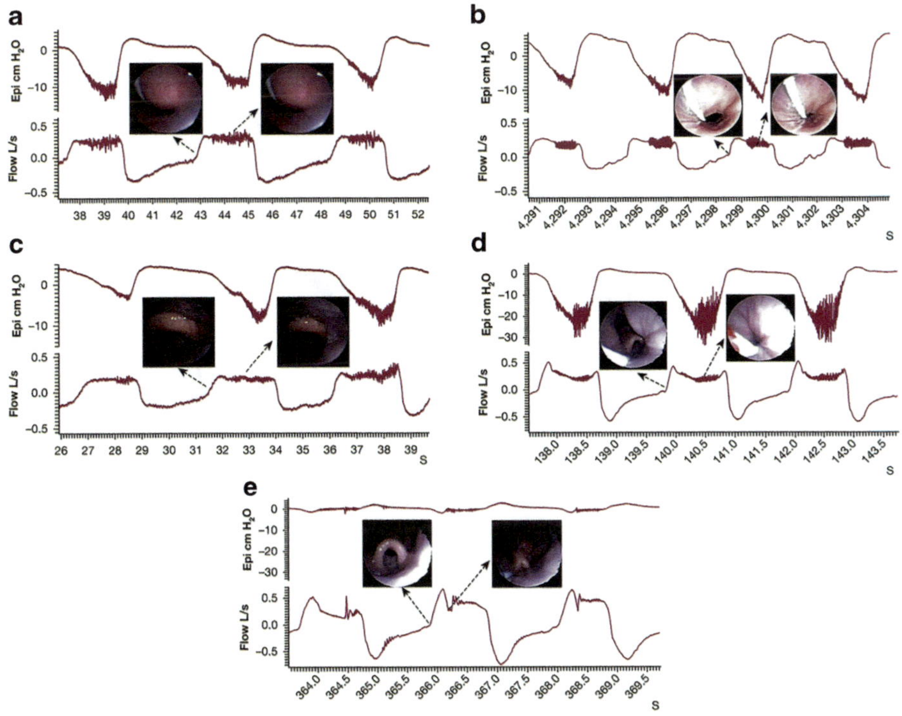

Fig. 2.6 Representation of flow shape and endoscopic images at different stages of respiration. (**a**, **b**) Velopharynx (**a**) and oropharynx (**b**) views of the same patient demonstrating retro-lingual collapse. (**c**, **d**) Isolated retro-palatal (**c**) and lateral wall (**d**) collapse in separate patients. (**e**) Epiglottic collapse with large and abrupt airflow changes (from Genta PR et al. Airflow Shape Is Associated With the Pharyngeal Structure Causing OSA. *Chest*. 2017, with permission)

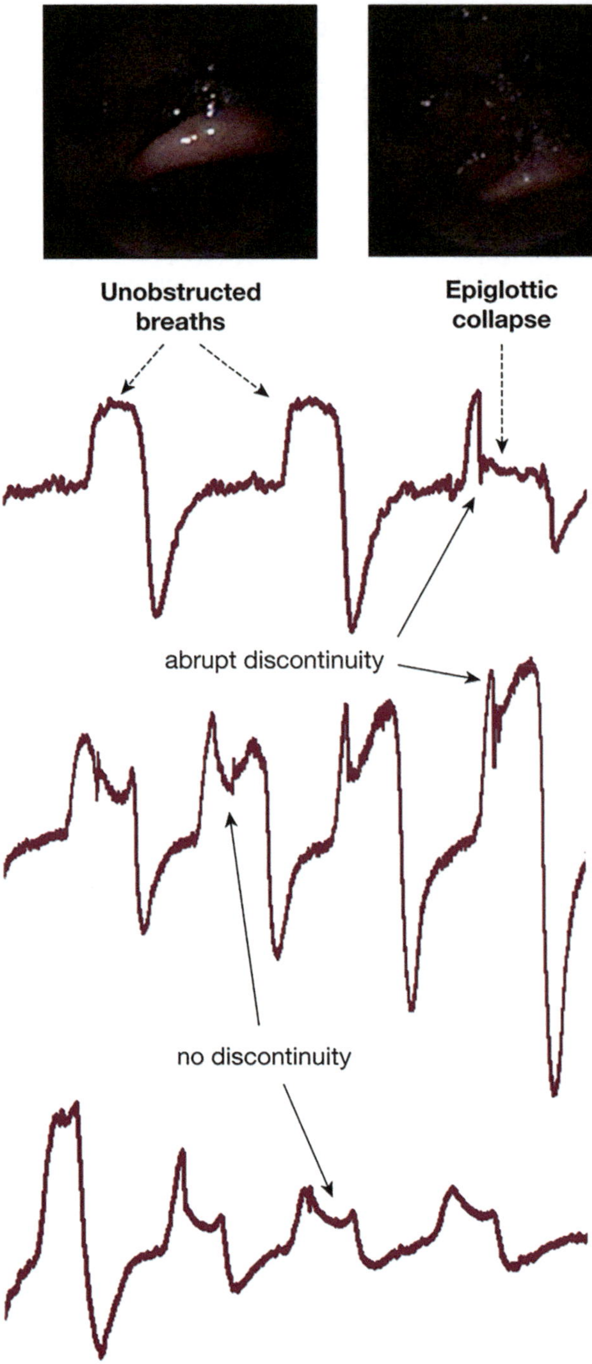

Fig. 2.7 Epiglottic collapse in different patients demonstrating a sudden abrupt discontinuity of airflow (from Genta PR et al. Airflow Shape Is Associated With the Pharyngeal Structure Causing OSA. *Chest*. 2017, with permission)

tracings are an important discovery, single versus multi-level collapse was not studied therefore the airflow patterns discovered in this paper may not yet be translatable into routine clinical practice. Nevertheless, they provide an important finding for future research in this area.

2.5 Conclusions

While single or multiple-site anatomical collapse is present to some extent in all OSA patients, muscle responsiveness, loop gain, and arousal threshold are key factors that contribute to OSA pathophysiology in at least 70% of patients. Individual patient phenotyping holds major future promise for identifying optimal treatment options and improving overall therapeutic outcomes.

References

1. Eckert DJ. Phenotypic approaches to obstructive sleep apnoea—new pathways for targeted therapy. Sleep Med Rev. 2018;37:45–59.
2. Pépin JL, Eastwood P, Eckert DJ. Novel avenues to approach non-CPAP therapy and implement comprehensive OSA care. Eur Respir J. 2021;59:2101788.
3. Dutta R, Delaney G, Toson B, et al. A novel model to estimate key obstructive sleep apnea endotypes from standard polysomnography and clinical data and their contribution to obstructive sleep apnea severity. Ann Am Thorac Soc. 2021;18(4):656–67.
4. Carney AS, Antic NA, Catcheside PG, et al. Sleep apnea multilevel surgery (SAMS) trial protocol: a multicenter randomized clinical trial of upper airway surgery for patients with obstructive sleep apnea who have failed continuous positive airway pressure. Sleep. 2019;04:04.
5. Brown EC, Cheng S, McKenzie DK, Butler JE, Gandevia SC, Bilston LE. Tongue stiffness is lower in patients with obstructive sleep apnea during wakefulness compared with matched control subjects. Sleep. 2015;38(4):537–44.
6. Eckert DJ, White DP, Jordan AS, Malhotra A, Wellman A. Defining phenotypic causes of obstructive sleep apnea. Identification of novel therapeutic targets. Am J Respir Crit Care Med. 2013;188(8):996–1004.
7. Joosten SA, Leong P, Landry SA, et al. Loop gain predicts the response to upper airway surgery in patients with obstructive sleep apnea. Sleep. 2017;40(7):01.
8. Hobson JC, Robinson S, Antic NA, et al. What is "success" following surgery for obstructive sleep apnea? The effect of different polysomnographic scoring systems. Laryngoscope. 2012;122(8):1878–81.
9. Ratnavadivel R, Chau N, Stadler D, Yeo A, McEvoy RD, Catcheside PG. Marked reduction in obstructive sleep apnea severity in slow wave sleep. J Clin Sleep Med. 2009;5(6):519–24.
10. Genta PR, Sands SA, Butler JP, et al. Airflow shape is associated with the pharyngeal structure causing OSA. Chest. 2017;152(3):537–46.

Current Diagnostics and Therapy Concept and Limitations

3

Simon D. Herkenrath and Winfried J. Randerath

3.1 Introduction

Obstructive sleep apnea (OSA) is a disease characterized by recurrent narrowing or complete collapse of the upper airway during sleep. These respiratory events cause repetitive hypoxemia, catecholamine release, an increase in sympathetic tone, and sleep fragmentation entailing long-term consequences, particularly of a cardiovascular nature. Depending on OSA severity, these may ultimately lead to an increased overall mortality. Growing evidence suggests that OSA is based on many different mechanisms, extending far beyond simple anatomic upper airway collapse. Furthermore, OSA shows different forms of manifestation with outcomes of varying clinical relevance. To account for this diversity and ultimately enable precision medicine, a fundamental and comprehensive understanding of the underlying pathomechanism, and their diagnosis and respective treatment options is essential.

S. D. Herkenrath
Department of Pneumology, Protestant Hospital, Bergisch Gladbach, Germany

W. J. Randerath (✉)
Internal Medicine, Cardiology and Sleep Medicine, Bethanien Hospitzal, Clinic of Pneumology and Allergology, Center for Sleep Medicine and Respiratory Care, Institute of Pneumology at the University of Cologne, Solingen, Germany

Internal Medicine, Pneumology, Allergology, Sleep Medicine, Palliative Medicine, Bethanien Hospital Clinic of Pneumology and Allergology, Center for Sleep Medicine and Respiratory Care, Institute of Pneumology at the University of Cologne, Solingen, Germany
e-mail: randerath@klinik-bethanien.de

M. Delakorda, N. de Vries (eds.), *The Role of Epiglottis in Obstructive Sleep Apnea*, https://doi.org/10.1007/978-3-031-34992-8_3

3.2 Definition of Obstructive Sleep Apnea

OSA is defined by repetitive episodes of complete or partial upper airway obstructions, leading to cessation or reduction of airflow, respectively. Corresponding single respiratory events associated with a complete or near-complete cessation of airflow are referred to as apneas, while those defined by reduced airflow are identified with the term hypopnea. These key respiratory events in OSA are defined by the globally established and regularly updated rules for the evaluation of sleep studies, published by the American Academy for Sleep Medicine [1]. To identify these events, a sleep study is required, which measures respiratory airflow. There are several types of sleep studies depending on the equipment's capacity to capture different biosignals. Full polysomnography allows for the most comprehensive evaluation of sleep and arousal, in addition to respiratory parameters. Obstructive apnea is characterized by a reduction in amplitude of the respiratory flow of ≥90% for at least 10 s, accompanied by continued respiratory muscle activity. An obstructive hypopnea is defined by a reduction of the respiratory flow of at least 30% with a minimum duration of 10 s. Typically, there is a flattening of the flow curve (plateauing) as well as an opposing movement of the thorax and abdomen (paradoxical effort). An additional mandatory criterion for hypopneas is the occurrence of either an oxygen desaturation ≥3% or arousal, i.e., a micro-awakening stimulus with an acceleration of the frequency of the electroencephalogram (EEG) and an increase in muscle tone. "Respiratory Effort Related Arousals" (RERA) indicate upper airway obstructions with the occurrence of arousal, not meeting the hypopnea criteria. They are, therefore, associated with only a small reduction in respiratory flow amplitude (<30%). The International Classification of Sleep Disorders (ICSD-3) defines sleep-related breathing disorders and provides 2 definitions for OSA [2].

1. Occurrence of 15 or more predominantly obstructive respiratory events per hour of sleep as measured by polysomnography or limited sleep study. Obstructive respiratory events include apneas, hypopneas, and RERA. When conducting a limited sleep study without recording sleep stages (i.e., without EEG), the extent of sleep apnea is usually underestimated because, on the one hand, the number of respiratory events is related to total recording time rather than total sleep time (TST), and, on the other hand, the lack of documentation of EEG arousals reduces the number of recorded hypopneas and RERAs.
2. Occurrence of at least five predominantly obstructive respiratory events per hour of sleep in combination with any of the following symptoms: (a) drowsiness, nonrestorative sleep, fatigue, or insomnia; (b) waking with shortness of breath or gasping for air at night; and (c) bed partner reports recurrent snoring, breathing pauses, or both. The presence of any of the following comorbidities is also sufficient to establish a diagnosis of OSA with a respiratory event index as low as 5 per hour: arterial hypertension, affective disorder, cognitive dysfunction, coronary artery disease, heart failure, atrial fibrillation, cerebral infarction, and type 2 diabetes mellitus. The limitations of using reduced sleep studies apply to definition 1.

3.3 Traditional Classification of Obstructive Sleep Apnea Severity

Traditionally, the number of respiratory disturbances defines OSA severity and is the basis of treatment. This approach is still valid according to national and international guidelines [2, 3]. The crucial parameter in this context is the apnea–hypopnea index (AHI), representing the mean number of apneas and hypopneas per hour of sleep. An AHI between 5.0 and 14.9/h indicates mild OSA, an AHI between 15.0 and 29.9/h indicates moderate OSA, and an AHI ≥30/h indicates severe OSA. However, more recent findings consider this traditional classification oversimplified and call for a much more differentiated approach.

Overall, the AHI correlates poorly with several outcome parameters. For example, it has recently been shown that only an AHI >20/h is independently associated with comorbidities [4]. Larger cohort studies also show that outcomes much more depend on the presence of daytime sleepiness and time with an oxygen saturation < 90% than on the AHI [5, 6]. Thus, for a clinically relevant severity classification of OSA, the underlying pathophysiology as well as the clinical presentation with regard to symptoms and end-organ damage have to be considered. These aspects can vary greatly from individual to individual and manifest in different phenotypes of OSA. The OSA severity classification is currently under discussion, but various proposals require prospective evaluation and have not yet resulted in a uniform revision of the severity classification [7]. Nevertheless, it is evident that the therapeutic approach should no longer depend solely on the AHI but should be based on the individual symptoms in combination with the number of respiratory disturbances, the hypoxic load, and the presence or absence of cardiovascular comorbidities.

3.4 Clinical Consequences of Obstructive Sleep Apnea

3.4.1 Symptoms of Obstructive Sleep Apnea

OSA symptoms vary largely interindividually and do not necessarily correlate with the extent of the respiratory disorder. On the one hand, about one quarter of OSA patients report classic symptoms, such as excessive daytime sleepiness (EDS), monotony intolerance, and performance deficits. Collateral history frequently reports snoring and pauses in breathing. Classic incidental findings include nocturnal awakening with short-term dyspnea, insomniac complaints, palpitations, nocturia, night sweats, nocturnal awakenings with retching or wheezing, morning drowsiness and headache, general fatigue, impotence, impaired memory, personality changes, and depressive episodes. On the other hand, OSA is not necessarily associated with these symptoms despite severe respiratory disturbances. An Icelandic prevalence study of the general population showed that the majority of OSA patients do not exhibit EDS [8]. This study also failed to show a significant correlation between OSA severity on the one hand and EDS or clinical symptoms on the other. Furthermore, a relationship between psychomotor vigilance and OSA severity was demonstrated in severe OSA only. People with cardiovascular comorbidities in particular often have few or no symptoms. Consequently, especially in this population, the likelihood of sleep-related breathing disorders should never be assessed solely on the basis of history or established questionnaires [9].

3.4.2 End-Organ Impact

Short-term effects of OSA include repetitive episodes of hypoxemia-reoxygenation, catecholamine release, an increase in sympathetic tone, sleep fragmentation, and pronounced intrathoracic pressure swings. In this context, fluctuations in blood pressure and cardiac output may also occur [10]. Repetitive hypoxia-reoxygenation triggers the upregulation of inflammatory mediators, such as tumor necrosis factor alpha and interleukin 6 [11]. These effects may contribute to the development of serious long-term sequelae. OSA is an independent risk factor for the occurrence of arterial hypertension, heart failure, and stroke [12–16]. In addition, there is a close association with metabolic syndrome, diabetes mellitus, atrial fibrillation, and coronary artery disease with acute coronary syndrome and sudden cardiac death [17–21]. In a large prospective cohort study, OSA was shown to be independently associated with all-cause mortality [22].

3.4.3 Risk of Accidents

Over the past decades, substantial evidence has accumulated, linking untreated OSA to an increased risk of accidents, motor vehicle accidents in particular. A previous meta-analysis considering 17 studies in professional and non-professional drivers established a clear association between sleepiness and motor vehicle accidents, with an odds ratio of 2.51 (95% CI 1.87–3.39) [23]. Another meta-analysis addressing the risk of occupational accidents in workers with OSA determined an odds ratio of 2.2 (95% CI 1.5–3.1) compared to controls [24]. EDS and decreased vigilance are a relevant part of the OSA symptom spectrum. However, there are controversial results on the relationship between subjective sleepiness as measured by the Epworth Sleepiness Scale and the extent of motor vehicle accidents in OSA patients [25, 26]. Nevertheless, EDS and impaired vigilance are considered key factors for the increased risk of accidents. The European Union Directive 2006/126/EC on driving licenses, in particular, amended by directive 2014/85/EU thus defines untreated moderate to severe OSA accompanied by excessive daytime sleepiness as an ineligibility factor for the issuance or renewal of a driver's license [27]. Furthermore, the directive demands that affected individuals under treatment undergo regular medical monitoring to assess treatment compliance and vigilance. This is supported by several studies that found effective OSA treatment to reduce the risk of motor vehicle accidents [28–31].

3.5 New Approaches for Obstructive Sleep Apnea Classification

Different approaches to OSA classification, beyond severity grading based on AHI, ultimately aim for individually tailored OSA precision medicine. In this context, the term "OSA phenotype" has been increasingly used in recent years. Although there is no strict and narrow definition, it has been used to differentiate OSA subtypes based on disease features of clinical relevance, such as symptoms, end-organ impact, and quality of life [32, 33]. Furthermore, in the pursuit of a yet more differentiated OSA classification, specific underlying pathophysiological disease features (upper airway anatomy, upper airway muscle responsiveness, ventilatory control, and arousal threshold) have been discriminated, which necessarily offer different therapeutic approaches [32, 34].

The determination of the individual OSA pathophysiology requires the use of different diagnostic tools, not all of which are widely available and easy to apply. Therefore, simplifications of specific methods are being pursued. For example, a signal analysis algorithm was presented by Sands and colleagues, allowing for the estimation of respiratory drive (loop gain) based on standard polysomnography [35]. Edwards and colleagues developed a regression model that also uses PSG variables to calculate the arousal threshold [36]. However, these simplified methods have not yet been sufficiently validated to be used widely.

Other proposals for OSA classification are based on symptoms and/or end-organ impact, thus defining different OSA phenotypes. Saaresranta and colleagues conducted a prospective cohort study, dividing OSA patients into four different clinical phenotypes based on the presence of excessive daytime sleepiness and insomnia symptoms [37]. They found that severe OSA as measured by AHI was most frequently associated with EDS, while insomnia was more often linked with cardiovascular comorbidity.

Adding parameters of end-organ impact alongside symptoms for OSA classification is a concept suggested by an ad hoc working group of the Sleep Disordered Breathing Group of the European Respiratory Society (ERS) and the European Sleep Research Society in 2018 (Baveno classification) [7]. In the proposed OSA multicomponent grading system, patients are classified into one of four categories (A–D) based on the presence or absence of defined symptoms and end-organ impacts (Fig. 3.1). Symptoms in this context include EDS, hypersomnia, and insomnia. End-organ effects comprise poorly controlled arterial hypertension, atrial fibrillation, heart failure, history of stroke, and diabetes mellitus. A recent prospective evaluation of this classification confirmed its relevance in guiding treatment decisions, as it may avoid unnecessary treatment in patients with moderate-to-severe OSA, who do not exhibit symptoms or relevant comorbidities. It may also help to identify missing treatments in symptomatic or comorbid OSA patients with low AHI [38].

However, the clinical application of these proposals for an alternative and more differentiated classification of OSA is still under discussion. It remains open to what extent professional societies will adopt them and whether the corresponding

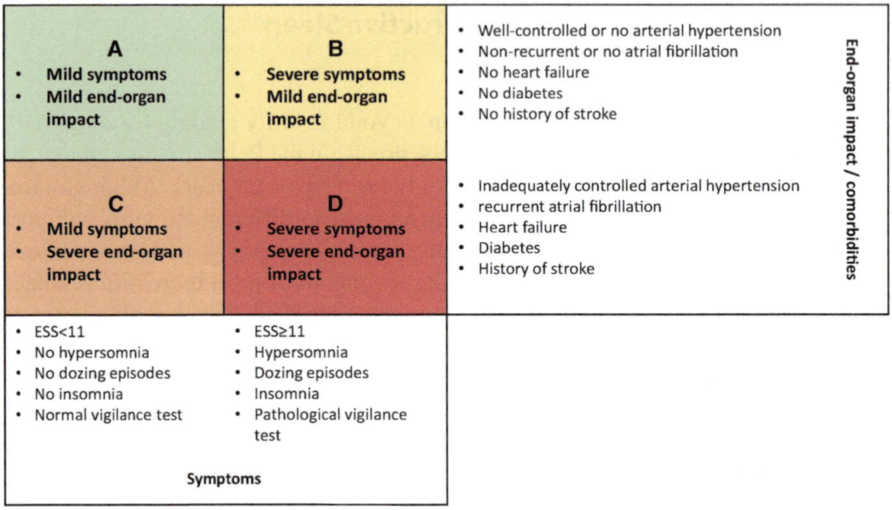

Fig. 3.1 Grading system for the severity of obstructive sleep apnea as proposed by the ERS Task Force (Baveno classification). (Adapted from Randerath et al [7])

classifications will be included in the guidelines. In any case, further prospective studies are necessary to evaluate the benefit of these concepts regarding consecutive therapeutic guidelines.

3.6 Clinical Diagnostics

In order to establish a precise diagnosis, determine the underlying pathophysiology, and select optimal treatment, symptoms and clinical signs need to be assessed using a broad spectrum of diagnostic methods.

3.6.1 Anamnesis

A detailed anamnesis including symptomatology, medical history, as well as collateral history is essential for the diagnosis and the therapeutic procedure. The anamnesis allows an early differentiation of other sleep-related, psychiatric, and organic diseases and should always be the first step in planning additional (differential) diagnostics. Typical and atypical symptoms of OSA should be evaluated specifically.

3.6.2 Physical Examination

The physical examination should include an assessment of the facial skull including the maxilla and mandible, oral cavity, soft palate, tonsils, tongue, and position of the hyoid bone. In particular, retrognathia and low-lying hyoid bone have been shown to be risk factors for OSA. The inspection of the pharynx allows for the assessment of the tonsils and has immediate therapeutic consequences in the event of tonsillar hyperplasia. There is a correlation between the visibility of the soft palate and the severity of OSA. In this regard, the Mallampati score (grades I-IV) represents an easy-to-survey clinical classification and allows an assessment of the upper airway diameter. Complementary technical examination modalities to assess upper airway anatomy include computed tomography of the neck and acoustic pharyngometry.

3.6.3 Questionnaires

Two groups of questionnaires must be fundamentally distinguished: Some have been developed to screen for the presence of OSA. Other questionnaires address OSA-associated symptoms but are not designed and validated for screening OSA.

The Berlin questionnaire and the STOP-BANG questionnaire are evaluated screening questionnaires. Although the latter was originally developed for the preoperative assessment of OSA likelihood, it is increasingly accepted clinically outside of surgical treatment measures due to its high sensitivity. In addition to information on snoring, sleepiness, breathing pauses observed by others, and treatment of arterial hypertension, anthropometric data, such as body mass index, age, gender, and neck circumference, are also included. However, it should be taken into account that these questionnaires do not seem to be particularly useful in the detection of sleep-related breathing disorders in patients with cardiovascular diseases [9].

The Epworth Sleepiness Scale is an evaluated instrument for assessing sleepiness. It captures the probability of falling asleep in eight different everyday situations (reading, watching TV, driving, etc.). A sum score > 10 is considered pathological.

3.6.4 Computer-Based Tests

Computer-based tests, such as the Carda, driving simulators, or pupillometry, evaluate selective or divided attention and vigilance. The Carda is a computer-based responsiveness test for evaluating selective attention [39]. Driving simulators also allow inference of divided attention. The pupillographic sleepiness test is based on the correlation between fluctuations in pupil diameter and daytime sleepiness [40]. An infrared camera is used to record pupillary behavior during the test. The target variables are the Pupillary Unrest Index (PUI) in millimeters per minute and the amplitude spectrum. The Quatember–Maly test, widely used in clinical settings, requires the patient to observe a circle consisting of dots. The dots of the circle light up sequentially. If a dot is skipped, the patient must respond by pressing a button. During the test, reaction time and the number of false positive or false negative responses are recorded. The Quatember–Maly test shows good sensitivity (61.9%) and specificity (72.2%) for detecting daytime sleepiness. In conclusion, all these tests can be considered useful, but they lack specificity and have been validated to varying degrees.

3.6.5 Sleep Studies

Attended polysomnography (level 1 PSG) is the gold standard in the diagnosis of sleep-related breathing disorders and includes a minimum of 7 and a maximum of 9 biosignals. An unattended PSG is a level 2 sleep study. Level 1 and level 2 PSGs record neurological, cardiac, and respiratory parameters. These include electroencephalography (EEG), electrooculography (EOG), electromyography (EMG), thoracic and abdominal movements, respiratory flow (via nasal cannula or thermistor), pulse oximetry, heart rate, electrocardiography, microphone (snoring), and body position. A level 3 (cardiorespiratory polygraphy) sleep study includes at least four biosignals, and a level 4 sleep study includes at least one. Levels 3 and 4 sleep studies do not include recording of the EEG, EOG, and EMG and, therefore, do not allow assessment of sleep and sleep-related movement disorders. A level 3 study includes respiratory biosignals, electrocardiogram, and pulse oximetry, whereas a level 4 sleep study includes only respiratory flow and/or pulse oximetry. Depending on the patient's medical history, the results of the questionnaires and vigilance tests, and the suspected diagnosis, the scope of the sleep study is determined. The reference method, especially in the context of differential diagnostic considerations, is the level 1 PSG. Especially in case of low pretest probability for OSA, the PSG is indispensable. Even in the presence of pulmonary, cardiac, psychiatric, and neurological comorbidities, reduced sleep studies are not able to provide a comprehensive assessment. Level 3 sleep studies either can be used as an alternative diagnostic if there is a high pretest probability for OSA or as an extended screening tool. Level 4 sleep studies, in contrast, are not sufficient as definitive diagnostic tests but may be helpful in screening asymptomatic patients. A high pretest probability is present in the case of the coexistence of snoring, EDS, as well as observed breathing pauses. Peripheral arterial tonometry also shows good evidence for the diagnosis and severity assessment of OSA, analogous to polygraphy, if the pre-test probability is high. In all other suspected cases, a PSG is indicated, especially in the presence of comorbidities and suspected sleep-related diseases other than OSA [3].

3.6.6 Carbon Dioxide Measurement

CO_2 measurement is necessary for evaluating (nocturnal) ventilation and, in particular, the occurrence of hypoventilation. While arterial blood gas analysis is the gold standard for the determination of $PaCO_2$ and thus for the assessment of hypoventilation, non-invasive surrogate methods for continuous CO_2 measurement are available. For this purpose, two different methods are established. On the one hand, end-tidal CO_2 can be measured via a capnograph, which requires the patient to wear an interface connected to the capnograph. Transcutaneous capnometry is yet another alternative, which continuously monitors the capillary CO_2 concentration photometrically using an ear clip or adhesive skin sensor. This allows for differentiating various forms of hypoventilation (Fig. 3.2). While end-tidal CO_2 measurement is only reliable in a purely diagnostic setting without the patient wearing a mask delivering positive airway pressure, transcutaneous capnometry may be applied without such restrictions.

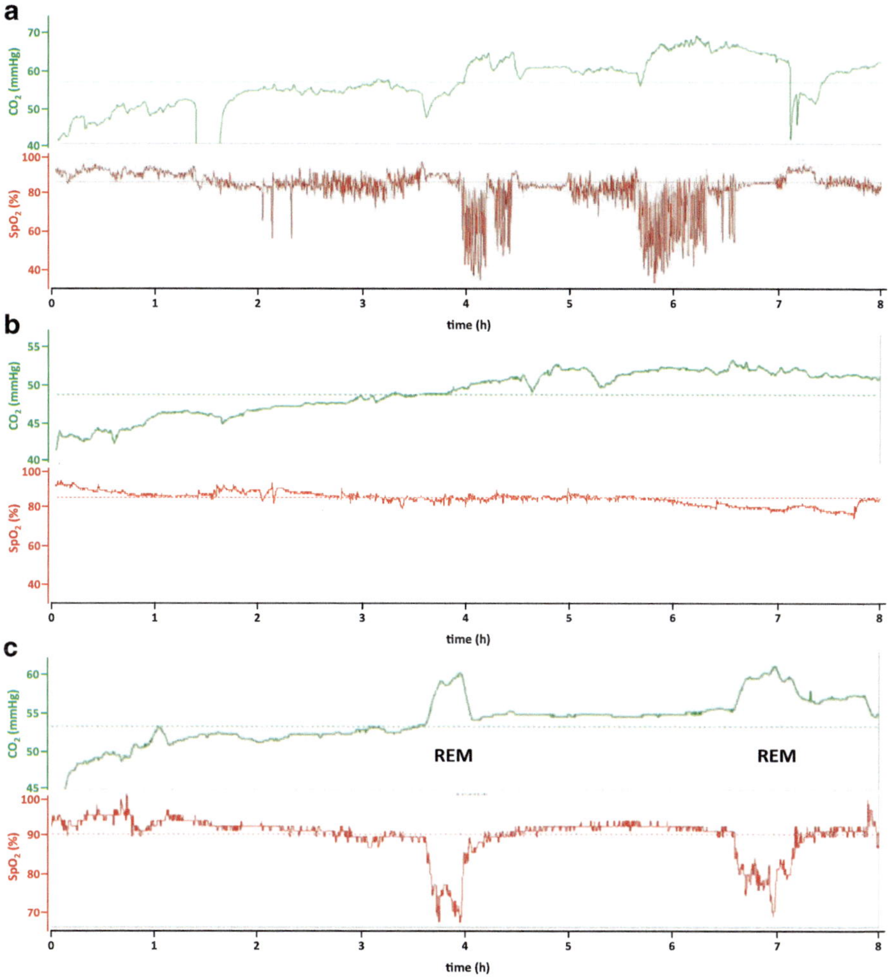

Fig. 3.2 Exemplary data from transcutaneous capnometry, which includes oximetry (green curves: transcutaneous carbon dioxide level and red curves: oxygen saturation [SpO_2]). (**a**) Obesity hypoventilation with the coexistence of predominant severe OSA and alveolar hypoventilation. (**b**) Severe sleep-related alveolar hypoventilation with successive carbon dioxide increase during the night without evidence of relevant comorbid sleep apnea. (**c**) REM sleep-dependent alveolar hypoventilation with subsequent compensation also moderate comorbid sleep apnea with short desaturations especially in the second half of the night

3.6.7 Electrophysiological Tests

The main electrophysiological tests used to assess central nervous activation and daytime sleepiness are the Multiple Sleep Latency Test (MSLT) and the Multiple Wakefulness Test (MWT). The MSLT assesses the extent of daytime sleepiness during five fixed time intervals during the day by measuring sleep latency based on

EEG, EOG, and EMG. Clinically, the test is used particularly to evaluate narcolepsy and hypersomnia but is also used to address specific issues related to sleep-disordered breathing and differential diagnosis. The MWT examines the patient's ability to stay awake in a sleep-promoting environment. The test results correlate with OSA severity and have been shown to improve with the initiation of positive airway pressure therapy. The MWT is important for assessing central tonic activation; although in isolation, it has limited evidence.

3.6.8 Drug-Induced Sedation Endoscopy

Drug-induced sedation endoscopy (DISE) may add important morphological information in patients with difficult-to-treat OSA. This procedure is usually performed with the patient in a supine position under sedation with propofol, midazolam, dexmedetomidine, or a combination, using a flexible endoscope and standard anesthesiological monitoring [41]. In patients with positional OSA, DISE may be performed in both the lateral and supine positions. It is primarily performed transnasally but may also be supplemented with a transoral examination. DISE allows for a comprehensive assessment of the shape and diameter of the upper airway on different levels (nasopharynx, oropharynx, and hypopharynx). Furthermore, the therapeutic success of mandibular advancement can be predicted by assessing the effect of different extents of mandibular protrusion during the examination [42]. A DISE is mandatory to evaluate a patient's eligibility for an inspiration-triggered selective stimulation of the hypoglossal nerve since a complete concentric collapse must be excluded. DISE also enables the detection of anatomical peculiarities, e.g. a so-called "floppy epiglottis" [41]. However, DISE has been criticized as drug-induced sleep differs from physiological sleep, and thus, the natural situation cannot be accurately recreated. In addition, various classifications have been devised in the past to accurately and uniformly represent DISE findings, of which the Nose oropharynx hypopharynx and larynx (NOHL) and the Velum oropharynx tongue base epiglottis (VOTE) classifications are commonly used [43, 44]. For full details on DISE, please review Chap. 8.

3.7 OSA Therapy

Basic OSA treatment options include weight reduction, sleep hygiene, and exercise training. However, these methods alone reduce breathing disturbances insufficiently. In recent years, the treatment portfolio has expanded substantially alongside the gold standard of positive airway pressure therapy. This allows for an individualized approach based on pathophysiological phenotypes and patient preferences [34]. Different therapeutic measures are described in more detail below, excluding surgical options for the treatment of OSA, which are addressed in separate chapters (Part 4).

3.7.1 Conservative OSA Treatments

Conservative treatment options for OSA comprise weight loss, exercise training, and upper airway muscle training. In a comprehensive meta-analysis by Gao et al., assessing the short-term (≤6 months) efficacy of different minimally invasive OSA treatments, exercise, and muscle training turned out to be effective, but more in terms of ESS reduction and less in AHI, while lifestyle modification (dietary control and weight loss) was by far least effective [45]. As is the case with other treatment modalities, the prediction of therapy effects requires the determination of the individual OSA phenotype. Weight loss can significantly improve the AHI, daytime sleepiness, and quality of life in obese OSA patients. Weight reduction alone might adequately treat mildly symptomatic OSA patients with an AHI < 15/h [46]. In addition, patients with moderate or severe OSA may benefit significantly from weight reduction in terms of AHI reduction but still usually do not reach a level justifying the abandonment of further more effective therapeutic measures [47].

Physical training can reduce the AHI and significantly improve quality of life and daytime sleepiness in moderate to severe OSA even without weight reduction [47]. However, it achieves a clinically relevant reduction in AHI only in individual cases but should generally be recommended as a basic therapy. Physical training reduces the nocturnal fluid shift in patients with coronary artery disease and at least moderate sleep apnea (OSA and central sleep apnea [CSA]), thereby widening the upper airway [48]. Different types of respiratory/upper airway muscle training, such as intraoral neuromuscular stimulation and normocapnic hyperpnea training, have limited effects on AHI, quality of life, and daytime sleepiness in OSA [49, 50]. Didgeridoo playing and targeted oropharyngeal muscle exercise can significantly improve AHI, snoring, and daytime sleepiness in moderate-severe OSA [51, 52]. Overall, the effect of targeted muscle training is limited and suitable as the sole therapy for mild to moderate asymptomatic OSA at best.

3.7.2 Positive Airway Pressure Therapy

OSA treatment by means of positive airway pressure (PAP) therapy primarily aims at restoring and maintaining upper airway patency by providing a pneumatic splint to the upper airway. Over several decades, different modes of PAP therapy have been developed, optimizing OSA treatment and addressing various sleep-related breathing disorders, which go beyond but may co-exist with OSA (Fig. 3.3).

3.7.3 Continuous Positive Airway Pressure

The standard therapy for OSA treatment is continuous positive airway pressure (CPAP). Regardless of the exact location of the upper airway collapse and functional pathophysiological characteristics, CPAP is able to suppress most obstructive

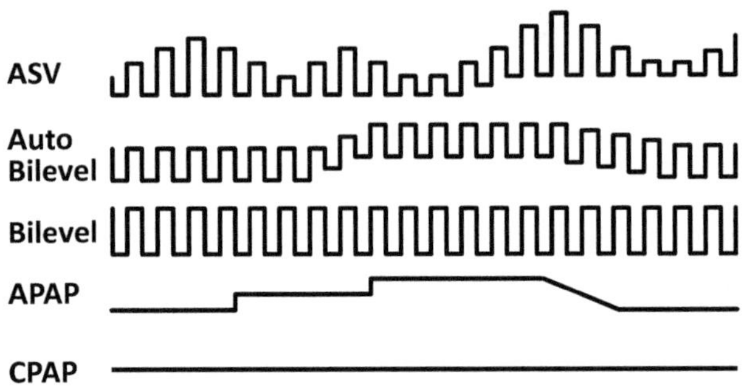

Fig. 3.3 Schematic representation of pressure curves according to different modes of positive airway pressure therapy. CPAP: continuous positive airway pressure, a constant pressure level is maintained throughout, which is set to overcome the critical occlusion pressure and thus keep the upper airway open. APAP: automatic continuous positive airway pressure, in addition to CPAP, the device automatically adapts the pressure level within pre-defined ranges, based on the detection of upper airway obstruction. Bilevel (BPAP): Applying different fixed pressure levels for end-expiration (positive end-expiratory pressure, PEEP) and inspiration (inspiratory positive airway pressure, IPAP). AutoBilevel (AutoBPAP): This enhanced Bilevel mode automatically adjusts the PEEP, while keeping the pressure support or tidal volume constant. ASV: adaptive servo-ventilation, adjusts pressure support during inspiration on a breath-by-breath basis in addition to an automatically adjusted PEEP, aiming at keeping minute ventilation on a constant and stable level

respiratory disturbances sufficiently. It prevents the collapse of the upper airway by increasing the intraluminal pressure over the ambient pressure. The therapy pressure level should, therefore, be slightly above the critical occlusion pressure in order to prevent upper airway obstruction on the one hand but also to prevent undesirable effects such as leakage due to inadequately high pressure levels. However, certain accompanying conditions such as epiglottis collapse might impair PAP therapy efficacy and even exacerbate obstructive events [53–55].

The optimal therapy pressure can be determined by individual titration during polysomnography. Automatic positive airway pressure (APAP) devices adapt the therapeutic pressure as required by the level of obstruction within predefined limits. They can provide an alternative in case of variable pressure demands depending on body position and sleep stage. APAP therapy should also be initiated during a sleep study to ensure an adequate pressure range and to avoid unintentional leakage, which potentially impairs correct pressure regulation. CPAP and APAP are considered equivalent and can be chosen according to individual therapy acceptance. If satisfactory suppression of the sleep-related breathing disorder is not achieved despite optimized settings, potential causes (e.g., anatomical malformations) must be identified, and alternative therapy measures or treatment combinations must be considered.

The evidence on CPAP efficacy is by far the highest among all forms of OSA therapy, mainly due to its long-term establishment. CPAP is able to effectively reduce symptoms, such as EDS and associated accidents, not only to improve quality of life but also to ameliorate a number of cardiovascular diseases, including a reduction in blood pressure, pulmonary arterial pressure, and risk of incident cerebral events [56, 57]. A large, prospective cohort study of patients hospitalized with acute heart failure found that newly diagnosed OSA at the time of admission is independently associated with mortality. Patients treated with PAP exhibited a 3-year survival similar to patients with no or minimal sleep-related breathing disorders [22]. On the other hand, one large prospective randomized controlled trial found no improved survival due to CPAP in a non-sleepy cardiovascular OSA cohort [58]. However, study participants in the CPAP group had a low long-term CPAP adherence of 3.3 h/night, which might have been insufficient to affect cardiovascular outcomes.

3.7.4 Bilevel

Bilevel therapy is a more advanced form of PAP and works with separate levels of inspiratory (IPAP) and expiratory pressure (EPAP). Three different forms of Bilevel are distinguished. Bilevel S (S = "spontaneous") is a variant in which the patient's spontaneous breathing triggers the device to switch to the IPAP level due to the onset of inspiratory flow. In Bilevel T ("timed") mode, the device cycles between EPAP and IPAP based on a preset fixed respiratory rate, thus providing ventilatory support. Bilevel S/T represents an intermediate form, in which the device is primarily triggered by spontaneous breathing but additionally ventilates the patient based on a defined minimum respiratory rate (or backup rate) when the spontaneous respiratory rate drops below this level. The use of Bilevel for the treatment of OSA in the absence of relevant hypoventilation is usually restricted to the S-mode. It may be applied in the case of high pressure demand, where the lower EPAP level compared to IPAP may facilitate therapy tolerance. The EPAP-IPAP difference applied in this context is usually in the range of 4 mbar.

3.7.5 Mandibular Advancement Device

Mandibular advancement devices (MADs) are clinically established as a primary alternative to PAP therapy. The overall treatment efficacy is inferior as compared to CPAP. However, MADs improve breathing disturbances and clinical symptoms in non-obese patients (BMI <30 kg/m^2) with mild to moderate sleep apnea equal to PAP [59, 60]. The therapeutic principle of MAD is based on a widening of the upper airway, especially in the lateral velopharyngeal segment, by advancing the mandible and tongue. In addition, the complementary tension on the supra-hyoidal tissue increases the airway diameter at the epiglottis level. A study in obese patients with severe OSA revealed that the critical occlusion pressure decreases with increasing mandibular advancement, whereas there is no systematic difference in genioglossus muscle function [61]. These findings suggest that the MAD effect is primarily due to improved passive pharyngeal anatomy. This also explains why patients with milder OSA are particularly suitable for MAD therapy, as they are characterized by less collapsible upper airway and lower critical occlusion pressure [62, 63]. A meta-analysis comprising a total of 743 patients with mild, moderate, or severe OSA found CPAP therapy to be more effective in terms of AHI reduction and improvement of oxygen saturation. The latter may be due to the fact that CPAP, in contrast to MAD, reduces ventilation-perfusion mismatch within the lungs and stabilizes the small airways in addition to providing a very effective upper airway splinting [64]. There were no significant differences in quality of life as well as cognitive performance. The treatment adherence was significantly higher in the MAD group by an average of 1.1 h per night. According to a meta-analysis comparing CPAP and MAD regarding the reduction of blood pressure, both therapy modalities were equally effective [65]. Other beneficial cardiovascular effects of MAD therapy have been described in relatively small studies not allowing for final conclusions. According to current studies, the MAD should be manufactured based on individual dental imprints, anchored bi-maxillary, and enable the practitioner to reproducibly adjust advancement in millimeter increments. Side effects following therapy initiation, such as temporomandibular pain, are often mild and transient. More severe side effects are rare, but after many years of use, changes in dental position may occur, often unnoticed, which may call for therapy adjustment [66–68]. For full details on MADs, please review Chap. 17.

3.7.6 Positional Therapy

Positional OSA (POSA) is generally diagnosed if the AHI in the supine position is at least twice as high as in the lateral position. A reliable assessment of this condition requires sufficient time spent in both supine and non-supine positions within a diagnostic sleep study. Several studies have found a high prevalence of POSA among OSA patients, ranging between 27 and 61% [69–72]. If patients suffer from predominant POSA (i.e., non-supine AHI < 10/h), positional therapy is a primary treatment option. Basically, two different treatment principles are available in this context. On the one hand, passive prevention of the supine position can be achieved purely mechanically via a vest or similar constructions referred to as "tennis ball technique." On the other hand, several electronic devices have been developed (sleep position trainers, SPT), which are worn on the body during sleep with the intention to actively keep the patient from entering the supine position by means of a vibration alarm. Several studies have demonstrated good efficacy of SPT therapy in terms of both symptomatic improvement and AHI reduction [73–75]. An analysis of effectiveness and compliance over 6 months using a chest-worn SPT in 106 patients showed a moderate reduction of subjective symptoms (median ESS 11 to 8, PSQI 8 to 6) and regular use (defined as >4 h usage over 5 nights per week) in 71% of the patients [73]. Another prospective clinical trial in 30 patients with a mean baseline AHI of 25/h showed a substantial reduction of the AHI to a mean value of 8/h at follow-up after 4 weeks of therapy using a neck-worn SPT [75]. However, subjective outcome measures, such as daytime sleepiness, were only mildly reduced by trend. A larger randomized controlled crossover trial in 117 patients with a mean baseline AHI of 21/h comparing SPT with APAP showed SPT to be equally effective in terms of AHI with higher treatment adherence [76]. The mean AHI after 6 weeks of therapy was 7.3 vs. 3.7/h, while mean nocturnal therapy adherence was 20% higher. Passive positional therapy is comparably effective but often lacks sufficient long-term adherence due to lack of comfort [74]. The effects of SPT therapy on cardiovascular comorbidity have not been investigated yet. For full details on positional therapy, please review Chap. 18.

3.7.7 Hypoglossal Nerve Stimulation

Hypoglossal nerve stimulation has recently been established as a second-line therapy for OSA. Different implantable devices are available, which differ regarding their specific mode of action but share the therapeutical principle of electric stimulation of the hypoglossal nerve to activate key muscles of the upper airway, thus achieving airway patency. The largest long-term multicenter trial for the investigation of hypoglossal nerve stimulation to date was the STAR trial, in which one specific device (Inspire® Upper Airway Stimulation) was implanted in 126 patients with CPAP failure, an initial AHI between 20 and 50/h and a BMI ≤32 kg/m^2, who were followed up over a period of up to 60 months. At the 12-month follow-up, this therapy achieved a reduction of the AHI by 16.4/h. Two-third of the participants met the success criteria defined as an AHI reduction >50% from baseline and an AHI <20/h [77]. About 97 of the STAR trial patients completed the 60-month follow-up and 71 of those underwent a PSG at that time point [78]. This revealed a sustained therapy effect in terms of AHI, oxygen desaturation index, and subjective outcomes with a success rate of 75% as defined above. Serious device-related adverse events occurred in 6% of the initial 126 participants within the 60-month follow-up. In a registry study on Inspire® therapy comprising 508 patients, a correlation between therapy success and BMI was demonstrated [79]. For each point increase in BMI, a 9% lower odds of treatment success were determined. Older age was also found to be a negative predictor of treatment success. Considering the invasive (but reversible) nature and the high costs of this therapy as compared to first-line OSA treatments as well as the experience from clinical trials, the indication for this type of OSA therapy must be carefully assessed and includes ensuring that other primary forms of therapy such as CPAP or MAD are not a viable option. The currently recommended criteria for hypoglossal stimulation include an AHI below 50/h and a BMI of <32 kg/m^2, a proportion of central respiratory disorders ≤25%, and an exclusion of concentric collapse at the level of the soft palate [80]. The collapse configuration should be assessed with drug-induced sleep endoscopy. For full details on hypoglossal nerve stimulation, please review Chap. 22.

3.7.8 Pharmacotherapy

Many different drugs have been investigated in clinical trials regarding their potential in OSA therapy, aiming at influencing different pathophysiological aspects of

OSA [81, 82]. These include anatomical features, upper airway muscle activity and response, arousal threshold, and ventilatory regulation (loop gain). A clinical aspect addressed by pharmacological treatment is residual EDS in treated OSA patients, for which sufficient evidence and different approved agents are available. These comprise modafinil/armodafinil, pitolisant, and solriamfetol, all aiming at the modulation of neurotransmitters implicated in sleep–wake regulation [83–88]. In the European Union, however, Pitolisant and Solriamfetol are approved for this indication. For the treatment of pathophysiological traits on the other hand, most trials to date were phase-II trials of small sample size and showed very limited effects on objective outcomes, with the AHI being the main outcome parameter. It is likely that the observed effects were also small because most of these clinical trials were conducted without specifically selecting certain OSA subgroups, matching the respective mechanisms of action of the investigated substance. Some promising results were seen with pharmaceuticals aimed at enhancing upper airway muscle responsiveness. A combination of two drugs, atomoxetine (a selective norepinephrine reuptake inhibitor) and oxybutynin (an anticholinergic agent), substantially reduced the AHI in 20 OSA patients [89]. The drug combination achieved a median AHI reduction of 63% from 28.5 (10.9–51.6) to 7.5 (2.4–18.6)/h. The treatment effect relies on blocking acetylcholine receptors on hypoglossal motor neurons and inhibiting norepinephrine re-uptake, thus increasing genioglossus responsiveness and consequently supporting upper airway patency. The various pharmacological substances that have been investigated in the context of OSA therapy to date each address different pathophysiological aspects. For this reason, and based on the often still insufficient data available, it currently seems unlikely that a single substance can represent an adequate OSA therapy. This would be most likely for very narrowly selected patient groups and only in the context of second-line therapy or supportive therapy. In addition, the combination of different drug classes is a therapeutic approach that seems worth investigating in larger studies, depending on the individual OSA pathophysiology.

3.7.9 Combination Therapy

Different therapy methods can be combined to enhance therapy success if necessary, again taking into account the particular OSA pathophysiology. However, the body of evidence regarding combinational therapies is limited. Several studies have investigated the combination of CPAP and MAD in recent years [90, 91]. Especially in more complex situations, MAD has proven to be a useful additive to reduce the need for very high pressure levels, to reduce potential side effects (aerophagia, leakage), and to improve therapy adherence. Under combination therapy, additive improvement in AHI can be expected, especially in the case of inadequate suppression of upper airway obstruction under single therapy regimens. The supine position exacerbates certain forms of obstruction and increases dynamic loop gain [92–94]. For this reason, therapy with a MAD, for example, may be insufficiently effective. A 2015 clinical study demonstrated that the combined use of an SPT and a MAD reduced the AHI from baseline significantly more than the respective single therapy modalities [95]. Combining first-line OSA therapy with pharmacological treatment can be considered for amelioration of persisting OSA-associated symptoms. For this purpose, solriamfetol and pitolisant are approved for the treatment of narcolepsy as well as residual excessive daytime sleepiness despite adequate OSA first-line therapy [87, 96].

References

1. Berry RB, Brooks R, Gamaldo CE. The AASM manual for the scoring of sleep and associated events: rules, terminology and technical specifications. Version 2.6. American Academy of Sleep Medicine: Darien, IL; 2020.
2. American Academy of Sleep Medicine. Diagnostic and coding manual, international classification of sleep disorders. 3rd ed. Westchester, IL: American Academy of Sleep Medicine; 2014.
3. Deutsche Gesellschaft für Schlafforschung, und Schlafmedizin (DGSM). S3-Leitlinie Nicht erholsamer Schlaf/Schlafstörungen—Kapitel "Schlafbezogene Atmungsstörungen". 2016.
4. Heinzer R, Vat S, Marques-Vidal P, Marti-Soler H, Andries D, Tobback N, et al. Prevalence of sleep-disordered breathing in the general population: the HypnoLaus study. Lancet Respir Med. 2015;3(4):310–8.
5. Xie J, Sert Kuniyoshi FH, Covassin N, Singh P, Gami AS, Wang S, et al. Nocturnal hypoxemia due to obstructive sleep apnea is an independent predictor of poor prognosis after myocardial infarction. J Am Heart Assoc. 2016;5(8):e003162.
6. Xie J, Sert Kuniyoshi FH, Covassin N, Singh P, Gami AS, Chahal CAA, et al. Excessive daytime sleepiness independently predicts increased cardiovascular risk after myocardial infarction. J Am Heart Assoc. 2018;7(2):e007221.
7. Randerath W, Bassetti CL, Bonsignore MR, Farre R, Ferini-Strambi L, Grote L, et al. Challenges and perspectives in obstructive sleep apnoea: report by an ad hoc working group of the sleep disordered breathing group of the European Respiratory Society and the European Sleep Research Society. Eur Respir J. 2018;52(3):1702616.
8. Arnardottir ES, Bjornsdottir E, Olafsdottir KA, Benediktsdottir B, Gislason T. Obstructive sleep apnoea in the general population: highly prevalent but minimal symptoms. Eur Respir J. 2016;47(1):194–202.
9. Reuter H, Herkenrath S, Treml M, Halbach M, Steven D, Frank K, et al. Sleep-disordered breathing in patients with cardiovascular diseases cannot be detected by ESS, STOP-BANG, and Berlin questionnaires. Clin Res Cardiol. 2018;107:1071.
10. Davies RJO. Cardiovascular aspects of obstructive sleep apnoea and their relevance to the assessment of the efficacy of nasal continuous positive airway pressure therapy. Thorax. 1998;53(5):416–8.
11. Kheirandish-Gozal L, Gozal D. Obstructive sleep apnea and inflammation: proof of concept based on two illustrative cytokines. Int J Mol Sci. 2019;20(3):459.
12. Arias MA, García-Río F, Alonso-Fernández A, Mediano O, Martínez I, Villamor J. Obstructive sleep apnea syndrome affects left ventricular diastolic function: effects of nasal continuous positive airway pressure in men. Circulation. 2005;112(3):375–83.
13. Shivalkar B, Van de Heyning C, Kerremans M, Rinkevich D, Verbraecken J, De Backer W, et al. Obstructive sleep apnea syndrome: more insights on structural and functional cardiac alterations, and the effects of treatment with continuous positive airway pressure. J Am Coll Cardiol. 2006;47(7):1433–9.
14. Arzt M, Young T, Finn L, Skatrud JB, Bradley TD. Association of sleep-disordered breathing and the occurrence of stroke. Am J Respir Crit Care Med. 2005;172(11):1447–51.
15. Redline S, Yenokyan G, Gottlieb DJ, Shahar E, O'Connor GT, Resnick HE, et al. Obstructive sleep Apnea–hypopnea and incident stroke. Am J Respir Crit Care Med. 2010;182(2):269–77.

16. Johnson KG, Johnson DC. Frequency of sleep apnea in stroke and TIA patients: a meta-analysis. J Clin Sleep Med. 2010;6(2):131–7.
17. Lyons OD, Bradley TD. Heart failure and sleep apnea. Can J Cardiol. 2015;31(7): 898–908.
18. Drager LF, Polotsky VY, O'Donnell CP, Cravo SL, Lorenzi-Filho G, Machado BH. Translational approaches to understanding metabolic dysfunction and cardiovascular consequences of obstructive sleep apnea. Am J Physiol Heart Circ Physiol. 2015;309(7):H1101–11.
19. Javaheri S, Drager LF, Lorenzi-Filho G. Sleep and cardiovscular disease: present and future. In: Kryger MH, Roth T, Dement WC, editors. Principles and practice of sleep medicine. 6th ed. Philadelphia, PA: Elsevier; 2017. p. 1222–8.
20. Bauters F, Rietzschel ER, Hertegonne KBC, Chirinos JA. The link between obstructive sleep apnea and cardiovascular disease. Curr Atheroscler Rep. 2016;18(1):1.
21. Baltzis D, Bakker JP, Patel SR, Veves A. Obstructive sleep apnea and vascular diseases. Compr Physiol. 2016;6(3):1519–28.
22. Khayat R, Jarjoura D, Porter K, Sow A, Wannemacher J, Dohar R, et al. Sleep disordered breathing and post-discharge mortality in patients with acute heart failure. Eur Heart J. 2015;36(23):1463–9.
23. Bioulac S, Micoulaud-Franchi J-A, Arnaud M, Sagaspe P, Moore N, Salvo F, et al. Risk of motor vehicle accidents related to sleepiness at the wheel: a systematic review and meta-analysis. Sleep. 2017;40(10):40. https://doi.org/10.1093/sleep/zsx134; [cited 2021 Jul 29].
24. Garbarino S, Guglielmi O, Sanna A, Mancardi GL, Magnavita N. Risk of occupational accidents in workers with obstructive sleep apnea: systematic review and meta-analysis. Sleep. 2016;39(6):1211–8.
25. Ellen RLB, Marshall SC, Palayew M, Molnar FJ, Wilson KG, Man-Son-Hing M. Systematic review of motor vehicle crash risk in persons with sleep apnea. J Clin Sleep Med. 2006;2(2):193–200.
26. Mulgrew AT, Nasvadi G, Butt A, Cheema R, Fox N, Fleetham JA, et al. Risk and severity of motor vehicle crashes in patients with obstructive sleep apnoea/hypopnoea. Thorax. 2008;63(6):536–41.
27. Consolidated text: directive 2006/126/EC of the European Parliament and of the Council of 20 December 2006 on driving licences. [cited 2021 Jul 29]. https://eur-lex.europa.eu/legal-content/EN/TXT/HTML/?uri=CELEX:02006L0126-20201101&from=EN#tocId66.
28. Findley L, Smith C, Hooper J, Dineen M, Suratt PM. Treatment with nasal CPAP decreases automobile accidents in patients with sleep apnea. Am J Respir Crit Care Med. 2000;161(3 Pt 1):857–9.
29. Karimi M, Hedner J, Häbel H, Nerman O, Grote L. Sleep apnea related risk of motor vehicle accidents is reduced by continuous positive airway pressure: Swedish traffic accident registry data. Sleep. 2015;38(3):341–9.
30. Antonopoulos CN, Sergentanis TN, Daskalopoulou SS, Petridou ET. Nasal continuous positive airway pressure (nCPAP) treatment for obstructive sleep apnea, road traffic accidents and driving simulator performance: a meta-analysis. Sleep Med Rev. 2011;15(5): 301–10.
31. Tregear S, Reston J, Schoelles K, Phillips B. Continuous positive airway pressure reduces risk of motor vehicle crash among drivers with obstructive sleep apnea: systematic review and meta-analysis. Sleep. 2010;33(10):1373–80.
32. Light M, Owens RL, Schmickl CN, Malhotra A. Precision medicine for obstructive sleep apnea. Sleep Med Clin. 2019;14(3):391–8.
33. Malhotra A, Mesarwi O, Pepin J-L, Owens RL. Endotypes and phenotypes in obstructive sleep apnea. Curr Opin Pulm Med. 2020;26(6):609–14.
34. Eckert DJ. Phenotypic approaches to obstructive sleep apnoea—new pathways for targeted therapy. Sleep Med Rev. 2018;37:45–59.
35. Sands SA, Edwards BA, Terrill PI, Taranto-Montemurro L, Azarbarzin A, Marques M, et al. Phenotyping pharyngeal pathophysiology using polysomnography in patients with obstructive sleep apnea. Am J Respir Crit Care Med. 2018;197(9):1187–97.

36. Edwards BA, Eckert DJ, McSharry DG, Sands SA, Desai A, Kehlmann G, et al. Clinical predictors of the respiratory arousal threshold in patients with obstructive sleep apnea. Am J Respir Crit Care Med. 2014;190(11):1293–300.
37. Saaresranta T, Hedner J, Bonsignore MR, Riha RL, McNicholas WT, Penzel T, et al. Clinical phenotypes and comorbidity in European sleep a pnoea patients. PLoS One. 2016;11(10):e0163439.
38. Randerath WJ, Herkenrath S, Treml M, Grote L, Hedner J, Bonsignore MR, et al. Evaluation of a multicomponent grading system for obstructive sleep apnoea: the Baveno classification. ERJ Open Res. 2021;7(1):00928–2020.
39. Gerdesmeyer C, Randerath W, Rühle K-H. Zeitliche Abhängigkeit der Fehlerzahl bei Messungen der Daueraufmerksamkeit mittels Fahrsimulator vor und nach nCPAP-Therapie bei Schlafapnoesyndrom. Somnologie. 1997;1(4):165–70.
40. Wilhelm B, Wilhelm H, Lüdtke H, Streicher P, Adler M. Pupillographic assessment of sleepiness in sleep-deprived healthy subjects. Sleep. 1998;21(3):258–65.
41. De Vito A, Carrasco Llatas M, Ravesloot MJ, Kotecha B, De Vries N, Hamans E, et al. European position paper on drug-induced sleep endoscopy: 2017 update. Clin Otolaryngol. 2018;43(6):1541–52.
42. Okuno K, Pliska BT, Hamoda M, Lowe AA, Almeida FR. Prediction of oral appliance treatment outcomes in obstructive sleep apnea: a systematic review. Sleep Med Rev. 2016;30:25–33.
43. Amos JM, Durr ML, Nardone HC, Baldassari CM, Duggins A, Ishman SL. Systematic review of drug-induced sleep endoscopy scoring systems. Otolaryngol Head Neck Surg. 2018;158(2):240–8.
44. Dijemeni E, D'Amone G, Gbati I. Drug-induced sedation endoscopy (DISE) classification systems: a systematic review and meta-analysis. Sleep Breath. 2017;21(4):983–94.
45. Gao Y-N, Wu Y-C, Lin S-Y, Chang JZ-C, Tu Y-K. Short-term efficacy of minimally invasive treatments for adult obstructive sleep apnea: a systematic review and network meta-analysis of randomized controlled trials. J Formos Med Assoc. 2019;118(4):750–65.
46. Tuomilehto HPI, Seppä JM, Partinen MM, Peltonen M, Gylling H, Tuomilehto JOI, et al. Lifestyle intervention with weight reduction: first-line treatment in mild obstructive sleep apnea. Am J Respir Crit Care Med. 2009;179(4):320–7.
47. Edwards BA, Bristow C, O'Driscoll DM, Wong A-M, Ghazi L, Davidson ZE, et al. Assessing the impact of diet, exercise and the combination of the two as a treatment for OSA: a systematic review and meta-analysis. Respirology. 2019;24(8):740–51.
48. Mendelson M, Lyons OD, Yadollahi A, Inami T, Oh P, Bradley TD. Effects of exercise training on sleep apnoea in patients with coronary artery disease: a randomised trial. Eur Respir J. 2016;48(1):142–50.
49. Randerath WJ, Galetke W, Domanski U, Weitkunat R, Ruhle K-H. Tongue-muscle training by intraoral electrical neurostimulation in patients with obstructive sleep apnea. Sleep. 2004;27(2):254–9.
50. Herkenrath SD, Treml M, Priegnitz C, Galetke W, Randerath WJ. Effects of respiratory muscle training (RMT) in patients with mild to moderate obstructive sleep apnea (OSA). Sleep Breath. 2018;22(2):323–8.
51. Puhan MA, Suarez A, Lo Cascio C, Zahn A, Heitz M, Braendli O. Didgeridoo playing as alternative treatment for obstructive sleep apnoea syndrome: randomised controlled trial. BMJ. 2006;332(7536):266–70.
52. Guimarães KC, Drager LF, Genta PR, Marcondes BF, Lorenzi-Filho G. Effects of oropharyngeal exercises on patients with moderate obstructive sleep apnea syndrome. Am J Respir Crit Care Med. 2009;179(10):962–6.
53. Andersen APD, Alving J, Lildholdt T, Wulff CH. Obstructive sleep apnea initiated by a lax epiglottis: a contraindication for continuous positive airway pressure. Chest. 1987;91(4):621–3.
54. Maurer JT, Stuck BA, Hein G, Hörmann K. Videoendoscopic assessment of uncommon sites of upper airway obstruction during sleep. Sleep Breath. 2000;4(3):131–6.
55. Verse T, Pirsig W. Age-related changes in the epiglottis causing failure of nasal continuous positive airway pressure therapy. J Laryngol Otol. 1999;113(11):1022–5.

56. Giles TL, Lasserson TJ, Smith BH, White J, Wright J, Cates CJ. Continuous positive airways pressure for obstructive sleep apnoea in adults. Cochrane Database Syst Rev. 2006;3:CD001106.
57. Javaheri S, Barbe F, Campos-Rodriguez F, Dempsey JA, Khayat R, Javaheri S, et al. Sleep apnea: types, mechanisms, and clinical cardiovascular consequences. J Am Coll Cardiol. 2017;69(7):841–58.
58. McEvoy RD, Antic NA, Heeley E, Luo Y, Ou Q, Zhang X, et al. CPAP for prevention of cardiovascular events in obstructive sleep apnea. N Engl J Med. 2016;375(10):919–31.
59. Holley AB, Lettieri CJ, Shah AA. Efficacy of an adjustable oral appliance and comparison with continuous positive airway pressure for the treatment of obstructive sleep apnea syndrome. Chest. 2011;140(6):1511–6.
60. Schwartz M, Acosta L, Hung Y-L, Padilla M, Enciso R. Effects of CPAP and mandibular advancement device treatment in obstructive sleep apnea patients: a systematic review and meta-analysis. Sleep Breath. 2018;22(3):555–68.
61. Bamagoos AA, Cistulli PA, Sutherland K, Ngiam J, Burke PGR, Bilston LE, et al. Dose-dependent effects of mandibular advancement on upper airway collapsibility and muscle function in obstructive sleep apnea. Sleep. 2019;42(6):zsz049; [cited 2019 Oct 21]. https://academic.oup.com/sleep/article/42/6/zsz049/5361366.
62. Edwards BA, Eckert DJ, Jordan AS. Obstructive sleep apnoea pathogenesis from mild to severe: is it all the same? Respirology. 2017;22(1):33–42.
63. Edwards BA, Andara C, Landry S, Sands SA, Joosten SA, Owens RL, et al. Upper-airway collapsibility and loop gain predict the response to oral appliance therapy in patients with obstructive sleep apnea. Am J Respir Crit Care Med. 2016;194(11):1413–22.
64. Herkenrath SD, Randerath WJ. More than heart failure: central sleep apnea and sleep-related hypoventilation. Respiration. 2019;10:1–16.
65. Bratton DJ, Gaisl T, Wons AM, Kohler M. CPAP vs mandibular advancement devices and blood pressure in patients with obstructive sleep apnea: a systematic review and meta-analysis. JAMA. 2015;314(21):2280–93.
66. Cohen-Levy J, Pételle B, Pinguet J, Limerat E, Fleury B. Forces created by mandibular advancement devices in OSAS patients. Sleep Breath. 2013;17(2):781–9.
67. Doff MHJ, Finnema KJ, Hoekema A, Wijkstra PJ, de Bont LGM, Stegenga B. Long-term oral appliance therapy in obstructive sleep apnea syndrome: a controlled study on dental side effects. Clin Oral Invest. 2013;17(2):475–82.
68. Perez CV, de Leeuw R, Okeson JP, Carlson CR, Li H-F, Bush HM, et al. The incidence and prevalence of temporomandibular disorders and posterior open bite in patients receiving mandibular advancement device therapy for obstructive sleep apnea. Sleep Breath. 2013;17(1):323–32.
69. Heinzer R, Petitpierre NJ, Marti-Soler H, Haba-Rubio J. Prevalence and characteristics of positional sleep apnea in the HypnoLaus population-based cohort. Sleep Med. 2018;48:157–62.
70. Mador MJ, Kufel TJ, Magalang UJ, Rajesh SK, Watwe V, Grant BJB. Prevalence of positional sleep apnea in patients undergoing polysomnography. Chest. 2005;128(4):2130–7.
71. Koh WP, Mok Y, Poh Y, Kam JW, Wong HS. Prevalence of positional obstructive sleep apnoea (OSA) among patients with OSA in a tertiary healthcare institution in Singapore. Singap Med J. 2020;61(12):665–6.
72. Oksenberg A, Silverberg DS, Arons E, Radwan H. Positional vs nonpositional obstructive sleep apnea patients: anthropomorphic, nocturnal polysomnographic, and multiple sleep latency test data. Chest. 1997;112(3):629–39.
73. van Maanen JP, de Vries N. Long-term effectiveness and compliance of positional therapy with the sleep position trainer in the treatment of positional obstructive sleep apnea syndrome. Sleep. 2014;37(7):1209–15.
74. Eijsvogel MM, Ubbink R, Dekker J, Oppersma E, de Jongh FH, van der Palen J, et al. Sleep position trainer versus tennis ball technique in positional obstructive sleep apnea syndrome. J Clin Sleep Med. 2015;11(2):139–47.
75. Levendowski DJ, Seagraves S, Popovic D, Westbrook PR. Assessment of a neck-based treatment and monitoring device for positional obstructive sleep apnea. J Clin Sleep Med. 2014;10(8):863–71.

76. Berry RB, Uhles ML, Abaluck BK, Winslow DH, Schweitzer PK, Gaskins RA, et al. NightBalance sleep position treatment device versus auto-adjusting positive airway pressure for treatment of positional obstructive sleep apnea. J Clin Sleep Med. 2019;15(7): 947–56.
77. Strollo PJ, Soose RJ, Maurer JT, de Vries N, Cornelius J, Froymovich O, et al. Upper-airway stimulation for obstructive sleep apnea. N Engl J Med. 2014;370(2):139–49.
78. Woodson BT, Strohl KP, Soose RJ, Gillespie MB, Maurer JT, de Vries N, et al. Upper airway stimulation for obstructive sleep apnea: 5-year outcomes. Otolaryngol Head Neck Surg. 2018;159(1):194–202.
79. Heiser C, Steffen A, Boon M, Hofauer B, Doghramji K, Maurer JT, et al. Post-approval upper airway stimulation predictors of treatment effectiveness in the ADHERE registry. Eur Respir J. 2019;53(1):1801405.
80. Randerath W, Verbraecken J, de Raaff C, Hedner J, Herkenrath S, Hohenhorst W, et al. European Respiratory Society guideline on non-CPAP therapies for obstructive sleep apnoea. Eur Respir Rev. 2021;30:210200.
81. Taranto-Montemurro L, Messineo L, Wellman A. Targeting Endotypic traits with medications for the pharmacological treatment of obstructive sleep apnea. A review of the current literature. J Clin Med. 2019;8(11):E1846.
82. Gaisl T, Haile SR, Thiel S, Osswald M, Kohler M. Efficacy of pharmacotherapy for OSA in adults: a systematic review and network meta-analysis. Sleep Med Rev. 2019;46:74–86.
83. Chapman JL, Vakulin A, Hedner J, Yee BJ, Marshall NS. Modafinil/armodafinil in obstructive sleep apnoea: a systematic review and meta-analysis. Eur Respir J. 2016;47(5):1420–8.
84. Dauvilliers Y, Verbraecken J, Partinen M, Hedner J, Saaresranta T, Georgiev O, et al. Pitolisant for daytime sleepiness in patients with obstructive sleep apnea who refuse continuous positive airway pressure treatment. A randomized trial. Am J Respir Crit Care Med. 2020;201(9):1135–45.
85. Pépin J-L, Georgiev O, Tiholov R, Attali V, Verbraecken J, Buyse B, et al. Pitolisant for residual excessive daytime sleepiness in OSA patients adhering to CPAP: a randomized trial. Chest. 2021;159(4):1598–609.
86. Wang J, Li X, Yang S, Wang T, Xu Z, Xu J, et al. Pitolisant versus placebo for excessive daytime sleepiness in narcolepsy and obstructive sleep apnea: a meta-analysis from randomized controlled trials. Pharmacol Res. 2021;167:105522.
87. Schweitzer PK, Rosenberg R, Zammit GK, Gotfried M, Chen D, Carter LP, et al. Solriamfetol for excessive sleepiness in obstructive sleep apnea (TONES 3). A randomized controlled trial. Am J Respir Crit Care Med. 2019;199(11):1421–31.
88. Subedi R, Singh R, Thakur RK, et al. Efficacy and safety of solriamfetol for excessive daytime sleepiness in narcolepsy and obstructive sleep apnea: a systematic review and meta-analysis of clinical trials. Sleep Med. 2020;75:510–21.
89. Taranto-Montemurro L, Messineo L, Sands SA, Azarbarzin A, Marques M, Edwards BA, et al. The combination of atomoxetine and oxybutynin greatly reduces obstructive sleep apnea severity. A randomized, placebo-controlled, double-blind crossover trial. Am J Respir Crit Care Med. 2019;199(10):1267–76.
90. Liu H-W, Chen Y-J, Lai Y-C, Huang C-Y, Huang Y-L, Lin M-T, et al. Combining MAD and CPAP as an effective strategy for treating patients with severe sleep apnea intolerant to high-pressure PAP and unresponsive to MAD. PLoS One. 2017;12(10):e0187032.
91. Tong BK, Tran C, Ricciardiello A, Donegan M, Chiang AKI, Szollosi I, et al. CPAP combined with oral appliance therapy reduces CPAP requirements and pharyngeal pressure swings in obstructive sleep apnea. J Appl Physiol (1985). 2020;129(5):1085–91.
92. Marques M, Genta PR, Sands SA, Azarbazin A, de Melo C, Taranto-Montemurro L, et al. Effect of sleeping position on upper airway patency in obstructive sleep apnea is determined by the pharyngeal structure causing collapse. Sleep. 2017;40(3):zsx005.
93. Lee CH, Kim DK, Kim SY, Rhee C-S, Won T-B. Changes in site of obstruction in obstructive sleep apnea patients according to sleep position: a DISE study. Laryngoscope. 2015;125(1):248–54.

94. Joosten SA, Landry SA, Sands SA, Terrill PI, Mann D, Andara C, et al. Dynamic loop gain increases upon adopting the supine body position during sleep in patients with obstructive sleep apnoea. Respirology. 2017;22(8):1662–9.
95. Dieltjens M, Vroegop AV, Verbruggen AE, Wouters K, Willemen M, De Backer WA, et al. A promising concept of combination therapy for positional obstructive sleep apnea. Sleep Breath. 2015;19(2):637–44.
96. Strollo PJ, Hedner J, Collop N, Lorch DG, Chen D, Carter LP, et al. Solriamfetol for the treatment of excessive sleepiness in OSA: a placebo-controlled randomized withdrawal study. Chest. 2019;155(2):364–74.

Redefining Outcome Measures

4

Madeline J. L. Ravesloot

4.1 Objective Outcome Measures

Sleep testing, in particular polysomnography (PSG), is the most important diagnostic tool in respiratory sleep medicine and is unique in measuring an abundance of simultaneously obtained objective measures such as sleep state, arousal, airflow, oxygen saturation, movements, and body position [1]. The data collected through the various components of a PSG result in the scoring of sleep and associated events [2]. The diagnosis and severity of obstructive sleep apnea (OSA) have been largely quantified by the numeric calculation of the number of obstructive, central, and mixed apneas and hypopneas per hour of sleep (AHI) [1]. Severity, spanning three levels is traditionally defined by the cut-offs 5–14, 15–29, and ≥30/h defining mild, moderate, and severe OSA, respectively, as suggested by the American Academy of Sleep Medicine (AASM) [3, 4]. For presenting daytime and night-time symptoms or cardiometabolic comorbidities caused by OSA, the term OSA syndrome (OSAS) is used. However, the terms "OSA" and "OSAS" are often used interchangeably in the medical literature [4]. It is important to realize that the AHI is a surrogate marker for disease severity and is not the only metric. Studies suggest that the oxygen desaturation index (ODI) would be more suited since clinical complications and mortality of OSA are more related to hypoxia during sleep [5–7]. ODI ≥ 3 or ≥4% is defined as the number of episodes of oxygen desaturation per hour of sleep with oxygen desaturation defined as a decrease in blood oxygen saturation (SpO_2) to lower than 3% and 4% below baseline. Other important metrics include apnea duration, SaO_2 nadir, length and depth of desaturations, and the time spent during sleep with an SaO_2 below 90% [8, 9]. Various guidelines and recommendations exist to

M. J. L. Ravesloot (✉)
Department of Otorhinolaryngology, OLVG, location West, Amsterdam, The Netherlands
e-mail: m.j.l.ravesloot@olvg.nl

M. Delakorda, N. de Vries (eds.), *The Role of Epiglottis in Obstructive Sleep Apnea*, https://doi.org/10.1007/978-3-031-34992-8_4

Table 4.1 Diagnostic criteria for obstructive sleep apnea, adult. (Adapted from ICSD-3; American Academy of Sleep Medicine, 2014)

(A and B) or C satisfy the criteria
A. The presence of one or more of the following
1. The patient complains of sleepiness, non-restorative sleep, fatigue, or insomnia symptoms
2. The patient wakes with breath holding, gasping, or choking voter
3. The bed partner or other observer reports habitual snoring, breathing interruptions, or both during the patient's sleep
4. The patient has been diagnosed with hypertension, a mood disorder, cognitive dysfunction, coronary artery disease, stroke congestive heart failure, atrial fibrillation, or type 2 diabetes mellitus
B. Polysomnography (PSG) or out-of-centre sleep testing (OCST) demonstrates:
1. Five or more predominantly obstructive respiratory events [obstructive and mixed apneas, hypopneas or respiratory effort-related arousals (RERAs)] per hour of sleep during a PSG or per hour of monitoring (OCST)
OR
C. PSG or OCST demonstrates:
1. Fifteen or more predominantly obstructive respiratory events (apneas, hypopneas, or RERAs) per hour of sleep during a PSG or per hour of monitoring (OCST

define OSA. The most commonly applied are the diagnostic criteria for adult obstructive sleep apnea defined in the International Classification of Sleep disorders (ISCD) of the AASM's manual of sleep disorders nosology as shown in Table 4.1 [10].

4.2 Variability of Objective Sleep Parameters

In both clinical practice and research it is important to realize that each sleep study is to a certain extent a "snapshot." Results may vary due to one of the following reasons:

- *Scoring rules:* Over time definitions of respiratory events, in particular for hypopnea scoring, have been reformulated. The scoring recommendations from the last AASM manual lead to increased AHI values, sometimes two-to three times greater [2, 11, 12].
- *Methodology (automated* versus *computer-assisted manual scoring), interrater variability, and level of expertise* [13–15].
- *Device use*: The most common sleep tests used in the diagnostic work-up of sleep disordered breathing are PSG and limited-channel polygraphy (PG). Since the latter does not measure actual sleep, the denominator of the AHI is recording time/time in bed, not total sleep time, and therefore invariably yields lower AHI results [4]. It is therefore mandatory not to mix up these two methods and to unequivocally discern AHI assessed by PSG (AHI_{PSG}) from AHI assessed by PG (AHI_{PG}). Peripheral arterial tonometry (PAT), a plethymographic technique, lacks registration of respiratory signals. An algorithm is used for analyzing the PAT signal together with oximetry and actigraphy [16, 17].

- *Night-to-night variability*: Night-to-night variability influences in particular the AHI, whereby the ODI is considered less susceptible and more robust. Factors influencing night-to-night variability include body sleeping position, first-night effect (FNE), unfamiliar environment, anxiety about the test, discomfort from wires and sensors, alcohol, or sedative use [16, 18, 19].
- To elaborate further, in positional patients (PP) with OSA, the overall severity of disease is dependent on the severity of disease in the various sleeping positions and even more so, on the time spent in the various sleeping positions. The longer a PP spends in the supine sleeping position, the greater the overall severity of disease and vice versa. Therefore sleeping position changes during sleep are considered a critical factor contributing to night-to-night variability of OSA severity, with a significant impact mainly among PP [18]. Another consideration is that studies suggest that while undergoing a PSG, patients spend a third more time in the supine position in comparison to habitual sleep. It is thought that the PSG apparatus leads to an increase in percentage of total time spent in the supine position [20]. This is of particular importance in PP, whereby the increased time spent in the supine position may cause overestimation in disease severity [18, 21].
- FNE is the alteration of sleep architecture observed on the first night of PSG studies. It is unclear whether the FNE reflects adaptation to the equipment, sleeping environment, or both and is characterized by a reduction in REM sleep and total sleep time, reduced sleep efficacy, increased wake time after sleep onset, and longer REM latency in the first night and is often amplified by a foreign sleep environment [22]. Furthermore, when one does not mimic normal sleep conditions at home, results may exacerbate or alleviate obstructive events. Neck position and elevation of the head in a different bed may impact the airway and influence results [4]. The same can be said concerning alcohol use for example. If a patient normally drinks alcohol, consumes caffeine, or uses certain medication which impact sleep such as sedatives at home, but not on the night of sleep test, the latter may be false negative.

4.3 Clinical Endpoints

Day- and night-time symptoms as well as comorbidities are extremely relevant in patients with OSA. Not only are they important when diagnosing the patient, but as physicians and surgeons we aim to improve quality of life, alleviate symptoms, comorbidities and behavioral, functional, and social consequences of the disorder, while not only focusing on improving respiratory disturbances during sleep. Polysomnographic variables can be considered intermediate outcomes, in particular, as they do not capture the impact of OSA on the cardiovascular, neurological, psychological, metabolic, and emotional aspects of the disease [9]. Furthermore conflicting results have been published concerning the correlation between PSG indexes and clinical endpoints [23, 24].

Alongside the patient medical interview, in general, questionnaires should be viewed as complementary and as useful tools to follow-up the impact of treatment of complaints. Questionnaires have been developed to structure and standardize evaluation and vary from more general to disease specific. TE Weaver in her two-part review titled "Outcome measures in sleep medicine practice and research" described measures to evaluate many of the outcomes as presented in Table 4.2 [25, 26]. She advocates that a comprehensive outcome assessment for sleep practice should include: (1) measure of subjective sleepiness; (2) disease-specific health-related quality of life (HRQoL) or functional status measures and optionally a generic instrument; (3) measure of mood; and (4) a measure of compliance to facilitate adequate interpretation of outcome responses. Although these additional parameters may be labor intensive for both research and the management of OSA, this stands in contrast to the oversimplification currently taking place with the use of the AHI alone [27].

The most common questionnaire applied in clinical practice and research is the Epworth Sleepiness Scale (ESS), a validated tool for the self-assessment of daytime sleepiness first introduced in 1990 [28]. It contains eight questions concerning the likelihood of dozing off or falling asleep in a variety of different situations. Unfortunately the ESS has a poor correlation with objective sleepiness as measured

Table 4.2 Clinical endpoints

Health-related consequences of OSA	Primarily cardiovascular and endocrine		
	Glaucoma		
Behavioral consequences of OSA	Excessive daytime sleepiness	Subjective sleepiness scales	Stanford Sleepiness Scale (SSS)
			Karolinska Sleepiness Scale (KSS)
			Epworth Sleepiness Scale (ESS)
			Sleep-Wake Activity Inventory (SWAI)
			Index of daytime sleepiness (ISS)
			Survey screen for sleep apnea (SSSA)
			Rotterdam Daytime Sleepiness Scale (RDSS)
		Objective sleepiness scales	Multiple sleep latency test (MSLT)
			Maintenance of wakefulness test (MWT)
			Oxford Sleep Resistance test (OSLER)
	Quality of Life	Generic instruments	Sickness Impact Profile Scale (SIP)
			Medical outcomes Study SF-36 (SF-36)
			Nottingham Health Profile (NHP)
			Functional Limitations Profile (FLP)
			Munich Life Quality Dimension List (MLQDL)
			WHOQOL-BREF
			EuroQoL (Eqol)
		Disease-specific instruments	Functional Outcome of Sleep Questionnaire (FOSQ)
			Calgary Sleep Apnea Quality of Life Index (SAQLI)
			OSA Patient-Orientated Severity Index (OS-APOSI)

Table 4.2 (continued)

Health-related consequences of OSA	Primarily cardiovascular and endocrine		
	Glaucoma		
Functional consequences of OSA	Performance	Cognitive	Digit Symbol Test (DST), Letter Cancellation, Block Design test, Object Assembly and Picture Arrangement from the gold standard Wechsler Intelligence Scale-Revised (WAIS-R)
			Paced Auditory Serial Addition Task (PASAT)
			Trailmaking A and B
		Memory	Probed recall memory task; Rey Auditory Verbal Learning Test (AVLT)
			Wechsler Memory Scale Story task [WMS stories]
			Rey-Osterrieth Complex Figure Test
		Mood	Profile of Mood States (POMS)
			Hospital Anxiety and Depression Scale (HADS)
			Beck Depression Inventory (BDI)
			Positive and Negative Affect Scale (PANAS)
			Minnesota Multiphasic Personality Inventory (MMPI)
			Zung Self-Rating Depression Scale Inventory (Zung)
			Geriatric Depression Scale (GDS)
			KDS self-rating scales for depression (KDS)
			Symptom Distress Check List (SCL-90-R)
			Freiburger Personality Inventory (FPI-R)
	Reaction time	Four Choice Reaction Time Test (FCRTT)	
		Psychomotor Vigilance Test (PVT)	
	Driving	Steer Clear	
		Divided Attention Driving Tests (DADT)	
Social consequences of OSA	Disruptive snoring and other OSA symptoms	Sleep Outcome Tool: Snore-25	
		Snoring Severity Scale (SSS)	
		Survey Screen for Sleep Apnea Index (SSSA)	
		Index of Sleep Apnea	
		Hawaii Sleep Questionnaire (HSQ)	
		Pittsburgh Sleep Quality index (PSQI)	

by the multiple sleep latency test (MSLT) [29]. Reporting on clinical endpoints in sleep disordered breathing, in particular in case of sleep surgery, is not yet common practice. To our best knowledge, besides the Stanford Sleepiness Scale (SSS) and the Sleep-Wake Activity Inventory (SWAI), no other subjective sleepiness scales have been evaluated in patients undergoing upper airway surgery for sleep apnea. Before applying these questionnaires in non-English speaking patients or countries it is important to check whether they have been validated into the specific language [30].

4.4 Treatment Success

In 1981, Fujita introduced uvulopalatopharyngoplasty (UPPP) as the first surgical procedure to treat OSA and reported an approximate 50% decrease in the apnea index (AI) from its preoperative value [31]. Thereafter a 50% reduction was used as a criterion for surgical response. Based on limited mortality data reported by He et al. indicating an acceleration of harm when the AHI rises above 20–25/h, others choose to define treatment success as a post-treatment respiratory disturbance index (RDI) of less than 20/h [32]. In surgical literature, Sher's criterion, a combination of both, is the most widely cited definition of success: an AI of less than 10/h or an RDI of less than 20/h and at least a 50% decrease from the baseline index, postoperatively [33]. Others have later proposed to tighten these criteria to a postoperative AHI to <15/h (regarded as a "clinically relevant" reduction), <10/h, and recently even <5/h [34]. Some have added "response" as reduction of the AHI between 20 and 50%. Without external validation, any arbitrary cut-off definition of success will be incorrect. Furthermore, the point at which the AHI becomes harmful remains unclear [35].

4.5 Therapeutic Effectiveness

In conservative treatment modalities such as continuous positive airway pressure (CPAP), oral devices (OA), and positional therapy (PT), it is common knowledge that a majority of patients are not compliant to the treatment during 100% of the total sleep time, under everyday non-laboratory conditions [36]. Patients seem to either tolerate the devices well or not at all—a bimodal distribution, with an average use of approximately 4 h/night [37]. Hence, the term "compliance" was introduced. Current trends define compliance as 4 h/night as an average over *all* nights observed [35]. This is a reach, but even the most effective medical devices are only effective when they are used. The effect may be 100% when always used, nil when never used, and partial when used sometimes but not always. This is particularly true for CPAP use in OSA [35]. In line with the theory that limited compliance leads to periods of sleep without effective treatment, studies have shown a positive relationship between hours of CPAP use and a favorable outcome; so the more hours a patient uses CPAP, the greater the therapeutic effect [38, 39]. To continue with this train of thought, the effectiveness of conservative treatment, regarding the reduction of AHI, depends both on its impact on airway obstruction and compliance [35, 40, 41]. Presently, the second aspect is often overlooked. Often when treatment effectiveness of CPAP is reported, this is in laboratory conditions, therefore insinuating an artificial compliance of 100% [41]. This is not only applicable for CPAP, but also for other conservative treatment modalities like OA therapy and PT. Various articles advocate that OSA treatment effects on the AHI should no longer be reported under conditions of artificial compliance only, but in consideration of the individual compliance to the treatment. This is of particular importance when different treatment options are compared [35, 40–42]. One method is to calculate the mean AHI with regard to treatment compliance. For example, taking CPAP as an example, using the total sleep time (TST), the hours of CPAP use in the treatment period as assessed with the devices' built-in counters (HOURSonCPAP), the AHI as assessed in the sleep lab before treatment (AHIoffCPAP), and while using CPAP (AHIonCPAP). In this way one can calculate the mean AHI using the following mathematical formula [35]:

$$\text{meanAHIforCPAP} = \frac{(\text{AHIonCPAP} \times \text{HOURSonCPAP}) + [\text{AHIoffCPAP} \times (\text{TST} - \text{HOURSonCPAP})]}{\text{TST}}$$

However, this formula is based on the assumption that the AHI will revert to baseline once the CPAP appliance is no longer used. It can be argued that after the termination of CPAP during night, the AHI may not completely revert to baseline. CPAP is thought to play a role in reducing edema resulting from snoring-associated vibrations and apnea-induced suction of the upper airway. It is thought that the baseline AHI may be reduced by a fraction in chronic CPAP use [43]. Another consideration is that one assumes that the AHI is uniform across night and matches the diagnostic sleep test. To illustrate, in a meta-analysis, pooling of data on the efficacy of maxillomandibular advancement (MMA), it was reported that the mean AHI decreased from 63.9 to 9.5/h following surgery [44]. In a study reporting on the effects of CPAP, taking individual compliance into account, the mean AHI decreased from 35.6 to 11.9/h. The mean AHI under CPAP was 2.4/h [45]. Juxtaposed, these treatment modalities seem to be equally effective in reducing the AHI when compliance is taken into account [41]. Another approach to the same concept is the mean disease alleviation (MDA), a measure of therapeutic effectiveness. The MDA is the product of therapeutic efficacy and adjusted compliance [40]. It is defined as the baseline AHI minus the AHI at follow-up, expressed as the percentage of baseline AHI. The adjusted compliance is defined as hours of use corrected for TST. This method was used to support findings that higher objective compliance with OA therapy translates into a similar adjusted effectiveness as compared with CPAP [40, 46]. Other suggestions on how to report therapeutic effectiveness include AHI "burden" and effectiveness of treatment AHI (ET-AHI) for example [42, 47].

4.6 Taking Body Position into Account

Another aspect to take into consideration, when reporting treatment effectiveness, is body position.

- As mentioned previously, in PP the overall severity of disease is dependent on the severity of disease in the various sleeping positions and even more so, on the time spent in the various sleeping positions [18].

Thus, when reporting on the results of OSA treatment:

- *Consider the effect of treatment on sleep study variables in various sleeping positions and take time spent in the various sleeping positions into account before and after treatment.*
- *Differentiate between pre-treatment PP and non-positional patients (NPP).*
- *Explore whether PP remain PP or become NPP and whether NPP remain NPP or become PP. Is there a post-operative shift in position-dependency?*
- *Is position-dependency a predictor for treatment success or failure?*

These considerations are applicable for the complete management armamentarium of OSA including UA surgery, bariatric surgery, or OA therapy, for example. A proposal on how to report these different results can be found in Tables 4.3, 4.4, 4.5, 4.6, and 4.7. Studies suggest that the effect of UA surgery and OA therapy could result in different outcomes in pre-treatment PP and NPP although they seem to report different outcomes and contradict each other [48].

Table 4.3 Framework for reporting on the role of sleeping position in the management of sleep apnea patients

	Framework for reporting	Rationale
Baseline characteristics (anatomical, morphological and physiologic factors, and sleep study data)	1. Total patient population	PP and NPP are a different phenotype
	2. Separately for PP and NPP	Baseline characteristics are associated with treatment outcome
Baseline sleep study data	1. P(S)G indices in various sleeping positions	Severity of disease in PP is totally dependent on the sleep time spent in supine position and severity of disease in the various sleeping positions
	2. Time spent in various sleeping positions	
	3. Separately for PP and NPP	
Post-treatment sleep study data	1. Total patient population	PP and NPP are a different phenotype
	2. Separately for PP and NPP	
	3. P(S)G indices in various sleeping positions	Baseline characteristics are associated with treatment outcome
	4. Time spent in various sleeping positions	
Treatment success	1. Total patient population	PP and NPP are a different phenotype
Responders and non-responders	2. Separately for PP and NPP	Baseline characteristics are associated with treatment outcome
	3. Separately for supine and non-supine sleeping position	
Therapeutic effectiveness of positional therapy	Mean AHI, mean disease alleviation, AHI "burden," and effectiveness of treatment AHI (ET-AHI), *including compliance*	Effectiveness of treatment requires both efficacy and compliance

Table 4.4 Framework for reporting on treatment success in the management of sleep apnea patients, considering the role of body sleeping position

	Analysis and statistical technique
Changes in outcomes	Comparison of pre- and post-treatment values:
	Continuous variables:
	Paired *t* test (normally distributed data)
	Wilcoxon signed rank test (non-normally distributed data)
	To correct for possible confounders, a multivariate logistic regression analysis can be applied
Comparison of changes in outcomes between pre-treatment NPP and PP	Changes in outcome measures within NPP and PP subgroups:
	Paired *t* test (normally distributed data)
	Wilcoxon signed rank test (non-normally distributed data)
	Compare changes in outcome measures between subgroups:
	Independent *t* test (normally distributed data)
	Mann–Whitney *U* test (non-normally distributed data)
Changes in position-dependency post-treatment	Descriptive statistics to analyze the occurrence of a shift in position-dependency post-treatment
Correlation position-dependency and treatment success	Regression techniques or Pearson's chi-squared test
	Correction for possible confounders: multivariate logistic regression analyses

Table 4.5 Example how to report baseline characteristics for total population and NPP and PP

	Total	NPP	PP	*p* Value*
Number of patients (*N*)				
Male: female				
Age (years)				
BMI (kg/m^2)				

Data presented as mean ± standard deviation or median [Q1, Q3]
NPP non-positional obstructive sleep apnea patients, *PP* positional obstructive sleep apnea patients, *BMI* body mass index
*p Value comparing baseline characteristics of NPP and PP

After UA surgery for OSA, studies report that 42–75% of NPP improve and become PP after UA surgery [48–57]. At the basis of these observations, the effect of surgery is greater in the lateral position than in the supine position, resulting in residual OSA in the supine position [48, 57]. Concerning preoperative PP, 50–90% remain positional after surgery [48, 51, 52, 54]. Studies report the beneficial effect of adjuvant PT in patients with postoperative persistent POSA [18, 54, 56, 58]. In the recent SAMS trial, a randomized controlled trial comparing multilevel surgery with medical management, MacKay et al. reported a similar favorable significant effect on the supine AHI (mean baseline adjusted between-group difference, −18.7 events/h [95% CI, −31.1 to −6.3] [51]; $P = 0.003$) and non-supine AHI (mean base line adjusted between-group difference, −18.4 events/h stoel; $P = 0.001$) [59]. It remains unsettled whether position-dependency is a predictor for surgical success [48]. Certain studies report no difference in surgical success rate between NPP and

Table 4.6 Example how to report sleep study data in various sleeping positions and time spent in various sleeping positions, reported for total patient population and for NPP and PP

		Sleep time (min)	AHI (events/h)	Obstructive AI (events/h)	Mixed AI (events/h)	Central AI (events/h)	ODI (events/h)	Average SpO_2 (%)	Minimum SpO_2
Total	Total								
	Supine								
	Non-supine								
	Left								
	Right								
	Prone								
PP	Total								
	Supine								
	Non-supine								
	Left								
	Right								
	Prone								
NPP	Total								
	Supine								
	Non-supine								
	Left								
	Right								
	Prone								

Data presented as mean ± standard deviation or median [Q1, Q3]
NPP non-positional obstructive sleep apnea patients, *PP* positional obstructive sleep apnea patients, *AHI* apnea–hypopnea index, *AI* apnea index, *ODI* oxygen desaturation index, SpO_2 saturation of peripheral oxygen

Table 4.7 Example how to report treatment success stratifying for the total AHI, the supine AHI, and non-supine AHI in total population, NPP and PP

Treatment success	Total population (N=)	NPP (N=)	PP (N=)	p value*
Total AHI	%	%	%	
Supine AHI	%	%	%	
Non-supine AHI	%	%	%	

AHI apnea–hypopnea index, *NPP* non-positional obstructive sleep apnea patients, *PP* positional obstructive sleep apnea patients
**p* Value comparing NPP and PP

PP undergoing UPPP [50], isolated tongue base or multilevel surgery [51], maxillomandibular advancement [57], and UA stimulation [60], while other studies suggest the opposite. Some report that PP have a greater chance of surgical success, whilst other are in favor of NPP [48, 53, 54, 61, 62]. The question whether position-dependency is a predictor for treatment success is also relevant for OA therapy. Two articles found that position dependency was not a predictor for treatment success, while Marklund et al. reported that position-dependency was a predictor [63–65]. Lee et al. reported that most PP remained positional after OA application, while half the NPP became PP after OA application [18, 66]. Some studies report a significant reduction in both supine AHI and in non-supine AHI after OA application [63, 64] whilst others report a greater decrease in supine AHI in PP in comparison to NPP [64, 67]. Others report better treatment outcomes in PP in comparison to NPP [66, 67] or in contrast lower treatment outcomes in PP in comparison to NPP [63], while others suggest that OA therapy is effective in reducing the AHI in both PP and NPP [18, 64]. A confusing topic that needs further investigating.

At a more complex but equally important level, one must keep confounders into consideration, for example the inverse relationship with BMI and AHI is not only related to PP, but also to surgical success [18]. Methods to exclude or control for confounding variables should be applied such as randomization or statistical testing and adjustment for potential confounders (Table 4.4).

References

1. Cielo CM, Tapia IE. Diving deeper: rethinking AHI as the primary measure of OSA severity. J Clin Sleep Med. 2019;15(8):1075–6.
2. Berry RB, Brooks R, Gamaldo CE, Harding SM, Marcus C, Vaughn BV. The AASM manual for the scoring of sleep and associated events. Rules, terminology and technical specifications. Darien: American Academy of Sleep Medicine; 2012. p. 176.
3. American Academy of Sleep Medicine. The report of an American Academy of sleep Medicine task force: sleep-related breathing disorders in adults; recommendations for syndrome definition and measurement techniques in clinical research. Sleep. 1999;22:667–89.
4. NVALT N. Richtlijn Obstructief Slaapapneu (OSA) bij Volwassenen; 2018.
5. Muraja-Murro A, Kulkas A, Hiltunen M, Kupari S, Hukkanen T, Tiihonen P, et al. The severity of individual obstruction events is related to increased mortality rate in severe obstructive sleep apnea. J Sleep Res. 2013;22(6):663–9.
6. Azarbarzin A, Sands SA, Taranto-Montemurro L, Redline S, Wellman A. Hypoxic burden captures sleep apnoea-specific nocturnal hypoxaemia. Eur Heart J. 2019;40(35): 2989–90.
7. Leppänen T, Kulkas A, Töyräs J. The hypoxic burden: also known as the desaturation severity parameter. Eur Heart J. 2019;40:2991.
8. Ravesloot MJ, De Raaff CA, Van De Beek MJ, Benoist LB, Beyers J, Corso RM, et al. Perioperative care of patients with obstructive sleep apnea undergoing upper airway surgery: a review and consensus recommendations. JAMA Otolaryngol Head Neck Surg. 2019;145(8):751–60.
9. Kezirian EJ, Weaver EM, Criswell MA, De Vries N, Woodson BT, Piccirillo JF. Reporting results of obstructive sleep apnea syndrome surgery trials. Otolaryngol Head Neck Surg. 2011;144(4):496–9.
10. Sateia MJ. International classification of sleep disorders. Chest. 2014;146(5):1387–94.

11. Duce B, Milosavljevic J, Hukins C. The 2012 AASM respiratory event criteria increase the incidence of hypopneas in an adult sleep center population. J Clin Sleep Med. 2015;11(12):1425–31.
12. Iber C. The AASM manual for the scoring of sleep and associated events: rules, terminology, and technical specification. 2007.
13. Danker-Hopfe H, Kunz D, Gruber G, Klösch G, Lorenzo JL, Himanen S-L, et al. Interrater reliability between scorers from eight European sleep laboratories in subjects with different sleep disorders. J Sleep Res. 2004;13(1):63–9.
14. Magalang UJ, Chen N-H, Cistulli PA, Fedson AC, Gíslason T, Hillman D, et al. Agreement in the scoring of respiratory events and sleep among international sleep centers. Sleep. 2013;36(4):591–6.
15. Malhotra A, Younes M, Kuna ST, Benca R, Kushida CA, Walsh J, et al. Performance of an automated polysomnography scoring system versus computer-assisted manual scoring. Sleep. 2013;36(4):573–82.
16. Kapur VK, Auckley DH, Chowdhuri S, Kuhlmann DC, Mehra R, Ramar K, et al. Clinical practice guideline for diagnostic testing for adult obstructive sleep apnea: an American Academy of Sleep Medicine clinical practice guideline. J Clin Sleep Med. 2017;13(3):479–504.
17. Yalamanchali S, Farajian V, Hamilton C, Pott TR, Samuelson CG, Friedman M. Diagnosis of obstructive sleep apnea by peripheral arterial tonometry: meta-analysis. JAMA Otolaryngol Head Neck Surg. 2013;139(12):1343–50.
18. Ravesloot M, Vonk P, Maurer J, Oksenberg A, de Vries N. Standardized framework to report on the role of sleeping position in sleep apnea patients. Sleep Breath. 2021;25:1–12.
19. Tkacova R, McNicholas WT, Javorsky M, Fietze I, Sliwinski P, Parati G, et al. Nocturnal intermittent hypoxia predicts prevalent hypertension in the European Sleep Apnoea Database cohort study. Eur Respir J. 2014;44(4):931–41.
20. Mueller CE, Li H, Begasse SM, Sommer JU, Stuck BA, Birk R. Sleep position, patient comfort, and technical performance with two established procedures for home sleep testing. Sleep Breath. 2021;26:1–9.
21. Vonk P, de Vries N, Ravesloot M. Polysomnography and sleep position, a Heisenberg phenomenon? HNO. 2019;67(9):679–84.
22. Roeder M, Bradicich M, Schwarz EI, Thiel S, Gaisl T, Held U, et al. Night-to-night variability of respiratory events in obstructive sleep apnoea: a systematic review and meta-analysis. Thorax. 2020;75(12):1095–102.
23. Weaver EM, Woodson BT, Steward DL. Polysomnography indexes are discordant with quality of life, symptoms, and reaction times in sleep apnea patients. Otolaryngol Head Neck Surg. 2005;132(2):255–62.
24. Kezirian EJ, Malhotra A, Goldberg AN, White DP. Changes in obstructive sleep apnea severity, biomarkers, and quality of life after multilevel surgery. Laryngoscope. 2010;120(7):1481–8.
25. Weaver TE. Outcome measurement in sleep medicine practice and research. Part 1: assessment of symptoms, subjective and objective daytime sleepiness, health-related quality of life and functional status. Sleep Med Rev. 2001;5(2):103–28.
26. Weaver TE. Outcome measurement in sleep medicine practice and research. Part 2: assessment of neurobehavioral performance and mood. Sleep Med Rev. 2001;5(3):223–36.
27. Pang KP, Baptista PM, Olszewska E, Braverman I, Carrasco-Llatas M, Kishore S, Chandra S, Yang HC, Chan YH, Pang KA, Pang EB, Rotenberg B. SLEEP-GOAL: a multicenter success criteria outcome study on 302 obstructive sleep apnoea (OSA) patients. Med J Malaysia. 2020;75(2):117.
28. Johns MW. Reliability and factor analysis of the Epworth Sleepiness Scale. Sleep. 1992;15(4):376–81.
29. Benbadis SR, Mascha E, Perry MC, Wolgamuth BR, Smolley LA, Dinner DS. Association between the Epworth sleepiness scale and the multiple sleep latency test in a clinical population. Ann Intern Med. 1999;130(4_Part_1):289–92.
30. Tsang S, Royse CF, Terkawi AS. Guidelines for developing, translating, and validating a questionnaire in perioperative and pain medicine. Saudi J Anaesth. 2017;11(Suppl 1):S80.

31. Fujita S, Conway W, Zorick F, Roth T. Surgical correction of anatomic azbnormalities in obstructive sleep apnea syndrome: uvulopalatopharyngoplasty. Otolaryngol Head Neck Surg. 1981;89(6):923–34.
32. He J, Kryger MH, Zorick FJ, Conway W, Roth T. Mortality and apnea index in obstructive sleep apnea. Experience in 385 male patients. Chest. 1988;94(1):9–14.
33. Sher AE, Schechtman KB, Piccirillo JF. The efficacy of surgical modifications of the upper airway in adults with obstructive sleep apnea syndrome. Sleep. 1996;19(2):156–77.
34. Elshaug AG, Moss JR, Southcott AM, Hiller JE. Redefining success in airway surgery for obstructive sleep apnea: a meta analysis and synthesis of the evidence. Sleep. 2007;30(4): 461–7.
35. Ravesloot MJ, de Vries N. Reliable calculation of the efficacy of non-surgical and surgical treatment of obstructive sleep apnea revisited. Sleep. 2011;34(1):105–10.
36. Weaver TE, Grunstein RR. Adherence to continuous positive airway pressure therapy: the challenge to effective treatment. Proc Am Thorac Soc. 2008;5(2):173–8.
37. Kribbs NB, Pack AI, Kline LR, Smith PL, Schwartz AR, Schubert NM, et al. Objective measurement of patterns of nasal CPAP use by patients with obstructive sleep apnea. Am Rev Respir Dis. 1993;147(4):887–95.
38. Weaver TE, Maislin G, Dinges DF, Bloxham T, George CF, Greenberg H, et al. Relationship between hours of CPAP use and achieving normal levels of sleepiness and daily functioning. Sleep. 2007;30(6):711–9.
39. Wozniak DR, Lasserson TJ, Smith I. Educational, supportive and behavioural interventions to improve usage of continuous positive airway pressure machines in adults with obstructive sleep apnoea. Cochrane Database Syst Rev. 2014;1:CD007736.
40. Vanderveken OM, Dieltjens M, Wouters K, De Backer WA, Van de Heyning PH, Braem MJ. Objective measurement of compliance during oral appliance therapy for sleep-disordered breathing. Thorax. 2013;68(1):91–6.
41. Ravesloot MJ, de Vries N, Stuck BA. Treatment adherence should be taken into account when reporting treatment outcomes in obstructive sleep apnea. Laryngoscope. 2014;124(1):344–5.
42. Boyd SB, Walters AS. Effectiveness of treatment apnea-hypopnea index: a mathematical estimate of the true apnea-hypopnea index in the home setting. J Oral Maxillofac Surg. 2013;71(2):351–7.
43. Ryan CF, Lowe AA, Li D, Fleetham JA. Magnetic resonance imaging of the upper airway in obstructive sleep apnea before and after chronic nasal continuous positive airway pressure therapy. Am Rev Respir Dis. 1991;144(4):939–44.
44. Holty J-EC, Guilleminault C. Maxillomandibular advancement for the treatment of obstructive sleep apnea: a systematic review and meta-analysis. Sleep Med Rev. 2010;14(5):287–97.
45. Stuck BA, Leitzbach S, Maurer JT. Effects of continuous positive airway pressure on apnea–hypopnea index in obstructive sleep apnea based on long-term compliance. Sleep Breath. 2012;16(2):467–71.
46. Ribeiro de Almeida F. Complexity and efficacy of mandibular advancement splints: understanding their mode of action. J Clin Sleep Med. 2011;7(5):447–8.
47. Bianchi MT, Alameddine Y, Mojica J. Apnea burden: efficacy versus effectiveness in patients using positive airway pressure. Sleep Med. 2014;15(12):1579–81.
48. Vonk P, Rotteveel P, Ravesloot M, den Haan C, De Vries N. The influence of position-dependency on surgical success in sleep apnea surgery—a systematic review. Sleep Breath. 2020;24(2):433–42.
49. Katsantonis GP, Miyazaki S, Walsh JK. Effects of uvulopalatopharyngoplasty on sleep architecture and patterns of obstructed breathing. Laryngoscope. 1990;100(10):1068–72.
50. Lee CH, Kim S-W, Han K, Shin J-M, Hong S-L, Lee J-E, et al. Effect of uvulopalatopharyngoplasty on positional dependency in obstructive sleep apnea. Arch Otolaryngol Head Neck Surg. 2011;137(7):675–9.
51. Van Maanen J, Ravesloot M, Witte B, Grijseels M, De Vries N. Exploration of the relationship between sleep position and isolated tongue base or multilevel surgery in obstructive sleep apnea. Eur Arch Otorhinolaryngol. 2012;269(9):2129–36.

52. Lee YC, Eun YG, Shin SY, Kim SW. Change in position dependency in non-responders after multilevel surgery for obstructive sleep apnea: analysis of polysomnographic parameters. Eur Arch Otorhinolaryngol. 2014;271(5):1081–5.
53. Li H-Y, Cheng W-N, Chuang L-P, Fang T-J, Hsin L-J, Kang C-J, et al. Positional dependency and surgical success of relocation pharyngoplasty among patients with severe obstructive sleep apnea. Otolaryngol Head Neck Surg. 2013;149(3):506–12.
54. van Maanen J, Witte B, de Vries N. Theoretical approach towards increasing effectiveness of palatal surgery in obstructive sleep apnea: role for concomitant positional therapy? Sleep Breath. 2014;18(2):341–9.
55. Kastoer C, Benoist L, Dieltjens M, Torensma B, de Vries L, Vonk P, et al. Comparison of upper airway collapse patterns and its clinical significance: drug-induced sleep endoscopy in patients without obstructive sleep apnea, positional and non-positional obstructive sleep apnea. Sleep Breath. 2018;22(4):939–48.
56. Benoist LB, de Ruiter MH, de Lange J, de Vries N. Residual POSA after maxillomandibular advancement in patients with severe OSA. In: Positional therapy in obstructive sleep apnea. Cham: Springer; 2015. p. 321–9.
57. Vonk PE, Rotteveel PJ, Ravesloot MJ, Ho J-PT, de Lange J, de Vries N. The influence of position dependency on surgical success in patients with obstructive sleep apnea undergoing maxillomandibular advancement. J Clin Sleep Med. 2020;16(1):73–80.
58. Benoist L, Verhagen M, Torensma B, van Maanen J, De Vries N. Positional therapy in patients with residual positional obstructive sleep apnea after upper airway surgery. Sleep Breath. 2017;21(2):279–88.
59. MacKay S, Carney AS, Catcheside PG, Chai-Coetzer CL, Chia M, Cistulli PA, et al. Effect of multilevel upper airway surgery vs medical management on the apnea-hypopnea index and patient-reported daytime sleepiness among patients with moderate or severe obstructive sleep apnea: the SAMS randomized clinical trial. JAMA. 2020;324(12):1168–79.
60. Steffen A, Hartmann JT, König IR, Ravesloot MJ, Hofauer B, Heiser C. Evaluation of body position in upper airway stimulation for obstructive sleep apnea—is continuous voltage sufficient enough? Sleep Breath. 2018;22(4):1207–12.
61. Lee CH, Shin H-W, Han DH, Mo J-H, Yoon I-Y, Chung S, et al. The implication of sleep position in the evaluation of surgical outcomes in obstructive sleep apnea. Otolaryngol Head Neck Surg. 2009;140(4):531–5.
62. Beyers J, Vanderveken OM, Kastoer C, Boudewyns A, De Volder I, Van Gastel A, Verbraecken JA, De Backer WA, Braem MJ, Van De Heyning PH, Dieltjens M. Treatment of sleep-disordered breathing with positional therapy: long-term results. Sleep and Breathing. 2019;23:1141–9.
63. Sutherland K, Phillips CL, Cistulli PA. Efficacy versus effectiveness in the treatment of obstructive sleep apnea: CPAP and oral appliances. J Dent Sleep Med. 2015;2(4):175–81.
64. Dieltjens M, Braem MJ, Van de Heyning PH, Wouters K, Vanderveken OM. Prevalence and clinical significance of supine-dependent obstructive sleep apnea in patients using oral appliance therapy. J Clin Sleep Med. 2014;10(9):959–64.
65. Marklund M, Persson M, Franklin KA. Treatment success with a mandibular advancement device is related to supine-dependent sleep apnea. Chest. 1998;114(6):1630–5.
66. Lee CH, Jung HJ, Lee WH, Rhee CS, Yoon IY, Yun PY, et al. The effect of positional dependency on outcomes of treatment with a mandibular advancement device. Arch Otolaryngol Head Neck Surg. 2012;138(5):479–83.
67. Chung JW, Enciso R, Levendowski DJ, Morgan TD, Westbrook PR, Clark GT. Treatment outcomes of mandibular advancement devices in positional and nonpositional OSA patients. Oral Surg Oral Med Oral Pathol Oral Radiol Endod. 2010;109(5):724–31.

Part II

Diagnosis of Epiglottis Collapse

Relevant Anatomy and Physiology of the Epiglottis

5

Matej Delakorda

5.1 Introduction

The nutritional and respiratory paths are joined in the upper aerodigestive tract that serves multiple functions. Due to the complex relationship between the skeletal frame and soft tissues, accurate neurological coordination is essential for maintaining adequate patency during breathing and for exerting effective constrictions during swallowing. A comprehensive knowledge of the anatomy of this region is fundamental for understanding pathophysiologic processes as well as performing safe and successful surgery.

The larynx is a cartilaginous segment of the respiratory tract, which is located in the anterior aspect of the neck. Phylogenetically, its primary function was to prevent ingested food and liquids from entering the trachea; the function of phonation developed with further evolution. Complete glottic closure is necessary for effective lung cleaning (coughing, sneezing) and for generating a positive intrathoracic pressure required for defecation, lifting heavy objects, body stabilization, and childbirth. The larynx also plays an important role in breathing and is actively involved in the regulation of respiration by a complex of sensory feedback loops. The epiglottis is a part of the supraglottic larynx and has an important function, especially in breastfeeding newborns and infants. It is exposed to many possible diseases, developmental anomalies, infections, and neoplasms. The role of epiglottis in obstructive sleep apnea (OSA) has only recently been observed and elucidated.

M. Delakorda (✉)
General Hospital Celje, Celje, Slovenia

M. Delakorda, N. de Vries (eds.), *The Role of Epiglottis in Obstructive Sleep Apnea*, https://doi.org/10.1007/978-3-031-34992-8_5

5.2 Embryology

The larynx begins to form during the third and fourth weeks of embryologic development as a morphogenetic component of the respiratory system, and by the 41st day, its cartilage and the intrinsic muscles are already observable. Its formation starts as a longitudinal ridge from the foregut caudal to the fourth pharyngeal pouch. Its lower portion grows inferiorly as a diverticulum to form the trachea and lungs, while the cephalic part forms a primitive laryngeal aditus covered by an endoderm lining—future epithelium. As it extends toward the caudal part of the embryo, it becomes invested by mesenchyme that gives rise to the cartilaginous and muscular structures. Antero-superior to this ridge is a hypobranchial eminence, a midline proliferation of mesenchyme anterior to third and fourth branchial arches visible as a swelling of the floor of the primitive hypopharynx. The epiglottis will develop from this structure and the ventral parts of the third and fourth arches. The latter will also give rise to the aryepiglottic folds and cuneiform cartilages. The arytenoids and corniculate cartilages are derived from the arytenoid swellings of the sixth branchial arches (Fig. 5.1).

The lesser cornu and the upper body of the hyoid are formed by the second pharyngeal arch, while the greater cornu and the lower portion of the body derive from the third pharyngeal arch. The process of hyoid chondrification begins in the fifth fetal week and is completed in the third and fourth months. Ossification in the greater cornu begins toward the end of the intrauterine life, in the hyoid body shortly before or after birth, and in the lesser cornu around puberty. The thyroid cartilage is

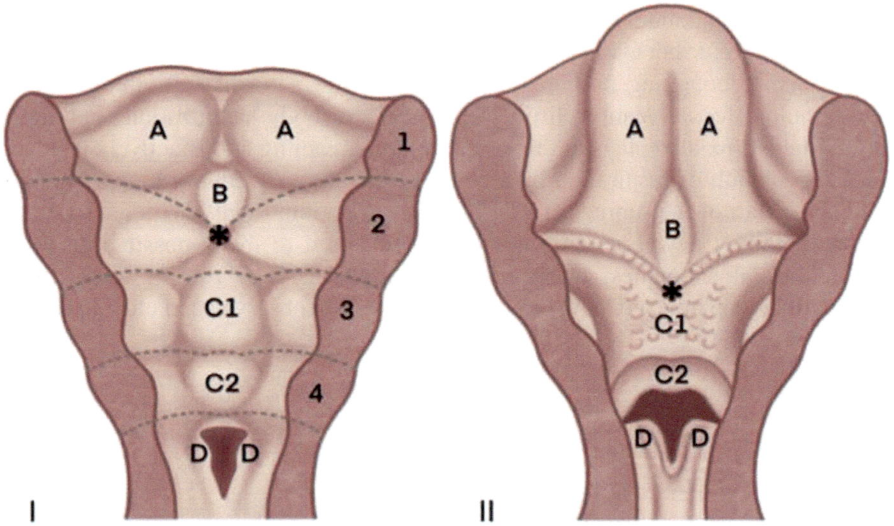

Fig. 5.1 The ventral part of the pharynx in the fourth week (I) and fifth month (II) of fetal life. *A* lateral lingual swellings, *B* medial lingual swelling, *C1* hypobranchial eminence, *C2* epiglottal swelling, *D* arytenoid swellings, and * foramen cecum

derived from the fourth pharyngeal arch. The future thyroid cartilage and hyoid are connected ventrally at the hypobranchial eminence and dorsally by a cartilaginous bar—the hypothyroid cartilage. At the third month of fetal development, the hyoid bone and thyroid cartilage separate, sometimes leaving a remnant of this connection in the form of a small oval-shaped hyaline cartilage called triticeal cartilage [1].

5.3 Developmental Anomalies

The incidence of congenital anomalies of the larynx and trachea is fairly low, reported at 1 in 10,000 to 50,000 live births, either as isolated occurrences or as synchronous lesions, frequently seen as part of syndromes such as short rib polydactyly, or tricho-rhino-phalangeal and lacrimo–auriculo-dental-digital syndromes [2]. The identification of such anomalies soon after birth, or prenatally, is often vital for the survival and growth of the infant. Laryngeal anomalies are commonly related to symptoms of aspiration and/or stridor, which can also be caused by dynamic conditions such as laryngomalacia (see Chap. 11).

Interruption before or during the embryological period during which the larynx is formed can result in aplasia, hypoplasia, and bifid epiglottis. The absence of the epiglottis can also be accompanied by severe glottic stenosis [3]. Patients with bifid epiglottis commonly experience symptoms of respiratory compromise caused by one or both of the cartilaginous halves being drawn into the glottic inlet with inspiration.

5.4 Maturation: Laryngeal Descent

The anatomy and position of the larynx in infants and children differ from that in adults [3]. From fetal to adult life, the epiglottis undergoes a considerable gradual descent in relation to the vertebral column as well as some morphologic changes [4, 5]. These anatomic changes of the upper respiratory tract probably evolved mainly to facilitate speech by enabling better articulation. An elevated laryngeal position enables contact between the epiglottis and soft palate, thus supporting nutrition by allowing breathing while sucking. It not only prevents aspiration but also makes newborns obligatory nasal breathers. Laryngeal descent is believed to be the anatomic basis predisposing humans to OSA as a developmental extension of the tongue backward and downward creates a compliant oropharynx prone to collapse [6–8].

At birth, the inferior margin of the cricoid cartilage is located at the level of the upper border of the C-4 vertebra, while the tip of the epiglottis is at the level of the C-1 vertebra. Usually, it can be visualized over the dorsum of the tongue in most infants. From birth, the larynx starts to descend with the most obvious changes taking place during puberty when the larynx lengthens rapidly. The cricoid cartilage descends to the level of the C-7 vertebra in men and the C-6 vertebra in women, and the tip of the epiglottis is opposite the C-3 vertebra.

The infant larynx has softer cartilage and laxer supporting ligaments. Epiglottis is omega- or tubular-shaped, and hence, it is more susceptible to collapse due to negative pressure during inspiration [9]. During maturation, the epiglottis becomes increasingly flat with the aryepiglottic folds in a more lateral position; but in most adults, it retains its curved shape. Additionally, an angle of the thyroid cartilage's laminae narrows from 110–120 to 90° in men after puberty but does not change significantly in women.

5.5 Skeletal Framework

An adult larynx is superiorly limited by the free end of the epiglottis and inferiorly by the lower edge of the cricoid cartilage. Its cartilaginous skeleton consists of multiple cartilage types: hyaline cartilage—specifically, thyroid, cricoid, arytenoid, and triticeal; elastic epiglottis; and fibroelastic corniculate (Santorini) and cuneiform (Wrisberg) cartilage. Together with the hyoid bone, they form a complex skeletal framework interconnected by numerous ligaments, fibrous membranes, and synovial joints that are moved by muscles in different directions.

The thyroid cartilage is the largest cartilage of the larynx. It is formed by two quadrangular alae that unite anteriorly and form a thyroid notch superiorly with the laryngeal prominence (Adam's apple) just below it, most obvious in males. On the lateral surface, there is an oblique line to which the sternothyroid, thyrohyoid, and inferior pharyngeal constrictor muscles attach [9]. Posteriorly, each ala has a superior and inferior horn. The inferior horn articulates with a facet on the cricoid cartilage to form the synovial cricothyroid joint that allows rotation of the cricoid cartilage. The superior horn attaches to the greater cornu of the hyoid bone with the lateral thyrohyoid ligament. In about one-third of the general adult population, this ligament contains small triticeal cartilages, which can cause symptoms such as dysphagia and odynophagia or can be mistaken for a foreign body when calcified [10–14]. The corniculate cartilages are housed on the apex of the arytenoids. The cuneiform cartilages, when present, are lateral to the corniculate cartilages embedded in the aryepiglottic fold. Although some feel that these cartilages are vestigial, they do appear to add rigidity to the aryepiglottic folds.

The epiglottis is a thin lamella of yellow cartilage, shaped like a leaf. It projects obliquely and vertically behind the base of the tongue and ventrally to the entrance of the larynx. Its broad and round free end, which is occasionally notched in the midline, is directed upward and sometimes bent anteriorly. Its lower part, called petioles, is like a stalk, long, and narrow and connected to the back of the thyroid cartilage. On the posterior surface of its lower half, there is a projecting part called the tubercle that, when prominent, can obscure the view of the anterior part of the vocal cords. The epiglottis is higher and wider in males with no significant changes observed with aging [15]. It can be divided into a suprahyoid and an infrahyoid portion. The suprahyoid portion protrudes into the laryngeal lumen, without any attachments, whereas on the infrahyoid part, only the posterior-laryngeal surface is exposed. Split lines in the epiglottic cartilage reflect the arrangement of its collagen bundles. On the posterior aspect, they run primarily in a horizontal direction throughout the upper one to two-thirds above the epiglottic tubercle and are most pronounced between the attachments of the lateral and median hyoepiglottic ligament. This area, approximately one-third of the way from the superior margin of the epiglottis, also referred to as the epiglottic folding plane, is important for the mechanism of epiglottic downfolding during swallowing [16]. The lower third, including the petiolus of the epiglottis, demonstrates a vertically directed orientation of split lines. The anterior aspect of each epiglottis shows a different, more complex orientation of split lines surrounding the holes and recesses formed by the mucous glands. The cartilage is also perforated by the branches of the internal laryngeal nerve.

It was traditionally believed that only structures composed of hyaline cartilage can undergo calcification (thyroid, cricoid, and arytenoid cartilages) [14, 17]. Enchondral calcification of these cartilages begins with skeletal maturity and progresses thereafter with aging. Based on macroscopic observations, the epiglottis had been considered a permanent elastic cartilage that does not undergo ossification [18]. However, a more detailed analysis of age-related changes in calcium deposition has shown that calcification increases with age and is more pronounced in males [15, 19, 20]. Laryngeal cartilage calcification may affect some mechanical properties and while it could theoretically add to its stability, it can also be a cause of different swallowing problems, such as dysphagia, foreign body sensations, or aspirations [21].

The hyoid bone is the central movable anatomical structure of the neck and functional part of the larynx. This U-shaped bone is located in the anterior midline and serves as an attachment for various muscles of the floor of the mouth, tongue, and pharynx. It is unique because in humans, unlike in other mammals, it does not articulate with any other bone or cartilage. Instead, it is suspended from the styloid processes by the bilateral stylohyoid ligaments, fibrous cords extending from the tip of the styloid processes to the lesser cornus of the hyoid bone. The hyoid position is determined by this suspension apparatus and the activity of muscles attached to it. Due to these connections, the hyoid position is closely related to pharyngeal airway dimensions and associated with critical closing pressure in OSA patients [22]. During inspiration, contraction of pharyngeal dilators causes anterior movement of the hyoid and increases the anteroposterior dimension of the retrolingual airway, contributing to upper airway (UA) patency. In resting state, it is positioned in the neck roughly parallel with the lower border of the mandible, and, when viewed in lateral projection, the tip of the greater cornue partially overlaps with the cervical spine [23].

The epiglottis has two anterior attachments. Inferiorly, at the petiolus, the epiglottis is attached to the inner surface of the laryngeal prominence of the thyroid cartilage, just above the level of the anterior commissure and below the thyroid notch, by the elastic thyroepiglottic ligament. At this point, bilateral vestibular ligaments and vocal ligaments are also attached, forming the Broyles' ligament that contains blood vessels and lymphatics [24, 25]. Superiorly, the epiglottis is attached to the hyoid bone by the paired lateral hyoepiglottic ligaments and a single medial hyoepiglottic ligament. The lateral hyoepiglottic ligaments are attached to the lateral edges of the upper portion of the epiglottis, running laterally to the tip of the greater horns of the hyoid bone forming the pharyngoepiglottic folds (lateral glossoepiglottic folds) [16]. The medial ligament is a fibrous fan-shaped band of tissue running in the midline from the upper border of the hyoid bone to the anterior surface of the epiglottis, forming the medial glossoepiglottic fold. The upper limit of its epiglottic attachment is at the level of the lower borders of the greater cornu of the hyoid bone and its lower attachment blends with the attachment of the thyroepiglottic ligament [26]. It had been traditionally believed that anteriorly the medial hyoepiglottic ligament attaches only to the hyoid bone, but a more recent anatomical study revealed that the hyoepiglottic ligament also extends to one of the intrinsic lingual muscles, most probably the genioglossus muscle [27, 28] (Fig. 5.2). Accordingly, two parts can be distinguished in the medial hyoepiglottic ligament: the lingual and the hyoid part. A significantly decreased number of elastic and collagen fibers has been found in these ligaments in elderly persons, which may put them at an increased risk of epiglottic instability [29, 30]. Taking into account the progressive flattening of epiglottis with aging, it is possible that this ligament maintains its anterior convexity.

The thyrohyoid membrane is a broad fibroelastic layer attached to the upper border and superior horn of the thyroid cartilage, the upper margin of the posterior surface of the body, and the greater horns of the hyoid bone. It thus ascends behind the concave posterior surface of the hyoid and is separated from its body by a bursa that facilitates the ascent of the larynx during speech and deglutition. The thickened portion of this membrane in the midline constitutes the thyrohyoid ligament. The aryepiglottic folds are paired structures arising from the apex and corniculate tubercle of the arytenoids and merging with the lateral margins of the epiglottis. Together with the laryngeal surface of the epiglottis, they enclose the space referred to as the laryngeal vestibule. The body of each aryepiglottic fold is composed of the

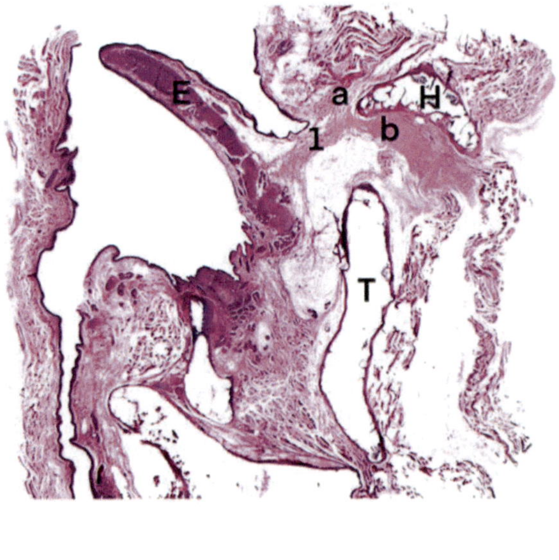

Fig. 5.2 Attachments of hyoepiglottic ligament. *1* hyoepiglottic ligament (*a* lingual part and *b* hyoid part), *E* epiglottis, *H* hyoid bone, and *T* thyroid cartilage

aryepiglottic muscle and quadrangular membrane, with its inferior margin terminating as a thickened ligamentous tissue, forming the ventricular ligament.

Behind, the thyrohyoid membrane lies a preepiglottic space (PES), which takes the shape of a triangular pyramid with an inferior apex and is divided into left and right sides by a thin sagittal membrane (septum) [31]. It is bounded by the medial hyoepiglottic ligament and valleculae superiorly; the hyoid bone, thyrohyoid membrane, and thyroid cartilage anteriorly; and the thyroepiglottic ligament and anterior surface of the epiglottic cartilage posteroinferiorly. The PES is continuous with the paraglottic space (PGS) that is laterally and posteriorly surrounded by the thyroid lamina and by the mucosa of the hypopharynx (piriform sinus), respectively. At the supraglottic level, it lies postero-inferiorly to the PES and medial to the lamina of the thyroid cartilage. The PES and PGS are composed of adipose tissue and loose elastic and collagen fibers [32]. Preepiglottic adipose tissue, sometimes referred to as "laryngeal fat body," plays an important role in the process of swallowing. PES also contains one or two lymph nodes, while the PGS is a space for the main laryngeal arteries and allows interrupted blood flow within it [33].

5.6 Muscles

There is a large number of skeletal muscles that have to act in a coordinated way to enable important physiological processes taking place in the larynx and pharynx (breathing, deglutition, phonation, and articulation). Many of them influence the UA patency and are sometimes referred to as accessory respiratory muscles. They can dilate and open or stiffen the airway to make it less prone to collapse by the negative inspiratory pressure. Describing all muscles involved in pharyngeal and laryngeal functions is beyond the scope of this work. Their characteristics and functions are presented in Table 5.1. Pharyngeal dilators and muscles that affect the distance between the thyroid cartilage and the hyoid bone, as well as their orientation, can also affect the position and shape of the epiglottis. That is why we believe these muscles are the most relevant for the development of obstructive respiratory events at the level of the tongue base and epiglottis.

Although many anatomic studies have evaluated the function of pharyngeal muscles during swallowing, a complete understanding of their role in sleep-disordered breathing still needs to be established. The pharyngeal muscles are anatomically and functionally connected and do not act as simple individual structures but rather move and function together in a very coordinated way. It is important to realize that a particular pharyngeal muscle can have different mechanical effects on the UA depending on the size and shape of the airway at the time of muscle activation, muscle fiber orientation, simultaneous activation of other muscles, and the timing of activation relative to the phase of respiration. This may help explain how pharyngeal muscles can play a role in such disparate functions as respiration, deglutition, and phonation [34].

The pharynx is a tube-like muscular structure that comprises three external circular muscles (the superior, middle, and inferior constrictor muscles) and three

Table 5.1 Pharyngeal muscles

Muscle name	Origin	Insertion	Function	Innervation
Tensor veli palatini	Medial pterygoid plate of the sphenoid bone	Palatine aponeurosis	Moves soft palate up and posterior	V
Levator veli palatini	The petrous part of the temporal bone, the cartilaginous part of the auditory tube	Palatine aponeurosis	Moves soft palate up	V
Palatoglossus	Palatine aponeurosis	Tongue	Moves tongue up and posterior	XII
Palatopharyngeus	Palatine aponeurosis and hard palate	The upper border of thyroid cartilage	Moves soft palate down, pharynx up	XI
Styloglossus	Styloid process of temporal bone	Tip and sides of the tongue	Moves tongue up and posterior	XII
Genioglossus	The superior part of the mental spine of the mandible	Underside of tongue and body of hyoid	Moves tongue down and anterior	XII
Hyoglossus	Hyoid	Side of the tongue	Moves tongue down and posterior	XII
Salpingopharyngeus	The lower part of the cartilage of the auditory tube	Blends with palatopharyngeus muscle	Elevates pharynx, opens auditory tube during swallowing	X
Stylopharyngeus	Styloid process	Thyroid cartilage	Moves pharynx up and widens it	IX
Constrictor pharyngis superior	Medial pterygoid plate, pterygomandibular raphe, alveolar process	Pharyngeal raphe, pharyngeal tubercle	Stiffens posterior pharyngeal wall, reduces pharyngeal lumen, swallowing	X
Constrictor pharyngis medius	Hyoid bone	Pharyngeal raphe	Stiffens posterior pharyngeal wall, reduces pharyngeal lumen, pulls hyoid backward, swallowing	X

Table 5.1 (continued)

Muscle name	Origin	Insertion	Function	Innervation
Constrictor pharyngis inferior	Thyropharyngeal part: Oblique line of thyroid cartilage	Thyropharyngeal part: Median pharyngeal raphe	Stiffens posterior pharyngeal wall, reduces pharyngeal lumen, sphincteric function, swallowing	X
	Cricopharyngeal part: Cricoid cartilage	Cricopharyngeal part: Blends inferiorly with circular esophageal fibers		
Digastric v. anterior	Digastric fossa of mandible	Body of hyoid bone	Moves hyoid anterior	VII
Digastric v. posterior	The mastoid notch of the temporal bone	Body of hyoid bone	Moves hyoid posterior	V
Geniohyoideus	Inferior mental spine of mandible	Body of hyoid bone	Moves tongue and hyoid up	XII
Stylohyoideus	Styloid process	Greater cornu of the hyoid bone	Moves hyoid up and posterior	VII
Mylohyoideus	Mylohyoid line of mandible	Body of hyoid bone and median ridge	Stiffens floor of the mouth	V
Omohyoideus	Inferior belly: Superior border of scapula near the suprascapular notch	Inferior belly: Intermediate tendon	Moves hyoid down	C1–3 via XII
	Superior belly: Intermediate tendon	Superior belly: the body of the hyoid bone		
Thyrohyoideus	Oblique line of the thyroid cartilage	Greater horn of the hyoid bone	Approximates hyoid in thyoroid	C1–3 via XII
Sternohyoideus	Manubrium of sternum, medial end of clavicle	The inferior border of the body of the hyoid bone	Moves hyoid down	C1–3 via XII
Sternothyroideus	The posterior surface of the manubrium of the sternum, costal cartilage of rib 1	Oblique line of thyroid cartilage	Moves thyorid down	C1–3 via XII
Crycothyroideus	Anterolateral part of cricoid cartilage	Oblique part: Inferior horn of thyroid cartilage	Tenses vocal cords	X
		Straight part: Inferior margin of thyroid cartilage		

(continued)

Table 5.1 (continued)

Muscle name	Origin	Insertion	Function	Innervation
Crycoarytenoideus posterior	The posterior part of the cricoid	Posterior surface of muscular process of the arytenoid cartilage	Abducts and laterally rotates arytenoid cartilage, pulling vocal ligaments away from the midline and forward and opening rima glottidis	X
Crycoarytenoideus lateralis	The lateral part of the arch of the cricoid	Muscular process of the arytenoid cartilage	Adducts and medially rotates the cartilage, pulling the vocal ligaments towards the midline and backwards and so closing off the rima glottidis	X
Arytenoideus transversus	Arytenoid cartilage on one side	Arytenoid cartilage on the opposite side	Approximates the arytenoid cartilages	X
Arytenoideus obliquus	Posterior surface of muscular process of arytenoid cartilage	The posterior surface of the apex of the adjacent arytenoid cartilage extends into the aryepiglottic fold	Sphincter of the laryngeal inlet	X
Thyroarytenoideus	The angle of the thyroid cartilage and adjacent cricothyroid ligament	The anterolateral surface of arytenoid cartilage	Relaxes vocal cords	X
Vocalis	Lateral surface of vocal processes of arytenoid cartilage	Anterior part of ipsilateral vocal ligament	Tenses anterior part and relaxes posterior part of vocal ligament	X
Aryepiglotticus	Apex of arytenoid	The lateral border of the epiglottis	Closes the inlet	X

(continued)

Table 5.1 (continued)

Muscle name	Origin	Insertion	Function	Innervation
Thyroepiglotticus	The inner surface of the thyroid cartilage is in common with the thyroarytenoideus muscle	Aryepiglottic fold and margin of epiglottis	Depresses base of epiglottis	X

internal longitudinal muscles (the stylopharyngeal, palatopharyngeal, and salpingopharyngeal muscles). It has been established that the activity of the three external circular muscles, which mutually overlap, produces a sphincteric and peristaltic action and that the three internal longitudinal muscles elevate the pharynx and larynx. The muscles attached to the epiglottis are weak and do not have much effect on its position [29]. Therefore, it depends mainly on the surrounding structures to which the epiglottis is attached by a complex suspension apparatus. Among them, the anterior ligaments that connect the epiglottis to the tongue and the hyoid bone are probably the most important for the movement and its shape [16]. The position of the epiglottis also depends on the relationship between the thyroid cartilage and the hyoid bone, and the position of the tongue base, which is related to the activity of the m. genioglossus, the main pharyngeal dilator.

The soft palate is composed of several integrated muscles: palatopharyngeus, palatoglossus, levator veli palatini, tensor veli palatini, and musculus uvulae. They control the stiffness and position of the palate, tongue, and pharynx. As such, these muscles are important in the maintenance of UA patency, and a comprehensive understanding of their action is necessary for successful surgical procedures of the soft palate and the lateral pharyngeal walls. The tensor palatini muscle makes the soft palate more rigid. Together with the levator palatini, which is an antagonist of the palatopharyngeus, it enables its proper functioning. The palatopharyngeal muscle originates from either the superior (nasal) or inferior (oral) surface of the palatine aponeurosis or the medial part of the soft palate. In its upper course, it has vertically and horizontally oriented fibers. After forming the palatopharyngeal arch, the palatopharyngeus continues infero-posteriorly toward the lateral part of the epiglottis spreading radially on the inner aspect of the pharyngeal wall, merging with the salpingopharyngeal and stylopharyngeal muscles. In most cases, the palatopharyngeus does not attach to the epiglottis but is in continuation with the sparse fibers of the aryepiglottic muscle [16]. From here, it passes behind the arytenoids as the continuation of the oblique arytenoids attaching to the posterior surface of the contralateral arytenoid cartilage. In its inferior part, the aryepiglottic muscle fibers continue and connect to the inner surface of the inferior pharyngeal constrictor where they help with opening the upper esophageal sphincter by pulling it in the superolateral direction [35]. It is believed that the palatopharyngeus muscle acts as a sphincter encircling the pharyngeal isthmus. It also holds the epiglottis in contact with the soft palate, providing a direct air channel from the nose to the larynx in newborns [36]. In about 25% of cases, the descending longitudinal muscles of the palatopharyngeus insert into the epiglottis and contribute to the formation of the pharyngoepiglottic fold [37–39]. According to an anatomic study performed by Vandaele et al., the only muscle fibers that consistently insert into the epiglottis are the continuation of the thyroarytenoid muscle; alternatively, they may originate from the anterolateral surface of the arytenoid cartilage as distinct muscle bundles. They are all attached to the epiglottic petiolus and contribute to the narrowing of the laryngeal vestibule [16]. All other muscles affect the position and movement of the epiglottis indirectly, through the movement of structures to which the epiglottis is attached by ligaments or membranes.

Because of its role in OSA pathogenesis, the genioglossus muscle (GG) is probably the most extensively studied UA dilator muscle. It is an extrinsic tongue muscle and the largest of the pharyngeal dilator muscles. The GG originates from the mental spine of the mandible and fans out with a bulk of fibers inserted into the body of the tongue. The lowermost fibers extend backward and downward into the hyoid bone, while the uppermost fibers extend upward and anteriorly into the tip of the tongue. [40] Its function is to move the tongue downward and anteriorly, thus widening the retroglossal space. The thyrohyoid, geniohyoid, and mylohyoid muscles are believed to be the primary effectors of anterior hyoid bone movement and thus are the principal muscles affecting epiglottic movements and position [41]. Based on structural properties, the geniohyoid muscle has the most potential to displace the hyoid in the anterior direction, and the mylohyoid has the most potential to displace the hyoid in the superior direction [42]. Other muscles such as the anterior belly of the digastric contribute less to the anterior motion of the hyoid [43].

OSA is thought to be associated with changes in the contractile properties of UA muscles. Several studies have shown remodeling of the UA muscles in patients with OSA with an increase in type II fast-twitch fibers that are more likely to fatigue than type I fibers, making patients with OSA more susceptible to fatigue than those of normal subjects [44–46].

5.7 Blood Vessels and Lymphatics

Sound knowledge of the vascular supply is important in order to avoid damage to major blood vessels during surgery, which may cause life-threatening complications due to potential aspiration and hypoxia. ENT surgeons undertaking surgery in the pharyngeal and supraglottic region must be aware that bleeding complications during endoscopic procedures are potentially more problematic than those in traditional open surgery [47].

The arterial blood supply to the supraglottic larynx comes mainly from the superior laryngeal artery (SLA). Usually, it is a branch of the superior thyroid artery, but in about one-third of the cases, it originates directly from the external carotid artery above the superior thyroid artery [9, 48]. From its origin, it passes horizontally toward the posterior portion of the thyrohyoid membrane together with the internal branch of the superior laryngeal nerve (SLN) and pierces the membrane below the nerve, anterior to the superior cornu of the thyroid cartilage, to enter the larynx. Here, it runs between the intrinsic laryngeal muscles and thyroid cartilage in the PGS and splits into several ascending and descending branches. An "aberrant" SLA is present in up to 20% of larynx dissections. It enters the PGS through the thyroid foramen in the posterior portion of the thyroid cartilage lamina; the same foramen can also serve as a passage for anastomosis of the external and internal laryngeal nerves [49]. Even in such cases, the intralaryngeal branching is similar to the normal SLA [48, 50]. The ascending branch runs upward tortuously until the level of the pharyngoepiglottic fold where it splits into smaller vessels. The most relevant for epiglottic surgery are the superior and anterior branches. The superior branch runs superficially on the lingual surface of the epiglottis and valleculae where it forms a vascular network with the dorsal branches of the lingual artery (Fig. 5.3). Some vessels from this plexus reach the upper part of the epiglottis and run over its edge or pierce the cartilage. The anterior branch runs toward the superior border of the thyroid cartilage and laryngeal prominence supplying the laryngeal ventricle. Collateral branches fan out of the ascending branch toward the lower half of the epiglottis cartilage, reaching its dorsal surface through

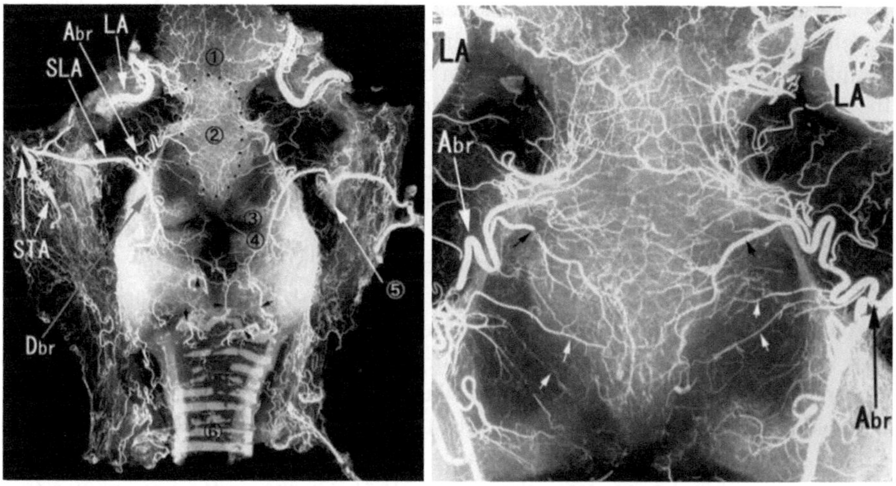

Fig. 5.3 Stereographic angiograms of the larynx with the surrounding tissue. The superior laryngeal artery (SLA), derived from the superior thyroid artery (STA), splits into ascending (Abr) and descending branches (Dbr). *1* base of the tongue, *2* epiglottis (dotted circle), *3* vestibular fold, *4* vocal fold, *6* trachea, *LA* lingual artery, *left: small black arrows* distal portions of the superior thyroid artery, *right: small white arrows* inferior vessels of Abr, and *small black arrows* superior vessels of Abr. (Adapted from Ref. [51]. Source: https://www.jstage.jst.go.jp/article/ofaj/86/2/86_2_61/_article/-char/en)

the aryepiglottic fold [48, 51]. The descending branch turns its course inferiorly approximately 1 cm anterior to the base of the superior horn of thyroid cartilage and continues deep to the thyroid cartilage lamina in the PGS, ending at the superior border of the lateral cricoarytenoid muscle. At this level, the anterior terminal branches anastomose with the cricothyroid artery and the posterior branches anastomose with the inferior laryngeal artery.

The lingual artery is the second branch of the external carotid artery from which it branches at the level of the hyoid bone. It courses laterally to the middle pharyngeal constrictor muscle where it is crossed by the hypoglossal nerve, and then, it passes deep to the hyoglossus muscle where it runs on the superior surface of the hyoid bone. It is this location where it is vulnerable to injury during transoral tongue base surgery. The lingual artery then gives off a suprahyoid branch, a dorsal lingual artery that passes to the dorsum of the tongue, the sublingual artery, and the deep lingual artery that passes between the genioglossus muscle and the inferior intrinsic tongue musculature [52]. Throughout the larynx, including the epiglottis, there is an abundant arterial anastomotic network with bilateral perfusion [53].

The laryngeal veins accompany the arteries and drain into the superior thyroid and inferior thyroid veins that drain into the internal jugular and the subclavian veins, respectively [52]. The tongue is drained by lingual veins that pass to the internal jugular vein directly or via the facial and retromandibular veins. Laryngeal lymphatics are numerous, except over the area of the true vocal cords. Due to different developmental origins, supraglottic and infraglottic regions drain separately and no lymphatic communication exists between these two regions. Lymphatic vessels of the supraglottic area are very dense and run through the floor of the piriform sinus with the SLA, and drain into the upper jugular nodes [9].

With the advancement of endoscopic approaches, there was also a need to understand the anatomy from an "inside-out" perspective, i.e., to visualize the structures as they are encountered when approaching through the lumen of the upper respiratory tract. Important work in this area has been done by robotic surgery instructors [52]. Due to the variability between individuals, most anatomical landmarks are unreliable, and a surgeon must rely on a meticulous and careful technique of tissue preparation. In the case of tongue-based surgery, special care should be taken due to the proximity of the larger branches of the lingual artery that can get medialized because of outward tongue retraction. Most authors agree that it is possible to avoid contact with the hypoglossal-lingual artery neurovascular bundle if the dissection is carried out within 1.5 cm from the midline [54]. During endoscopic preparation close to the lateral wall, the main trunk of the intralaryngeal SLA can be identified just inferior to the greater cornu of the hyoid bone in the PGS, right after piercing the thyrohyoid membrane (Fig. 5.4) [55].

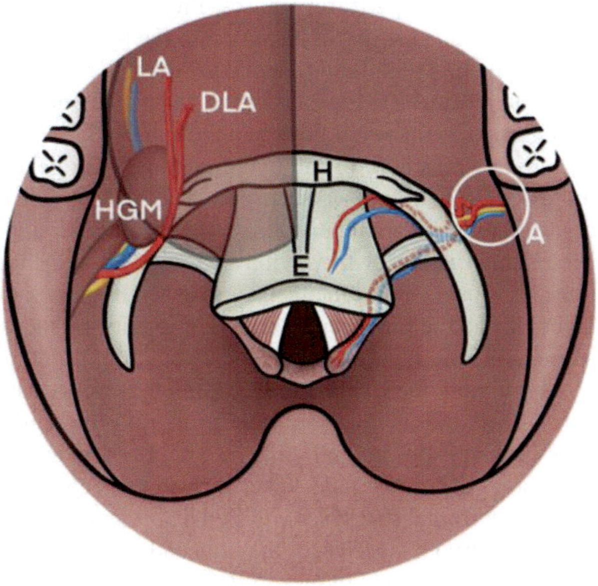

Fig. 5.4 Endoscopic view of supraglottic anatomy. *A* superior laryngeal bundle, *LA* lingual artery, *DLA* dorsal lingual artery, *E* epiglottis, *H* hyoid bone, and *HGM* hyoglossal muscle

5.8 Innervation

Most muscles of the pharynx, including the soft palate, receive motor innervation from the pharyngeal plexus overlying the posterior surface of the middle pharyngeal constrictor. This structure's detailed anatomy and functional mechanism are still not entirely understood [56]. It is formed by pharyngeal branches of the glossopharyngeal and vagal nerve, and sympathetic fibers from the superior cervical ganglion. The pharyngeal branches of the vagal nerve provide motor innervation to most muscles of the pharynx and palate, except the stylopharyngeus muscle and the tensor veli palatini muscle, which are supplied by the glossopharyngeal nerve and the mandibular branch of the trigeminal nerve, respectively. All tongue muscles except for the palatoglossus muscle, which is innervated by the glossopharyngeal nerve, are innervated by the hypoglossal nerve [52].

The larynx is supplied by the vagal laryngeal branches, the superior laryngeal nerve (SLN), and the recurrent laryngeal nerve (RLN). The SLN arises from the inferior (nodose) ganglion of the vagal nerve, and it is accompanied by branches from the superior cervical ganglion of the sympathetic trunk. After descending between the carotid arteries and the pharyngeal wall, it reaches the larynx and splits into an internal and external branch just below the hyoid bone. The external branch runs close to the superior thyroid artery and provides motor innervation to the inferior constrictor and cricothyroid muscle. The internal branch passes the thyrohyoid membrane with the SLA and splits into several branches. The upper branches provide sensation to the epiglottis, valleculae, laryngeal vestibule, and vestibular (false vocal) folds, while the lower branches provide sensation to mucosa below the vestibule and the pyriform sinuses. Preserving the lower branches during surgical resection spares sensory innervation to the hypopharynx and larynx below the vestibule, which is important to avoid aspiration [52]. The RLN provides motor innervation to all intrinsic muscles of the larynx except the cricothyroid muscle as well as sensation to the vocal folds and the subglottis.

Muscles attaching to the hyoid have a heterogeneous innervation, and precise motor control differs for each one. The mylohyoid muscle and anterior belly of digastric muscles are innervated by the mandibular division of the trigeminal nerve. Motor innervation of the stylohyoid muscles and the posterior belly of digastric muscles is provided by the facial nerve. Motor innervation to the infrahyoid muscles comes from the ansa cervicalis. The activity of the geniohyoid, mylohyoid, and sternohyoid are reported to change with respiration (Table 5.1) [57].

Throughout the UA, the mucosal lining is richly supplied with a dense plexus of nerve fibers that is in close association with the epithelium. Sensory nerve terminals, heterogenous in their embryological origin and functionality, are essential for respiratory regulation and lower airway protection. They can be associated with different terminal structures within the airway wall, such as mucosal glands, vasculature, or smooth muscles, or they can end as free nerve endings in mucosal, submucosal, or parenchymal tissues [58]. The posterior epiglottic surface is perforated by branches of the internal laryngeal nerve and fibrous tissue, so the posterior, i.e., laryngeal surface of the epiglottis, is in continuity through these perforations with the pre-epiglottic space.

5.9 Mucosa

The mucosa of the UA is not just a uniform and homogeneous tube for gas transmission and exchange, but a complex and heterogeneous organic system that allows monitoring of the air environment and physiological responses to changes in it [59]. Most of the larynx, including the posterior surface of the epiglottis, is covered by a ciliated, pseudostratified respiratory epithelium that provides a ciliary clearance mechanism shared with most of the respiratory tract. The anterior surface of the epiglottis is covered by non-keratinized, stratified squamous epithelium protecting the underlying tissues from mechanical stress [13]. The transition zone between both epithelia is located at the lower half of the posterior surface of the epiglottis, medial to the aryepiglottic folds [9]. The epiglottic epithelium is reflected onto the base of the tongue and the lateral pharyngeal walls as a medial glossoepiglottic, and two lateral glossoepiglottic (pharyngoepiglottic) folds. The submucosal tissue of the epiglottis is fascial and continuous laterally with the internal pharyngeal fascia overlying the middle and inferior constrictor muscles and medially with the submucosa of the laryngeal vestibule. Superiorly, it is continuous with the submucosa of the tongue [16].

In the squamous epithelium of the epiglottis, aryepiglottic folds, arytenoid regions, the interarytenoid notch, and the membranous portion of the vocal folds, the Langerhans cells are present [33]. These tissue-resident macrophages are an important part of the human immune system. As a part of the dendritic antigen-presenting system, they have an ability to capture antigens and initiate T cell-mediated immunity, which is essential for the defense of the UA mucosa [60, 61]. Laryngeal secretions also contain IgG, IgA, and IgE antibodies and lactoferrin, all important in the local immune system [62]. The posterior surface of the epiglottis cartilage is pitted by small mucous glands. Like other secretory glands in the UA, they produce a liquid lining of the respiratory epithelium consisting of a periciliary liquid layer and a superficial mucous component. Its properties, i.e., thickness and viscosity, influence surface tension and wall shear stress. Additionally, they appear to have an effect on the response of the pharyngeal dilator muscles to stimulation of the mechanoreceptors and thus pharyngeal collapsibility [63]. Overstimulation of UA secretion makes a collapsed airway more difficult to open, while application of the substances with surface tension-lowering properties is associated with a reduction in airflow resistance [64]. Age-related changes in the laryngeal glands influence the local immunity and mucociliary transport of the larynx. The concentration of laryngeal glands decreases with age; moreover, the ratio of mucous versus serous glands tends to increase. This affects not only the amount but also the quality and viscosity of secretions. A similar effect can be observed in the laryngeal mucosa of irradiated patients [33, 65, 66].

The larynx is a highly reflexogenic area with many different types of receptors that respond to mechanical and chemical stimuli. Sensory information from the UA is transmitted by the trigeminal, glossopharyngeal, and internal branches of the SLN [67]. While the role of reflex arches in the protective mechanism against aspiration has been extensively researched, their role in OSA pathogenesis has not been definitively elucidated. Chemoreceptors similar to taste buds of the tongue are found on the epithelium of the soft palate, aryepiglottic folds, and laryngeal surfaces of the epiglottis. They are adapted for the detection of chemicals that are not saline-like in composition and thus do not respond to normal mucus secretions. Electrophysiological recordings from SLN fibers in response to stimulation of the epiglottis have demonstrated the highest response to NaCl solutions higher or lower than saline with a U-shaped response-concentration function [68–70]. Accordingly, their role is not the gustation but prevention of aspiration of food and liquids [71, 72]. Morphologically diverse and highly sensitive mechanoreceptors are located within the UA mucosa, near muscles, and joints [73]. Recordings from their afferent fibers have revealed that some of them are spontaneously active whereas others are silent until stimulated. They respond to negative pressure, mechanical deformation, and high-frequency vibrations, like those generated during snoring. [67, 74, 75] The majority are located in the nose, larynx, and upper trachea. Their effect is abolished when topical anesthetic is applied and may be altered after radiotherapy of the neck. Efferent actions include alterations in the rate and depth of breathing as well as increasing or decreasing autonomic flow to the airway's smooth muscle, glands, and vasculature [76]. Moreover, these reflex arches regulate the response of the pharyngeal dilator muscles, a mechanism that mediates the increased genioglossal activity observed in patients with inadequate pharyngeal anatomy during wakefulness. How these mechanisms are modulated by sleep is just beginning to be understood, but it seems it might have an important implication in the pathophysiology of OSA [57, 59, 77, 78]. Studies indicate that there is a subset of laryngeal receptors sensitive to intralaryngeal CO_2, which are not responsive to changes in systemic pCO_2 [79, 80]. Many candidates for CO_2 reception have been identified, namely the taste buds, pressure receptors, as well as intraepithelial free nerve endings. It appears that there are two processes involved in the CO_2 effect on laryngeal receptors; one is topical stimulation, and the other is modulation of sensitivity to other stimuli. It is speculated that intralaryngeal CO_2 is hydrated by the epithelium; however, the relationship or conduction process between the epithelial cells and the end receptorial organ is not clear [81, 82]. Animal studies showed that these effects ultimately cause a reflex excitation of the UA dilator muscles and a decrease in ventilation [83]. The impact of these receptors and their possible role in OSA treatment is still to be determined.

5.10 The Role of the Epiglottis in OSA

The function of the epiglottis has been debated since ancient times when it was already described as a structure protecting the larynx by covering it during deglutition [84, 85]. Since then, it has long been established that it allows for comfortable breathing, combined with laryngeal competence. Its role is particularly important in breastfeeding infants as it separates the breathing and respiratory path to allow simultaneous nutritive sucking with swallowing and breathing, which is not possible in adults. While adults with mature swallowing reflexes compensate for its absence by other mechanisms, neonates with congenital aplasia or hypoplasia of the epiglottis are often tracheostomy and gastrostomy dependent [86, 87].

Most of our knowledge on possible epiglottis moving patterns comes from analysis of swallowing. From numerous studies, it is now clear that the position and interrelationship between the hyoid bone, thyroid cartilage, lower jaw, and tongue play a decisive role in the position and different shapes of the epiglottis [23, 88]. The advancement of ingested bolus requires an approach of the thyroid cartilage and hyoid bone, as well as the movement of both structures upward and forward, toward the mandible. The described sequence causes a specific movement of the epiglottis: downward into a horizontal position, followed by a downfold to below the horizontal plane, which results in obstruction of the laryngeal entrance. While its role in dysphagia has long been clarified, the epiglottis was largely ignored in the early research on obstructive sleep breathing disorders. More recent studies, however, have shown that it plays an important role as obstructions occur at this level more often than previously assumed. It cannot be simply assumed that the different patterns in which the epiglottis moves during swallowing also apply to obstructive respiratory events. Taking into account that the same structures affect and limit their positions, we can still use this information when trying to explain some phenomena at this level of the UA.

Obstructions at the level of the epiglottis can occur in two ways: in primary (isolated) obstruction, the epiglottis closes the airway independently of the tongue;

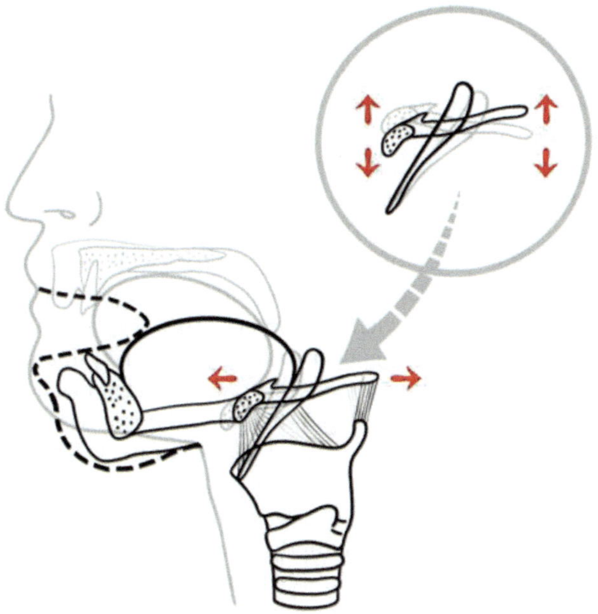

Fig. 5.5 Effect of mouth closure and hyoid inclination on epiglottis position

while in case of secondary obstruction, the epiglottis is pushed posteriorly by the tongue base. The distinction is important as therapeutic approaches are different in each case [89]. Secondary epiglottis obstructions are the consequence of tongue base collapse. The stability of the tongue during sleep is directly affected by the function of pharyngeal dilators, especially m. genioglossus that controls its position. Epiglottis is connected with intrinsic muscles of the tongue via the medial part of the hyoepiglottic ligament. This ligament responds to the protrusor (genioglossus) and retrusor (hyoglossus) muscle movement, and this co-activation is influenced by the position of the epiglottis during respiration [29]. This means that tongue position can also influence the position of the epiglottis and the cross-sectional area behind it. At the same time, gravity acts on the tongue base and the epiglottis, pushing both structures toward the posterior pharyngeal walls. When the mouth opens, the lower jaw and the tongue are displaced even more posteriorly, further contributing to the narrowing behind the epiglottis and adding to its instability (Fig. 5.5).

The importance of neuromuscular control on UA patency is most evident when taking into account that obstructive respiratory events in OSA patients only occur during sleep. Studies have shown that the transition from wakefulness to sleep in both OSA patients and control groups increases the resistance in the upper respiratory tract four- to five-fold [90–93]. Most patients with OSA have some periods of sleep with stable breathing, indicating that they can overcome their anatomic abnormality some of the time. In such periods, at least one UA dilator muscle, m. genioglossus, is highly active [94–96]. The pharyngeal tube acts as a collapsible resistor with each part having its own critical pressure (the pressure at which airflow is terminated). As the airflow through the narrowed UA segment increases, airway pressure decreases as a consequence of an increase in kinetic energy. This progressively limits the airflow, which is in accordance with the dynamic tube law. Further increase in the inspiratory effort commonly produces a progressive reduction of the limited inspiratory flow (negative effort dependence). Once an obstructive event develops, an increase in airflow can no longer be achieved by increased activity of inspiratory muscles but only through changes in pharyngeal dilators' activity and their ability to stiffen or dilate the pharynx [97]. While usually passive during quiet breathing, many of the 20 or more skeletal muscles surrounding the pharyngeal airway are phasically activated during more vigorous inspiration [98]. Under conditions of increased chemoreceptory drive, their role is indispensable. Motor neurons of the UA dilators appear to have a higher systemic CO_2 threshold for activation than inspiratory pump muscles [94, 98]. This means that during increased respiratory work, due to the lag of the muscular response of pharyngeal dilators, a rise in negative pressure can cause a collapse of the UA structures.

Unlike the pharynx, in cases of isolated antero-posterior epiglottis collapse, the epiglottis behaves as a one-way valve with infinite collapsibility, with obstructions at this level occurring abruptly, intermittently, and exclusively during the inspiratory phase [99–101]. Its stability is affected by its mass, angle, and the pressure difference between anterior and posterior epiglottis surfaces [101]. In contrast to secondary epiglottis collapse, it can be noticed in the case of isolated epiglottis collapse that the tongue remains static or even moves anteriorly while the epiglottis collapses. Due to the mentioned complex ligamentous connections, the epiglottis cannot be viewed as an isolated structure. Ligament attachments provide information about the static relationships between the epiglottis and other structures, while the internal fiber architecture of the epiglottis cartilage provides us with clues as to the effects of those attachments on the epiglottis [16]. We speculate that in such cases, epiglottis stability might be affected by the position or relationship between the hyoid bone and thyroid cartilage.

The epiglottis consists of elastic cartilage that allows diverse changes in shape and position in various planes. The epiglottis is attached with ligaments to the circumference of the hyoid bone, like a puppet on a string, and responds to the changes in the hyoid bone position and inclination, as well as to its position relative to other structures in the neck (Fig. 5.5). In their anatomical study, Ardran and Kemp point out that the approximation of the thyroid cartilage to the hyoid bone, and the change in the alignment of the hyoid bone relative to the thyroid cartilage, permits a wide range of epiglottis positions, while also causing compression of the hyo-thyroid fat. Such compression, however, cannot entirely explain the resulting changes in the size of the laryngeal vestibule. They observe that when the thyroid cartilage passively approximates the hyoid bone and the greater cornu of the hyoid bone is parallel to the upper border of the ala of the thyroid cartilage, the epiglottis moves backward relative to the thyroid cartilage. This movement is greatest when the hyoid bone is displaced slightly backward relative to the thyroid cartilage and the least extensive when the hyoid bone is displaced forward. If the body of the hyoid was tilted forward over the anterior surface of the thyroid cartilage, the pre-epiglottic fat was not significantly compressed, and the epiglottis was straight and erect [23]. Interesting results come from studies of articulation in which they find that in the production of certain sounds, the epiglottis can move completely independently of the tongue and act as a separate articulator, i.e., it folds toward the pharyngeal wall in some consonants. Additionally, in a whisper, the epiglottis is generally more retracted than in normal speech [102].

Because of all the above, it is unlikely that the epiglottis in OSA acts as an isolated structure that passively responds to pressure changes. The introduction of new technologies, i.e., computer fluid dynamics, airflow analysis, mechanical models, machine-learning, and artificial intelligence, could accelerate our understanding and bring new insights into the role of the epiglottis in obstructive respiratory events. Further research will be needed to elucidate the pathophysiological mechanisms leading to epiglottic collapse and possible new individualized OSA treatment strategies.

Acknowledgments The author wishes to thank Katarina Dimnik, DMD, PhD, Institute of Pathology, University of Ljubljana, for providing laryngeal specimens and preparing some of the figures included.

References

1. Grossman JW. The triticeous cartilages. Am J Roentgenol Radium Ther. 1945;53(2):166–70.
2. Watters K, Rahbar R. Congenital anomalies of the larynx and trachea. In: Wackym PA, Snow BJ, editors. Ballenger's otorhinolaryngology head and neck surgery. Shelton: People's Medical Publishing House; 2016. p. 995–1011.
3. Holinger PH, Brown WT. Congenital webs, cysts, laryngoceles and other anomalies of the larynx. Ann Otol Rhinol Laryngol. 1967 [cited 2021 Aug 8];76(4):744–52. http://www.ncbi.nlm.nih.gov/pubmed/6059212.
4. Symington J. The relations of the larynx and trachea to the vertebral column in the foetus and child. J Anat Physiol. 1885 [cited 2021 Aug 8];19(Pt 3):286–91. http://www.ncbi.nlm.nih.gov/pubmed/17231581.
5. Schwartz DS, Keller MS. Maturational descent of the epiglottis. Arch Otolaryngol Head Neck Surg. 1997;123(6):627–8. http://www.ncbi.nlm.nih.gov/pubmed/9193225.
6. Davidson TM, Sedgh J, Tran D, Stepnowsky CJ. The anatomic basis for the acquisition of speech and obstructive sleep apnea: evidence from cephalometric analysis supports The Great Leap Forward Hypothesis. Sleep Med. 2005;6(6):497–505.
7. Malhotra A, Huang Y, Fogel RB, Pillar G, Edwards JK, Kikinis R, et al. The male predisposition to pharyngeal collapse. Am J Respir Crit Care Med. 2002 [cited 2021 Aug 8];166(10):1388–95. http://www.atsjournals.org/doi/abs/10.1164/rccm.2112072.
8. Yamashiro Y, Kryger M. Is laryngeal descent associated with increased risk for obstructive sleep apnea? Chest. 2012;141(6):1407–13. https://doi.org/10.1378/chest.10-3238.
9. Janfaza P, Nadol JB, Galla R, Fabian RL, Montgomery WW. Surgical anatomy of the head and neck. Cambridge: Harvard University Press; 2011. p. xi–xii. http://www.jstor.org/stable/10.2307/j.ctvjf9vjb.4.
10. Alsarraf R, Mathison S, Futran N. Symptomatic presentation of an enlarged, ossified triticeal cartilage. Am J Otolaryngol. 1998 [cited 2021 Aug 14];19(5):339–41. http://www.ncbi.nlm.nih.gov/pubmed/9758185.
11. Munir Turk L, Hogg DA. Age changes in the human laryngeal cartilages. Clin Anat. 1993;6:154–62.

12. Wilson I, Stevens J, Gnananandan J, Nabeebaccus A, Sandison A, Hunter A. Triticeal cartilage: the forgotten cartilage. Surg Radiol Anat. 2017 [cited 2021 Aug 9];39(10):1135. http://link.springer.com/10.1007/s00276-017-1841-z.
13. Anatomy G. 39th Edition: the anatomical basis of clinical practice. Am J Neuroradiol. 2005;26(10):2703–4. http://www.ajnr.org/content/26/10/2703.
14. Last R. Tissues and structures: anatomy, regional and applied. New York: Churchill Livingstone; 1966. p. 1–20.
15. Kano M, Shimizu Y, Okayama K, Igari T, Kikuchi M. A morphometric study of age-related changes in adult human epiglottis using quantitative digital analysis of cartilage calcification. Cells Tissues Organs. 2005;180(2):126–37.
16. Vandaele DJ, Perlman AL, Cassell MD. Intrinsic fibre architecture and attachments of the human epiglottis and their contributions to the mechanism of deglutition. J Anat. 1995;186:1–15.
17. Hatley W, Samuel E, Evison G. The pattern of ossification in the laryngeal cartillages: a radiological study. Br J Radiol. 1965 [cited 2021 Aug 9];38:585–91. http://www.ncbi.nlm.nih.gov/pubmed/14326459.
18. Ajmani ML, Jain SP, Saxena SK. A metrical study of laryngeal cartilages and their ossification. Anat Anz. 1980 [cited 2021 Aug 9];148(1):42–8. http://www.ncbi.nlm.nih.gov/pubmed/7212281.
19. Günbey HP, Günbey E, Sayit AT. A rare cause of abnormal epiglottic mobility and dyspagia: calcification of the epiglottis. J Craniofac Surg. 2014 [cited 2021 Aug 9];25(6):e519–21. http://www.ncbi.nlm.nih.gov/pubmed/25347598.
20. Fernández-Rodríguez A, Benito-Orejas JI, Jiménez-Pérez AE, Morais-Pérez D. [Calcification of the epiglottis]. Acta Otorrinolaringol Esp. 2009 [cited 2021 Aug 9];60(3):215–6. http://www.ncbi.nlm.nih.gov/pubmed/19558912.
21. Jeph S, Aidi M, Shah A, Ly T-T, Bronov O. Calcification of the epiglottis presenting as foreign body sensation in the neck. J Radiol Case Rep. 2017 [cited 2021 May 10];11(6):1–5. http://www.ncbi.nlm.nih.gov/pubmed/29299092.
22. Genta PR, Schorr F, Eckert DJ, Gebrim E, Kayamori F, Moriya HT, et al. Upper airway collapsibility is associated with obesity and hyoid position. Sleep. 2014 [cited 2020 Feb 15];37(10):1673. http://www.ncbi.nlm.nih.gov/pubmed/25197805.
23. Ardran GM, Kemp FH. The mechanism of the larynx. II. The epiglottis and closure of the larynx. Br J Radiol. 1967;40(473):372–89.
24. Wu J, Zhao J, Wang Z, Li Z, Luo J, Liao B, et al. Study of the histopathologic characteristics and surface morphologies of glottic carcinomas with anterior vocal commissure involvement. Medicine (Baltimore). 2015 [cited 2021 Aug 14];94(29):e1169. http://www.ncbi.nlm.nih.gov/pubmed/26200618.
25. Mor N, Blitzer A. Functional anatomy and oncologic barriers of the larynx. Otolaryngol Clin North Am. 2015 [cited 2021 Aug 14];48(4):533–45. http://www.ncbi.nlm.nih.gov/pubmed/26111895.
26. Fink BR, Martin RW, Rohrmann CA. Biomechanics of the human epiglottis. Acta Otolaryngol. 1979;87(5–6):554–9. http://www.ncbi.nlm.nih.gov/pubmed/463526.
27. Pernkof. Head and neck. In: Pernkof anatomy. 4th ed. Baltimore: Urban & Schwarzenberg; 1989. p. 323, 325.
28. Sobotta. Head, neck, upper limb. In: Putz R, Pabst R, editors. Atlas of human anatomy. 12th ed. Baltimore: Williams & Wilkins; 1997. p. 121–6.
29. Sawatsubashi M, Umezaki T, Kusano K, Tokunaga O, Oda M, Komune S. Age-related changes in the hyoepiglottic ligament: functional implications based on histopathologic study. Am J Otolaryngol. 2010;31(6):448–52. https://linkinghub.elsevier.com/retrieve/pii/S019607090900163X.
30. Irvine LE, Yang Z, Kezirian EJ, Nimni ME, Han B. Hyoepiglottic ligament collagen and elastin fiber composition and changes associated with aging. Laryngoscope. 2018;128(5):1245–8. Available from: https://pubmed.ncbi.nlm.nih.gov/29330863/.

31. Lutz JC, Clavert P, Wolfram-Gabel R, Kahn JL. The laryngeal fat body. Morphologie. 2010;94(305):13–9. https://doi.org/10.1016/j.morpho.2009.12.002.
32. Reidenbach MM. The periepiglottic space: topographic relations and histological organisation. J Anat. 1996 [cited 2020 Apr 2];188(Pt 1):173–82. http://www.ncbi.nlm.nih.gov/pubmed/8655405.
33. Sato K. Functional histoanatomy of the human larynx. Berlin: Springer; 2018. p. 1–331.
34. Hudgel DW, Harasick T. Fluctuation in timing of upper airway and chest wall inspiratory muscle activity in obstructive sleep apnea. J Appl Physiol. 1990;69(2):443–50.
35. Fukino K, Tsutsumi M, Nimura A, Miwa K, Ono T, Akita K. Anatomy of inferior end of palatopharyngeus: its contribution to upper esophageal sphincter opening. Eur Arch Otorhinolaryngology. 2020;278(3):749–54. https://doi.org/10.1007/s00405-020-06437-2.
36. Cave A. The nature and function of the mammalian epipharynx. J Zool. 1967 [cited 2021 Sep 18];153(3):277–89. https://onlinelibrary.wiley.com/doi/10.1111/j.1469-7998.1967.tb04063.x.
37. Meng H, Murakami G, Suzuki D, Miyamoto S. Anatomical variations in stylopharyngeus muscle insertions suggest interindividual and left/right differences in pharyngeal clearance function of elderly patients: a cadaveric study. Dysphagia. 2008;23(3):251–7.
38. Choi DY, Bae JH, Youn KH, Kim HJ, Hu KS. Anatomical considerations of the longitudinal pharyngeal muscles in relation to their function on the internal surface of pharynx. Dysphagia. 2014;29(6):722–30.
39. Sumida K, Yamashita K, Kitamura S. Gross anatomical study of the human palatopharyngeus muscle throughout its entire course from origin to insertion. Clin Anat. 2012;25(3):314–23.
40. Cori JM, O'donoghue FJ, Jordan AS. Sleeping tongue: current perspectives of genioglossus control in healthy individuals and patients with obstructive sleep apnea. Nat Sci Sleep. 2018;10:169–79.
41. Jordan AS, White DP, Lo Y-L, Wellman A, Eckert DJ, Yim-Yeh S, et al. Airway dilator muscle activity and lung volume during stable breathing in obstructive sleep apnea. Sleep. 2009 [cited 2020 Apr 1];32(3):361–8. http://www.ncbi.nlm.nih.gov/pubmed/19294956.
42. Pearson WG. Evaluating the structural properties of suprahyoid muscles and their potential for moving the hyoid. Dysphagia. 2011;26(4):345–51.
43. Hrycyshyn AW, Basmajian J V. Electromyography of the oral stage of swallowing in man. Am J Anat. 1972 [cited 2021 Sep 18];133(3):333–40. http://www.ncbi.nlm.nih.gov/pubmed/5026658.
44. Carrera M, Barbé F, Sauleda J, Tomás M, Gómez C, Agustí AG. Patients with obstructive sleep apnea exhibit genioglossus dysfunction that is normalized after treatment with continuous positive airway pressure. Am J Respir Crit Care Med. 1999 [cited 2021 Sep 29];159(6):1960–6. http://www.ncbi.nlm.nih.gov/pubmed/10351945.
45. Sériès F, Côté C, Simoneau JA, Gélinas Y, St Pierre S, Leclerc J, et al. Physiologic, metabolic, and muscle fiber type characteristics of musculus uvulae in sleep apnea hypopnea syndrome and in snorers. J Clin Invest. 1995 [cited 2021 Sep 29];95(1):20–5. http://www.ncbi.nlm.nih.gov/pubmed/7814616.
46. Friberg D, Ansved TOR, Borg K, Carlsson-nordlander B, Larsson H, Svanborg EVA. Histological indications of a progressive snorers disease in an upper airway muscle. Am J Respir Crit Care Med. 1998 [cited 2021 Aug 3];157(2):586–93. http://www.ncbi.nlm.nih.gov/pubmed/9476877.
47. Souvirón R, Maranillo E, Vázquez T, Patel N, McHanwell S, Cobeta I, et al. Proposal of landmarks for clamping neurovascular elements during endoscopic surgery of the supraglottic region. Head Neck. 2013 [cited 2021 Sep 7];35(1):57–60. https://sci-hub.se/10.1002/hed.22902.
48. Rusu MC, Nimigean V, Banu MA, Cergan R, Niculescu V. The morphology and topography of the superior laryngeal artery. Surg Radiol Anat. 2007 [cited 2021 Sep 6];29(8):653–60. http://www.ncbi.nlm.nih.gov/pubmed/17938847.

49. Sañudo JR, Maranillo E, León X, Mirapeix RM, Orús C, Quer M. An anatomical study of anastomoses between the laryngeal nerves. Laryngoscope. 1999 [cited 2021 Sep 19];109(6):983–7. http://www.ncbi.nlm.nih.gov/pubmed/10369294.
50. Liu JL, Liang CY, Xiang T, Wang F, Wang LH, Liu SX, et al. Aberrant branch of the superior laryngeal artery passing through the thyroid foramen. Clin Anat. 2007;20(3): 256–9.
51. Imanishi N, Kondoh T, Kishi K, Aiso S. Angiographic study of the superior laryngeal artery. Okajimas Folia Anat Jpn. 2009;86(2):61–5.
52. Dallan I. Surgical anatomy in transoral robotic procedure: basic fundamentals. In: Vicini C, Hoff PT, Montevecchi F, editors. Robotic surgery in otolaryngology: head and neck surgery. Berlin: Springer; 2016. p. 91–109. http://link.springer.com/10.1007/978-3-319-34040-1.
53. Anthony JP, Argenta P, Trabulsy PP, Lin RY, Mathes SJ. The arterial anatomy of larynx transplantation: microsurgical revascularization of the larynx. Clin Anat. 1996;9(3):155–9.
54. Lin HS, Rowley JA, Badr MS, Folbe AJ, Yoo GH, Victor L, et al. Transoral robotic surgery for treatment of obstructive sleep apnea-hypopnea syndrome. Laryngoscope. 2013;123(7):1811–6.
55. Goyal N, Yoo F, Setabutr D, Goldenberg D. Surgical anatomy of the supraglottic larynx using the da Vinci robot. Head Neck. 2014;36(8):1126–31. http://www.ncbi.nlm.nih.gov/pubmed/23804224.
56. Shoja MM, Oyesiku NM, Shokouhi G, Griessenauer CJ, Chern JJ, Rizk EB, et al. A comprehensive review with potential significance during skull base and neck operations, part II: glossopharyngeal, vagus, accessory, and hypoglossal nerves and cervical spinal nerves 1-4. Clin Anat. 2014 [cited 2022 Jan 6];27(1):131–44. https://onlinelibrary.wiley.com/doi/10.1002/ca.22342.
57. Kubin L, O. Davies R. Mechanisms of upper airway hypotonia. In: Pack AI, editor. Sleep apnea: pathogenesis, diagnosis and treatment. 2nd ed. London: Informa Healthcare; 2012. p. 155–78.
58. Mazzone SB, Undem BJ. Vagal afferent innervation of the airways in health and disease. Physiol Rev. 2016 [cited 2020 Dec 9];96(3):975–1024. http://www.ncbi.nlm.nih.gov/pubmed/27279650.
59. Kubin L. Neural control of the upper airway: respiratory and state-dependent mechanisms. Compr Physiol. 2016 [cited 2021 May 17];6(4):1801–50. https://www.ncbi.nlm.nih.gov/pmc/articles/PMC5242202/pdf/nihms-840493.pdf.
60. Romani N, Schuler G. The immunologic properties of epidermal Langerhans cells as a part of the dendritic cell system. Springer Semin Immunopathol. 1992 [cited 2021 Aug 17];13(3–4):265–79. http://www.ncbi.nlm.nih.gov/pubmed/1411898.
61. Steinman RM. The dendritic cell system and its role in immunogenicity. Annu Rev Immunol. 1991 [cited 2021 Aug 17];9:271–96. http://www.ncbi.nlm.nih.gov/pubmed/1910679.
62. Mogi G, Watanabe N, Maeda S, Umehara T. Laryngeal secretions. An immunochemical and immunohistological study. Acta Otolaryngol 1979 [cited 2021 Aug 17];87(1–2):129–41. http://www.ncbi.nlm.nih.gov/pubmed/367050.
63. Pirnar J, Širok B, Bombač A. Effect of airway surface liquid on the forces on the pharyngeal wall: experimental fluid–structure interaction study. J Biomech. 2017;63:117–24.
64. Kirkness JP, Christenson HK, Garlick SR, Parikh R, Kairaitis K, Wheatley JR, et al. Decreased surface tension of upper airway mucosal lining liquid increases upper airway patency in anaesthetised rabbits. J Physiol 2003 [cited 2021 Jul 26];547(Pt 2):603–11. http://www.ncbi.nlm.nih.gov/pubmed/12562967.
65. Tomita H, Nakashima T, Maeda A, Umeno H, Sato K. Age related changes in the distribution of laryngeal glands in the human adult larynx. Auris Nasus Larynx. 2006 [cited 2022 Mar 13];33(3):289–94. http://www.ncbi.nlm.nih.gov/pubmed/16580162.
66. Sato K, Hirano M. Age-related changes in the human laryngeal glands. Ann Otol Rhinol Laryngol. 1998 [cited 2022 Mar 13];107(6):525–9. http://www.ncbi.nlm.nih.gov/pubmed/9635464

67. Abdal Razaq AS, Mohamad I, Salim R. Mechanoreceptors in the nose. Egypt J Ear Nose Throat Allied Sci. 2015 1 [cited 2021 Sep 20];16(1):9–12. https://doi.org/10.1016/j.ejenta.2014.11.001.
68. Stedman HM, Bradley RM, Mistretta CM, Bradley BE. Chemosensitive responses from the cat epiglottis. Chem Senses. 1980 [cited 2021 Aug 23];5(3):233–45. https://academic.oup.com/chemse/article-lookup/doi/10.1093/chemse/5.3.233.
69. Bahgat AY. Effect of cooling irrigating saline in tongue base ablation in obstructive sleep apnea. OTO Open. 2021 [cited 2021 Feb 25];5(1):2473974X21989599. http://journals.sagepub.com/doi/10.1177/2473974X21989599.
70. Smith D V, Hanamori T. Organization of gustatory sensitivities in hamster superior laryngeal nerve fibers. J Neurophysiol. 1991 [cited 2021 Aug 23];65(5):1098–114. http://www.ncbi.nlm.nih.gov/pubmed/1869907.
71. Bradley RM. Sensory receptors of the larynx. Am J Med. 2000;108(4 Suppl 1):47–50.
72. Bradley RM. The role of epiglottal and lingual chemoreceptors: a comparison. In: Steiner JE, Ganchrow JR, editors. Determination of behaviour by chemical stimuli. London: IRL Press; 1982. p. 37–45.
73. Wirth KJ, Steinmeyer K, Ruetten H. Sensitization of upper airway mechanoreceptors as a new pharmacologic principle to treat obstructive sleep apnea: investigations with AVE0118 in anesthetized pigs. Sleep. 2013;36(5):699–708.
74. Zhang S, Mathew OP. Response of laryngeal mechanoreceptors to high-frequency pressure oscillation. J Appl Physiol. 1992 [cited 2021 Sep 20];73(1):219–23. http://www.ncbi.nlm.nih.gov/pubmed/1506373.
75. Kubin LDR. Mechanisms of airway hypotonia. In: Pack A, editor. Sleep apnea: pathogenesis, diagnosis and treatment. New York: Marcel Dekker; 2011. p. 99–154.
76. Hwang JC, St John WM, Bartlett D. Respiratory-related hypoglossal nerve activity: influence of anesthetics. J Appl Physiol Respir Environ Exerc Physiol. 1983 Sep [cited 2021 Aug 23];55(3):785–92. https://pubmed.ncbi.nlm.nih.gov/6629915/.
77. Akahoshi T, White DP, Edwards JK, Beauregard J, Shea SA. Phasic mechanoreceptor stimuli can induce phasic activation of upper airway muscles in humans. J Physiol. 2001 [cited 2021 Jul 17];531(Pt 3):677–91. http://www.ncbi.nlm.nih.gov/pubmed/11251050.
78. White DP. Airway reflexes Sleep, changes with sleep. In: Pack AI, editor. Sleep apnea: pathogenesis, diagnosis, and treatment. 2nd ed. London: Informa Healthcare; 2012. p. 155–78.
79. Nishijima K, Tsubone H, Atoji Y. Contribution of free nerve endings in the laryngeal epithelium to CO2 reception in rats. Auton Neurosci. 2004 [cited 2020 Dec 9];110(2):81–8. http://www.ncbi.nlm.nih.gov/pubmed/15046731.
80. Coates EL, Knuth SL, Bartlett D. Laryngeal CO2 receptors: influence of systemic PCO2 and carbonic anhydrase inhibition. Respir Physiol. 1996 [cited 2020 Dec 9];104(1):53–61. http://www.ncbi.nlm.nih.gov/pubmed/8865382.
81. Lyall V, Feldman GM, Heck GL, DeSimone JA. Effects of extracellular pH, PCO2, and HCO3- on intracellular pH in isolated rat taste buds. Am J Physiol. 1997 [cited 2022 Mar 13];273(3 Pt 1):C1008–19. http://www.ncbi.nlm.nih.gov/pubmed/9316422.
82. Kusakabe T, Yoshida T, Matsuda H, Yamamoto Y, Hayashida Y, Kawakami T, et al. Changes in the immunoreactivity of substance P and calcitonin gene-related peptide in the laryngeal taste buds of chronically hypoxic rats. Histol Histopathol. 2000 [cited 2021 Sep 21];15(3):683–8. http://www.ncbi.nlm.nih.gov/pubmed/10963111.
83. Bartlett D, Knuth SL, Knuth SL. Responses of laryngeal receptors to intralaryngeal CO2 in the cat. J Physiol. 1992 [cited 2022 Mar 13];457:187–93. http://www.ncbi.nlm.nih.gov/pubmed/1297833.
84. May M. Galen on the usefulness of the parts of the body, vol. 1. Ithaca: Cornell University Press; 1968. p. 372.
85. Bowman L. Historical perspective. In: Matthew O, editor. Respiratory function of the upper airway. New York: Marcel Dekker; 1980. p. 23.

86. Dritsoula AK, Thevasagayam MS. Congenital aplasia/hypoplasia of the epiglottis-a case report and a review of the literature. Int J Pediatr Otorhinolaryngol. 2015;79(10):1609–12. https://doi.org/10.1016/j.ijporl.2015.07.031.
87. Reyes BG, Arnold JE, Brooks LJ. Congenital absence of the epiglottis and its potential role in obstructive sleep apnea. Int J Pediatr Otorhinolaryngol. 1994;30(3):223–6.
88. Garon BR, Huang Z, Hommeyer S, Eckmann D, Stern GA, Ormiston C. Epiglottic dysfunction: abnormal epiglottic movement patterns. Dysphagia. 2002;17(1):57–68.
89. Lan MC, Liu SYC, Lan MY, Modi R, Capasso R. Lateral pharyngeal wall collapse associated with hypoxemia in obstructive sleep apnea. Laryngoscope. 2015;125(10):2408–12.
90. Fogel RB, Trinder J, White DP, Malhotra A, Raneri J, Schory K, et al. The effect of sleep onset on upper airway muscle activity in patients with sleep apnoea versus controls. J Physiol. 2005 [cited 2020 Mar 13];564(Pt 2):549–62. http://www.ncbi.nlm.nih.gov/pubmed/15695240.
91. Pierce R, White D, Malhotra A, Edwards JK, Kleverlaan D, Palmer L, et al. Upper airway collapsibility, dilator muscle activation and resistance in sleep apnoea. Eur Respir J. 2007 [cited 2021 Sep 5];30(2):345–53. http://www.ncbi.nlm.nih.gov/pubmed/17459896.
92. Katz ES, White DP. Genioglossus activity during sleep in normal control subjects and children with obstructive sleep apnea. Am J Respir Crit Care Med. 2004 [cited 2021 Sep 5];170(5):553–60. http://www.ncbi.nlm.nih.gov/pubmed/15172891.
93. White DP. Pathogenesis of obstructive and central sleep apnea. Am J Respir Crit Care Med. 2005 [cited 2021 Sep 5];172(11):1363–70. http://www.ncbi.nlm.nih.gov/pubmed/16100008.
94. Jordan AS, White DP. Pharyngeal motor control and the pathogenesis of obstructive sleep apnea. Respir Physiol Neurobiol. 2008 [cited 2020 Apr 1];160(1):1–7. http://www.ncbi.nlm.nih.gov/pubmed/17869188.
95. Younes M. Role of arousals in the pathogenesis of obstructive sleep apnea. Am J Respir Crit Care Med. 2004 [cited 2020 Feb 11];169(5):623–33. http://www.ncbi.nlm.nih.gov/pubmed/14684560.
96. Jordan AS, Wellman A, Edwards JK, Schory K, Dover L, MacDonald M, et al. Respiratory control stability and upper airway collapsibility in men and women with obstructive sleep apnea. J Appl Physiol. 2005 [cited 2022 Feb 22];99(5):2020–7. http://www.ncbi.nlm.nih.gov/pubmed/15994243.
97. Younes M. Role of respiratory control mechanisms in the pathogenesis of obstructive sleep disorders. J Appl Physiol. 2008;105(5):1389–405.
98. Sériès F. Upper airway muscles awake and asleep. Sleep Med Rev. 2002;6(3):229–42.
99. Genta PR, Sands SA, Butler JP, Loring SH, Katz ES, Demko BG, et al. Airflow shape is associated with the pharyngeal structure causing OSA. Chest. 2017 [cited 2019 Mar 29];152(3):537–46. http://www.ncbi.nlm.nih.gov/pubmed/28651794.
100. Azarbarzin A, Marques M, Sands SA, Op de Beeck S, Genta PR, Taranto-Montemurro L, et al. Predicting epiglottic collapse in patients with obstructive sleep apnoea. Eur Respir J. 2017 [cited 2021 Jul 13];50(3):1700345. https://doi.org/10.1183/13993003.00345.
101. Isono S. Two valves in the pharynx. Eur Respir J. 2017;50(3):7–9. https://doi.org/10.1183/13993003.01496-2017.
102. Laufer A, Condax ID. The function of the epiglottis in speech. Lang Speech. 1979;24(Pt 1):39–62. http://www.ncbi.nlm.nih.gov/pubmed/7266191.

Clinical Assessment of OSA Patients

6

Matej Delakorda and Blaz Maver

6.1 Introduction

Clinical assessment is an important component of obstructive sleep apnea (OSA) patient evaluation. Traditionally, the main purpose of otorhinolaryngological (ENT) examination is to identify anatomical structures or levels at which obstructions occur, and which can be modified by surgery. Considering the recent insight regarding the multifactorial etiology of OSA, sleep surgeons should also be able to understand the non-anatomical causes of OSA and possible ways to address them [1]. Among all specialists, ENT are best suited to comprehensively evaluate the upper airway (UA), and possess the knowledge on how to modify it effectively. Nevertheless, their role should not be limited to mastering various surgical techniques; rather, they should also be familiar with other treatment modalities. Additionally, they must be able to identify some of the other most common sleep disorders that can cause symptoms similar to sleep-disordered breathing, i.e., insomnia and narcolepsy.

As a rule, most OSA patients are still examined by sleep specialists, usually pulmonologists and neurologists, who make the decision regarding referral to other clinics or specialists. Given the high prevalence of OSA, these referrals are relatively rare, and in our clinical practice, we mostly see patients who do not tolerate or do not wish to try positive pressure therapy. Such an approach can be problematic, since a significant share of patients who use this therapy in a suboptimal

Supplementary Information The online version contains supplementary material available at https://doi.org/10.1007/978-3-031-34992-8_6. The videos can be accessed individually by clicking the DOI link in the accompanying figure caption or by scanning this link with the SN More Media App.

M. Delakorda (✉) · B. Maver
General Hospital Celje, Celje, Slovenia

M. Delakorda, N. de Vries (eds.), *The Role of Epiglottis in Obstructive Sleep Apnea*, https://doi.org/10.1007/978-3-031-34992-8_6

manner could be successfully treated in other ways [2–5]. In any case, patients coming from a sleep specialist are diagnostically evaluated with qualitative and quantitative assessment of sleep-disordered breathing. A technically adequate and manually scored sleep study record can provide information on OSA severity, point to the number and level of obstructions and positional dependence, and possibly yield other important information. However, potential shortcomings of sleep studies and the resulting possibility of misjudging a patient's condition when relying solely on them should be kept in mind.

The training of ENT specialists emphasizes the morphological rather than the functional assessment of UA. Recognizing the extent to which both of these factors are present in each individual patient might be the key to successful treatment but is often difficult to determine. When gathering information about a patient's clinical condition, we usually consider the possibility of surgical treatment. In this regard, the key question to be constantly kept in mind is whether we can significantly improve or cure OSA and its consequences; if not, we should aim to facilitate or enable other treatments. As surgical procedures are irreversible and associated with possible complications, non-surgical approaches have, as a rule, traditionally taken precedence over surgical ones. In recent years, protocols have been on the rise that take into the account the heterogeneity of OSA and encourage the identification of specific phenotypes, i.e., sets of morphological and other characteristics that may allow a more personalized approach. In certain cases, invasive procedures are preferred, based on the claim that anatomic considerations should be taken as the true prognosis factor for OSA surgery, rather than merely the severity of the disease [6–8].

Routine pre-operative drug induced sleep endoscopy (DISE) investigations have confirmed that obstructions often occur at the level of the epiglottis and it is now recognized as one of the predominant sites affecting treatment success [9]. Nevertheless, to date, no reliable system has been established that could help us identify patients with obstruction at this level during clinical examination. As a relatively recently discovered entity, epiglottis obstructions are still associated with many unresolved issues related to classification, diagnosis, and treatment.

6.2 History

History taking remains a fundamental part of OSA patient assessment. It can take place in different clinical settings, often during routine appointment when other complaints are being evaluated and OSA symptoms or typical clinical features are detected. Sometimes, only a few simple screening questions can start revealing an undiagnosed OSA. These patients might need more extensive workup, and the ENT specialist sets the sequence of medical treatment. A systematic approach to history taking should be established to acquire all necessary information. In this respect, tools like sleep questionnaires can be very helpful. With high clinical suspicion, the patient is sent to a sleep study and is expected to return for further workup. In this case, a sleep surgeon should be familiar with the contraindications for unattended sleep studies—severe pulmonary disease, neuromuscular disease, congestive heart failure, hypoventilation, chronic opioid use, history of stroke, or severe insomnia. [10] An alternative clinical setting is when the patient is suspected to have OSA or has already been positively tested and is referred to an ENT specialist. Once again, a full comprehensive history is required, even though we anticipate that a thorough assessment has already been performed. With growing incidence and awareness of the disease, we can expect a substantial increase in OSA patient influx to clinics. An effort should be made to educate colleagues of other specialties about the disease, since their role in recognizing sleep disorders is not negligible.

OSA patients are usually not able to evaluate their own respiratory events. Therefore, it is helpful if their bed partner is present at the office while taking history or during follow-up. Quite often, the main reason a patient seeks help is socially disruptive snoring leading to partner's sleep deprivation. They can provide information on snoring loudness, disturbance, position dependency, breathing route, etc. Such observations are valuable in evaluating the outcome of any potential treatment, and it is therefore advisable to describe and quantify them with questionnaires employing a visual analogue scale. To avoid bias, these questionnaires should be filled out in advance and without the presence of medical staff.

OSA-oriented history involves the evaluation of typical symptoms, divided into daytime and nighttime. The most common symptoms are presented in Table 6.1. Pang et al. found a strong correlation between patient's self-perception and OSA severity [11]. However, we must be cautious when assessing objectivity of self-reported symptoms. A precise description of the sleeping pattern is important, so it is advisable for the patient to keep a sleep diary documenting sleep and its features over a period of several weeks. We must also address abnormal behavior during sleep (e.g., strange movements of limbs, catathrenia), personal habits (drinking, smoking, and consumption of stimulants), drugs abuse (sedatives, antidepressants, anxiolytics), and occupational and social history.

Many questionnaires were developed for the assessment of sleep quality, OSA symptoms, and risk factors. In the English literature alone there are already more than 30. The Epworth Sleepiness Scale (ESS), Pittsburgh Sleep Quality Index (PSQI), and STOP BANG are among the most commonly used. The ESS is used to assess excessive daytime sleepiness in different sleep disorders. Patients rate the probability of falling asleep in diverse real-life scenarios [12]. It is regularly used in clinical practice; however, with low test–retest reliability and poor sensitivity (46%)

Table 6.1 Daytime and nighttime OSA symptoms

Daytime symptoms	Nighttime symptoms
Unrefreshing sleep[a]	Snoring[a,b]
Morning headache and dry/sore throat	Witnessed apneas[a,b]
Excessive daytime sleepiness or fatigue[a,b,c]	Gasping and choking sounds[a]
Cognitive deficits	Insomnia[a]
Decreased vigilance	Restless sleep[a]
Sexual dysfunction	Nocturia[a]
Irritability	

[a] PSQI
[b] STOP, BANG
[c] ESS

and specificity (60%), it is not a good OSA predictor [13–15]. PSQI is a good tool for assessing sleep quality, although it is not specific to any primary sleep disorders and it is not indicated for screening patients with a high risk of OSA [16–18]. It focuses on sleep quality, efficiency, duration and latency, daytime symptoms, and the use of sleeping medications. Currently, the most utilized questionnaire is the STOP BANG; the abbreviations stand for snoring (S), tiredness (T), observed apnea (O), high blood pressure (P), body mass index (B), age (A), neck circumference (N), and male gender (G) [19]. It is easy to use and shows a high sensitivity (90%) and moderate specificity (46%) for detecting OSA [20]. In contrast to other questionnaires, it can be used as an efficient screening tool for OSA [21].

It is important to recognize the risk factors for OSA, such as obesity, increased neck circumference, airway abnormalities, hypertension, and family history of OSA, and therefore, relevant questions addressing them should not be omitted. The points of interest include cardiovascular (arterial hypertension, congestive heart failure, arrhythmias, ischemic heart disease, pulmonary hypertension), endocrine (hypothyroidism), metabolic (diabetes type 2, gout), neurological (epilepsy, stroke, headaches), pulmonary (asthma, emphysema, chronic bronchitis), gastroesophageal, and psychiatric diseases (depression, anxiety, bipolar disorder) [22, 23]. All signs, symptoms, and OSA-related comorbidities should be recorded to aid our diagnostic process and to provide therapy outcome measures for re-evaluation in addition to sleep studies' results.

6.3 BMI

Excess body weight is the most important risk factor for the development of OSA with incidence increasing rapidly at values of body mass index (BMI) above 30 kg/m^2 [24]. At such values, the likelihood of multilevel obstructions increases as well [25]. Changes in BMI affect OSA severity in both positive and negative ways [26, 27]. Fat accumulation in soft tissues of the neck, especially in the tongue, causes reduction of the pharyngeal lumen and greater collapsibility of the walls [28]. Paradoxically, according to some studies, lower BMI patients are more prone to obstructions at the level of the tongue base and epiglottis when compared to others [29–31]. On the other hand, Kuo et al. observed no difference in BMI between epiglottis collapse and non-epiglottic collapse groups [32].

6.4 Gender

Historically, OSA has always been considered a male disease [33]. Previous estimations showed that male-to-female ratio of OSA prevalence in general population ranged from 3:1 to 5:1, while in clinical study groups, the ratio was between 8:1 and 10:1 [34–36]. It is believed that sex difference in OSA prevalence is linked to different fat distribution, length of the upper airway, pharyngeal collapsibility, neuromuscular control, arousal threshold, and sex hormones [37]. Women tend to express differently when describing symptoms, and according to Young, 40% of women with an apnea–hypopnea index greater than 15 did not report any typical OSA symptoms, while in men this share was 20% [38]. The difference in collapsibility of retroglossal airway in women and men has not been proven, although Whittle et al. have shown by means of MR imaging that women have greater fat deposition and a narrower airway in this area [39]. Significant differences in the epiglottis cross-sectional area (CSA) and oropharyngeal airway length (OPAL) between men and women with severe OSA were noticed in a study by Ma et al. OSA males had increased CSA and longer OPAL [40]. Another study showed that male gender is positively related to a thicker epiglottis, which could attribute to its collapsibility [41].

6.5 Age

Aging is a risk factor for OSA, although the mechanisms are still not elucidated completely. A study by Zhao showed that aging increases the probability of multilevel obstructions [42]. On the other hand, some authors observed no correlation between age and obstruction at the level of the epiglottis [29, 31, 32]. Two anatomic studies have confirmed age-related changes in the medial hyoepiglottic ligament with decreased level of elastin and collagen fibers that could cause the posterior displacement of the epiglottis as well as its instability during breathing [43, 44]. Additionally, it was discovered with electromyography that age-related weakening with remodeled motor units is present in the genioglossus muscle of individuals above 55 years, which may have implications in tongue base collapsibility [45].

6.6 Craniofacial Features and Cephalometry

A physician should be aware of the connection between certain craniofacial skeletal features and OSA, as they can be an important predisposing factor for the development of the disease [46–48]. Mandibular and maxillary hypoplasia, inferior position of the hyoid bone, narrowed posterior air space, and a greater flexion of the cranial base are the most frequently observed features linked to OSA [49–51]. We must also not forget about the importance of narrowed maxilla in the transverse plane [52]. For objectivization we can use the multi-detector computer tomography or 2D lateral cephalogram, with the latter being simpler, cheaper, and less harmful due to the radiation. Probably the most important feature in assessing/diagnosing an OSA patient is the position of the hyoid bone. In a study by Neelapu, it was shown that inferiorly placed hyoid bone in relation to the mandible and sella, strongly correlated to OSA patients [51]. It also plays a role in EC, as it determines the position of the tongue and epiglottis.

6.7 Upper Airway Evaluation

After we use medical history and initial clinical evaluation to identify patients with a high risk for OSA, a detailed physical examination of UA should be the next step. Most clinicians dealing with surgical treatment of OSA agree that determining the level and configuration of obstructions are important to help in planning adequate treatment and identify patients who could benefit from surgery [53–55]. In this regard, information obtained from sleep and radiologic studies can be very helpful (see Chaps. 7 and 9). While observing the anatomy, we should keep in mind that at least 70% of OSA patients have multilevel obstructions and that the number of obstructions tends to increase with OSA severity [56–58]. When describing observations during UA assessment, it makes sense to use classification systems, as they enable standardized reporting, improved interpretation, and comparison of research results. Many grading systems are available for describing and scoring the affected sites during office examination, although their actual clinical value is still questionable.

Inferring the importance of different observations during clinical examination is complicated by the fact that UA characteristics can differ considerably between wakefulness and sleep. This is especially true for the level of the larynx and hypopharynx, where awake assessment frequently underestimates the degree of obstructions [59, 60]. Despite this fact, traditional methods of UA examination are regularly performed by sleep surgeons when they tend to rely on anatomical traits. Such evaluations are performed in a relatively static airway, but some techniques to evaluate dynamic changes have been introduced. Muller's maneuver was first described by Borowiecki and Sassin in 1983 with an initial intent to select patients suitable for uvulopalatopharyngoplasty [61]. Although still used by many clinicians, there are many controversies about the investigation [11, 62]. After literature review, Mattos Soares et al. came to a conclusion that Muller's maneuver has low reproducibility, that it is not a good predictor of disease severity or oropharyngeal surgery success, and that it does not reliably detect the site of upper airway collapse [63]. In a study from Sung et al., no epiglottis collapse was noted during the Muller's maneuver in any of the patients with isolated epiglottis collapse detected with DISE [30].

Radiological methods allowed the first clear conclusions that patients with OSA have, on average, smaller pharyngeal cross-sections compared to the healthy population [64]. A clear proof that obstructive respiratory events during the sleep should be viewed as dynamic phenomena is the fact that they never occur in wakefulness. In accordance with this, it makes sense to distinguish visible sites of UA narrowing (obstructions) from collapses resulting from increased tissue compliance and/or intraluminal pressure. The pharyngeal airway collapse follows the principle of the "tube law," with gradual lumen narrowing dependent on transmural pressure and tissue compliance. Unlike these structures, the epiglottis behaves as a one-way valve with obstructions occurring abruptly and intermittently, exclusively during inspiratory phase [65–67]. The displacement of such valve-like structures is determined by the driving pressure, as well as the shape and position (angle). The epiglottis is located low in the upper respiratory tract and therefore, when assessing its stability, it is necessary to look for the primary flow-limiting site that may be located at a higher UA level [68]. This multifactorial dependency is probably one of the reasons why it is difficult to predict the success of epiglottis surgery [69, 70].

In most studies, the determination of the level of obstruction (topodiagnosis) is based on and confirmed with DISE. It is known that some medications used for sedation can affect the tone of the genioglossus muscle, the main pharyngeal dilator, and thus affect the position of the tongue base and consequently also the epiglottis [71, 72]. This might explain the disagreement between surgical plans based on the DISE findings and those based on awake techniques, with epiglottis surgery being more frequently indicated after DISE [73, 74]. Also, the prevalence of epiglottis obstructions requiring surgery seems to be lower than that found during DISE [70]. Therefore, we can reasonably suspect that at least a part of obstructions detected at this level may be due to the effect of sedating agents. Accordingly, results of DISE should be evaluated with some care and interpreted with a degree of doubt. It also means that DISE should be combined with awake examination as a complementary method.

6.7.1 The Nose

The role of the nose in the development of obstructive sleep disorders has not been definitively elucidated. Nasal patency can influence OSA pathogenesis in several ways. Although nasal resistance represents around half of the total airway resistance in the awake state, this share is much lower during sleep. While many studies have confirmed that treating nasal obstruction does not substantially affect OSA severity in terms of respiratory events, it has an important effect on subjective outcome measures [75–78]. Consequently, a complete sinonasal symptoms evaluation and thorough exam of the nasal cavity are necessary in any patient with OSA. Nasal obstruction can affect the epiglottis in two ways: either through posterior displacement of the tongue base during oral breathing or by contributing to higher downstream negative pressures (see Chap. 12).

When examining the patient, we should obtain information on nasal patency, discharge, previous facial trauma, or surgery (endoscopic sinus surgery, esthetic rhinoplasty, septoplasty, turbinate reduction, adenoidectomy). Tools like the Nasal Obstruction Symptom Evaluation scale (NOSE) can be of great help when evaluating a patient's perception of nasal obstruction or treatment outcome [79]. Some authors even consider it a screening tool for patients with a high risk of OSA [80]. Assessment begins with the inspection of the outer nose. In case of a collapsible nasal alae, we can perform Cottle's maneuver to assess nasal valves' collapse. In our experience, patients with a long soft palate often complain of sensations of nasal obstruction when in the supine position. The examiner should also be aware of the negative effects of the supine body position on nasal congestion [81]. We proceed with anterior rhinoscopy and systematically evaluate the nasal mucosa, turbinates, and septum. Any pathological discharge, septal deviation, perforation, synechiae, crusting, nasal polyps, and turbinate hypertrophy should be described. In case of clinical suspicion, we can additionally perform endoscopy that can reveal pathologic processes in the nasopharynx, such as enlarged adenoids, antrochoanal polyps, and neoplasms.

6.7.2 The Oral Cavity (Skeletal Frame)

There are several important skeletal characteristics in the dental/maxillofacial area that a sleep surgeon should notice when assessing a patient [47, 82]. OSA is a known risk factor for bruxism, so teeth should be checked for signs of dental wear [83]. Then, one should proceed with the assessment of the upper and lower jaws. Angle's classification of malocclusion is widely accepted and divides the patient into three groups (classes I, II, and III). Retrognathia (class II) is a condition where the mandible is deficient in growth and lies more posteriorly (Fig. 6.1). It is commonly associated with a narrower airway at the retroglossal area [83–85]. Cephalometric studies have shown that in addition to mandible position, other factors in OSA etiopathogenesis include retro-positioned maxilla, extrusion of teeth, proclined incisors, and open bite [50]. Another important feature is the shape of the hard palate. The narrow maxilla and high-arched hard palate are associated with a history of mouth breathing, and are commonly seen in people with OSA [52]. Often, a long and ptotic soft palate is co-observed (Fig. 6.2). Discrepancy between the size of the tongue and bony skeletal frame can result in a scalloped tongue that in turn may be a useful clinical indicator for OSA [86]. Oral devices are widely used, but we should assess the appropriate candidates for such treatment. Suitable patients should have stable dentition and usually at least six healthy teeth per arch with adequate jaw mobility, with the ability to protrude the mandible for at least 6 mm [87].

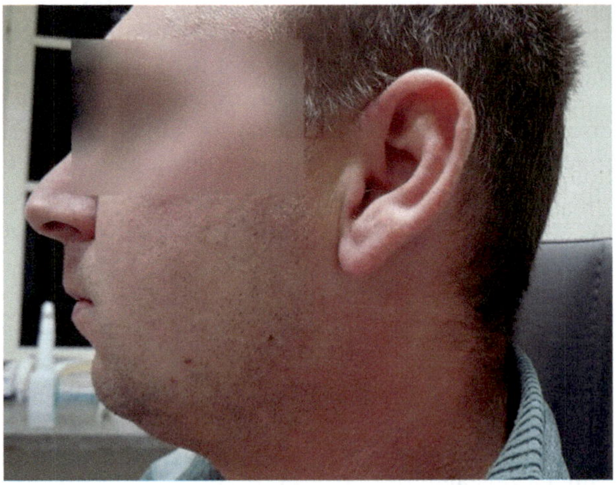

Fig. 6.1 OSA patient with class II malocclusion

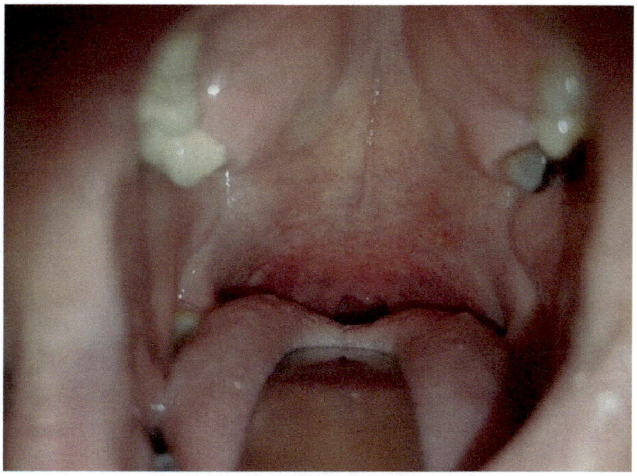

Fig. 6.2 OSA patient with a high-arched hard palate and a long, ptotic soft palate

6.7.3 The Pharynx

The pharynx lacks skeletal support and is the primary obstruction site in OSA patients, so a clinical evaluation of this part is an essential part of UA inspection. When accessing the tongue base, one should keep in mind that obstructions at the level of the epiglottis can be primary, where the epiglottis closes the airway independently (trap door or floppy epiglottis), or secondary, where it is pushed back by the base of the tongue. Identifying the difference between both options is important as it affects the choice of treatment [88].

The tongue base and larynx can be examined either indirectly or by means of endoscopy that can be either transnasal flexible or transoral rigid. Each of these techniques has its advantages and disadvantages. Indirect examination with a laryngeal mirror can be quite demanding in people with pronounced pharyngeal reflex, as it can cause the tongue base and the epiglottis to move forward. Due to the activation of the pharyngeal muscles, an altered shape of some soft tissues, e.g., tongue base position, the curvature of the epiglottis, or their interrelationship may occur. Additionally, when the patient is asked to regulate breathing or hold a breath, variable degrees of laryngeal closure can be noticed [89]. Some authors suggest to evaluate UA at end expiration to eliminate the possible effect of dynamic collapse from negative intraluminal pressure [90]. During early inspiration in the awake state, a small increase of the pharyngeal lumen occurs, but during the rest of the respiration cycle, it remains constant, which points to phasic dilator activity [91]. All of the above may affect our assessment of UA; therefore, a gentle use of transnasal flexible endoscopy is advisable in sensitive patients.

When examining the tongue base and the larynx, we should be aware that the head position can also have an impact on the pharyngeal lumen and hence influence our judgement on possible obstruction sites. With indirect laryngoscopy, using laryngeal mirror, the patient's head is usually tilted backward, i.e., the neck is extended. This position makes the retroglossal pharyngeal lumen wider.

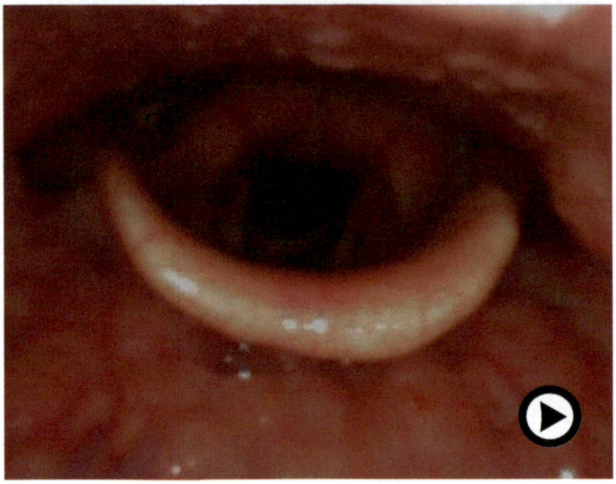

Fig. 6.3 (Video 6.1) Video showing the effect of oral positioning on UA (▶ https://doi.org/10.1007/000-bf4)

Contrary, any head flexion with the chin tucked in, which can occur during transnasal laryngoscopy, causes a posterior shift of anterior pharyngeal structures in combination with shortening of the distance from the epiglottis to the posterior pharyngeal wall. Mouth opening has a similar effect on the size of the pharyngeal lumen. While opening the jaw slightly can increase the size of the pharynx by providing more space for the tongue, progressive opening leads to a posterior movement of the mandible, the tongue, and hyoid, thereby narrowing the pharyngeal airway [91, 92]. A similar effect on the enlargement of the lumen behind the epiglottis can sometimes be noticed with the protrusion of the tongue. Nevertheless, paradoxical patterns can occur in a substantial share of patients [93] (Fig. 6.3).

When assessing a patient preoperatively, the pharynx is one of the anatomical regions where we can use well-established grading systems. Fujita was the first to classify upper airway obstructions, as follows: type 1 (soft palate), type 2 (soft palate and tongue base), and type 3 (tongue base and hypopharynx) [94]. Friedman's tongue position staging is used for the estimation of pharyngeal obstruction and describes tongue position relative to the soft palate and uvula. The staging system is based on the Mallampati score introduced in 1983. It was proposed as a non-invasive method for assessing difficult intubation [95]. In 1999 Friedman et al. added two parameters and named it the modified Mallampati score that was later renamed to the Friedman tongue position grade (FTP). Mallampati classification has three grades and evaluates the position of the protruded tongue relative to the soft palate [96]. So far, two classifications of lingual tonsils have been introduced, one by Friedman et al. and the second by Sung et al. Both consist of grades from 0 to 4, with 0 indicating absent lymphoid tissue and 4 hypertrophied lymphoid tissue spreading toward the epiglottis (Fig. 6.4) [97, 98].

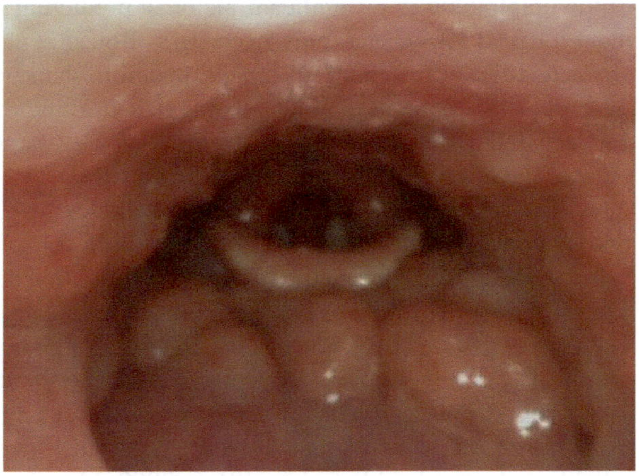

Fig. 6.4 Friedman grade 4 lingual tonsils

6.7.4 The Larynx

To date, quite a few clinical models for predicting the presence or the degree of OSA have been presented, but they generally do not include the epiglottis [11, 99]. On the other hand, considerable research has been conducted on the role of the base of the tongue and epiglottis in glottis visualization when assessing the difficulty of intubation. Majority of this research was performed by anesthesiologists who mostly concentrated on the position of the epiglottis relative to the tongue base during examination under general anesthesia [100, 101]. In 1984, Cormack and Lehane were the first to describe the laryngeal view during direct laryngoscopy to predict the ease of endotracheal intubation. Since then, the grading system they proposed became the anesthesiologist's gold standard for UA classification, with some modifications [102, 103]. However, despite the widespread use, some studies question its validity [104–106]. In a study conducted by Uzun et al. in 2005, a classification was proposed based on different types of epiglottis shapes evaluated during general anesthesia. They concluded that free edges of the omega-shaped epiglottis could prevent total obstruction at this level by leaning onto the posterior wall of the hypopharynx when the tongue base moves posteriorly. Additionally, they observed that leaf-shaped or flat epiglottises had a flexible character with a tendency to collapse and close the laryngeal inlet [107].

Nowadays, it is widely accepted that OSA and difficult intubation are related [108]. Moreover, a connection between some epiglottis characteristics and the presence of OSA has been established. Ma et al. conducted a study with magnetic resonance imaging of the upper airway in awake OSA patients lying in a supine position. They investigated the relation between epiglottis position and OSA severity. The distance between the hard palate and the tip of the epiglottis increased with OSA severity, while a significantly reduced cross-sectional area behind the tip of the epiglottis appeared only in severe OSA cases [40]. A similar conclusion on the connection of the lower laryngeal position and OSA severity was published by Yamashiro and Kryger. Airway length from the hard palate to vocal cords as well as to the base of the epiglottis was a significant factor in predicting AHI > 30 even after adjustment for BMI [109]. In a study from 2019, Bolzer et al. described some anatomical characteristics of the epiglottis (shape, position, shape of the retroepiglottic airway) by which OSA patients could be distinguished from others, and found a correlation between the presence of a mega-epiglottis—i.e., large epiglottis obstructing the view of the glottis—and severity of OSA [110].

A widely accepted grading system is still lacking for classifying OSA-relevant findings determined in the awake state at the level of the larynx. Additionally, in many OSA texts, the epiglottic obstructions are often described as part of the hypopharynx [111]. This makes reproducible and clinically relevant communication of the laryngeal status difficult. In 2018, Torre et al. conducted a study to assess the utility of adopting the existing Cormack–Lehane grading systems for vocal cord visualization during direct laryngoscopy in awake fiberoptic examination. They proposed the use of a 5-grade system to describe the hypopharyngeal airway in a reliable and reproducible fashion [9]. In 2002, Moore et al. proposed a modification of the Fujita clinical classification system to evaluate narrowing at the tongue base level in OSA patients. Using awake fiberoptic nasopharyngoscopy with Mueller's maneuver in both upright and supine positions, they described different types of obstructions based on the involvement of the tongue base and/or epiglottis. No statistical correlation was found between the obstruction pattern and severity of OSA, age, or facial skeletal pattern, but males had a higher percentage of type C pattern—isolated retro-epiglottic narrowing [112].

It would be very practical for every sleep surgeon to be able to anticipate possible sites of obstruction based on anatomical features in wakefulness. Unfortunately, examination in the awake state often underestimates the degree of laryngeal obstruction [59, 60]. Nevertheless, some anatomical features of OSA patients with obstruction at the epiglottis level have been presented in recent years. When examining the larynx, one should try to get an impression of the laryngeal position (high vs. low). It is important to assess the epiglottis position relative to the tongue base, its angle, consistency, and airspace behind it. Describing its shape (regular, flat, or omega-shaped) is needed since it affects the configuration of obstruction at this level. Surgical approach to lateral epiglottis obstructions that occur in patients with a closed, omega-shaped epiglottis, differs from the "trap door" type. Laryngeal motility should be evaluated and described. The assessment of aryepiglottic folds, subglottic area, and initial part of trachea is also important. We must pay attention to possible cysts, vascular formations, or other hyperplastic mucosal changes that can cause additional resistance to airflow (Fig. 6.5).

For a long time, it was considered that patients with obstruction at the level of the larynx cannot be distinguished from other OSA patients with awake clinical assessment. In a study by Woodson and Wooten, clinical examination results were compared to endoscopic and manometry findings. The absence of obstructing oropharyngeal features was the most characteristic feature of patients with collapse at the tongue base and epiglottis [59]. More recently, some studies have shown that certain epiglottis characteristics observed during awake examination could be used in clinical practice for a preliminary assessment of laryngeal obstructions. The omega-shaped

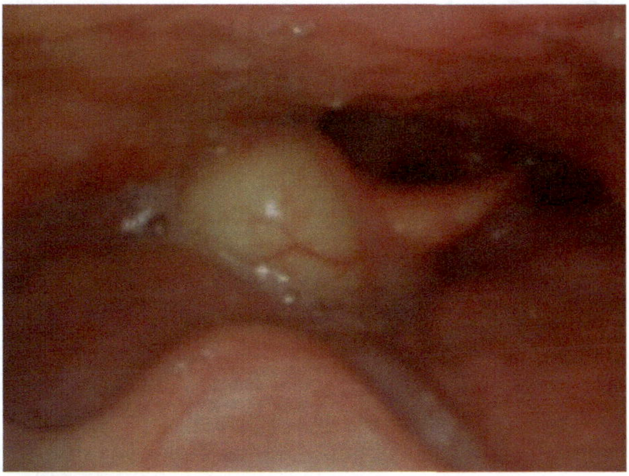

Fig. 6.5 Epiglottic retention cyst

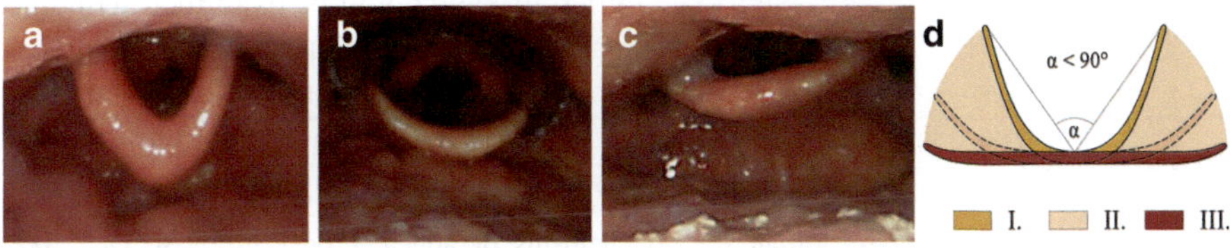

Fig. 6.6 Different shapes of epiglottis. Type 1—omega-shaped epiglottis (**a**); type 2—normal concave epiglottis shape (**b**); and type 3—flat epiglottis (**c**), graphic scheme (**d**)

epiglottis is present in about 30–50% of infants, but is much less common in adults, as it becomes flatter during growth [113, 114]. In a study by Li et al., it was established that spacing between the tongue base and epiglottis as assessed in the awake state in the supine position could predict glossopharyngeal obstructions detected with PSG and the nasopharyngeal tube inserted. The finding of obscured valleculae correlated well with some polysomnographic findings (AHI, lowest saturation). However, their method did not allow for distinction between obstructions at the base of tongue and isolated epiglottis obstructions [115]. In a recently published study, the authors described how epiglottis shape correlates to obstructions at the level of the tongue base and epiglottis as assessed during the DISE. They have also proposed a classification system based on epiglottis concavity as seen during the awake examination (Fig. 6.6). In the group of patients with flat epiglottises (type 3), obstructions at the level of the epiglottis and/or base of tongue—primary and secondary epiglottis collapse—occurred in most cases (94%) [116]. Another study analyzing the clinical characteristics of patients with isolated epiglottis collapse found a relation between such collapse and a shorter distance between mandible plane and hyoid, relative to the control group. However, no differences were observed between the two groups in terms of epiglottis shape or curvature, and the authors concluded that isolated epiglottic collapse could not be determined during awake endoscopy [30].

6.8 Conclusion

Although obstructions at the epiglottic level are present in a significant number of OSA patients, there are still many unresolved issues related to the role of this structure. Predicting the level of obstructions solely by clinical assessment is not yet adequately reliable. A widely accepted system for describing this part of the UA during awake laryngoscopy is currently lacking, and this makes communication difficult. The current body of evidence indicates some unique laryngeal characteristics by which OSA patients differ from others. Moreover, the connection between some clinical features and epiglottic collapse has been established. While the laryngeal position and some other cephalometric features are a known risk factor for epiglottic collapse, male gender, lower BMI, and OSA severity also seem to coincide with obstructions at this level. In cases of suspected epiglottic collapse, it is sensible to supplement the data obtained during clinical examination with other investigations, particularly DISE—although its results should be carefully interpreted. Further larger studies using uniform classification systems could shed more light on the role of clinical assessment in patients with epiglottic collapse.

References

1. Eckert DJ, Malhotra A, Jordan AS. Mechanisms of apnea. Prog Cardiovasc Dis. 2009 [cited 2020 Feb 11];51(4):313–23. http://www.pubmedcentral.nih.gov/articlerender.fcgi?artid=PMC3427748.
2. Weaver TE, Sawyer A. Management of obstructive sleep apnea by continuous positive airway pressure. Oral Maxillofac Surg Clin North Am. 2009 [cited 2020 Feb 23];21(4):403–12. http://www.ncbi.nlm.nih.gov/pubmed/19944340.
3. Weaver TE, Grunstein RR. Adherence to continuous positive airway pressure therapy: the challenge to effective treatment. Proc Am Thorac Soc. 2008 [cited 2020 March 3];5(2):173–8. http://www.ncbi.nlm.nih.gov/pubmed/18250209.
4. Weaver TE, Maislin G, Dinges DF, Bloxham T, George CFP, Greenberg H, et al. Relationship between hours of CPAP use and achieving normal levels of sleepiness and daily functioning. Sleep. 2007 [cited 2020 Feb 23];30(6):711–9. http://www.ncbi.nlm.nih.gov/pubmed/17580592.
5. Rotenberg BW, Murariu D, Pang KP. Trends in CPAP adherence over twenty years of data collection: a flattened curve. J Otolaryngol Head Neck Surg. 2016 [cited 2021 Aug 2];45(1):43. http://www.ncbi.nlm.nih.gov/pubmed/27542595.
6. Zinchuk A, Yaggi HK. Phenotypic subtypes of OSA: a challenge and opportunity for precision medicine. Chest. 2020 [cited 2021 Jun 25];157(2):403–20. http://www.ncbi.nlm.nih.gov/pubmed/31539538.
7. Rotenberg BW, Theriault J, Gottesman S. Redefining the timing of surgery for obstructive sleep apnea in anatomically favorable patients. Laryngoscope. 2014 [cited 2020 Feb 23];124 Suppl:1–9. http://doi.wiley.com/10.1002/lary.24720.
8. Friedman M, Ibrahim H, Bass L. Clinical staging for sleep-disordered breathing. Otolaryngol Head Neck Surg. 2002 [cited 2020 Feb 22];127(1):13–21. http://journals.sagepub.com/doi/10.1067/mhn.2002.126477.
9. Torre C, Zaghi S, Camacho M, Capasso R, Liu SY. Hypopharyngeal evaluation in obstructive sleep apnea with awake flexible laryngoscopy: Validation and updates to Cormack-Lehane and Modified Cormack-Lehane scoring systems. Clin Otolaryngol. 2018 [cited 2020 Feb 18];43(3):823–7. http://doi.wiley.com/10.1111/coa.13054.

10. Kapur VK, Auckley DH, Chowdhuri S, Kuhlmann DC, Mehra R, Ramar K, et al. Clinical practice guideline for diagnostic testing for adult obstructive sleep apnea: an American Academy of Sleep Medicine clinical practice guideline. J Clin Sleep Med. 2017 [cited 2020 March 10];13(3):479–504. http://www.ncbi.nlm.nih.gov/pubmed/28162150.
11. Pang KP, Oto F, Terris DJ, Podolsky R. Severity of obstructive sleep apnea: correlation with clinical examination and patient perception. Otolaryngol Head Neck Surg. 2006;135: 555–60.
12. Johns MW. A new method for measuring daytime sleepiness: the Epworth Sleepiness Scale. Sleep. 1991;14(6):540–5. https://pubmed.ncbi.nlm.nih.gov/1798888/.
13. Grewe FA, Roeder M, Bradicich M, Schwarz EI, Held U, Thiel S, et al. Low repeatability of Epworth Sleepiness Scale after short intervals in a sleep clinic population. J Clin Sleep Med. 2020 [cited 2021 Nov 14];16(5):757–64. http://www.ncbi.nlm.nih.gov/pubmed/32039756.
14. Lee SJ, Kang HW, Lee LH. The relationship between the Epworth Sleepiness Scale and polysomnographic parameters in obstructive sleep apnea patients. Eur Arch Otorhinolaryngol. 2012;269(4):1143–7. https://pubmed.ncbi.nlm.nih.gov/22037721/.
15. Ulasli SS, Gunay E, Koyuncu T, Akar O, Halici B, Ulu S, et al. Predictive value of Berlin Questionnaire and Epworth Sleepiness Scale for obstructive sleep apnea in a sleep clinic population. Clin Respir J. 2014;8(3):292–6.
16. Buysse DJ, Reynolds CF, Monk TH, Berman SR, Kupfer DJ. The Pittsburgh Sleep Quality Index: a new instrument for psychiatric practice and research. Psychiatry Res. 1989;28(2):193–213. https://pubmed.ncbi.nlm.nih.gov/2748771/.
17. Scarlata S, Pedone C, Curcio G, Cortese L, Chiurco D, Fontana D, et al. Pre-polysomnographic assessment using the Pittsburgh Sleep Quality Index questionnaire is not useful in identifying people at higher risk for obstructive sleep apnea. J Med Screen. 2013;20(4):220–6.
18. Nishiyama T, Mizuno T, Kojima M, Suzuki S, Kitajima T, Ando KB, et al. Criterion validity of the Pittsburgh Sleep Quality Index and Epworth Sleepiness Scale for the diagnosis of sleep disorders. Sleep Med. 2014;15(4):422–9. https://pubmed.ncbi.nlm.nih.gov/24657203/.
19. Chung F, Yegneswaran B, Liao P, Chung SA, Vairavanathan S, Islam S, et al. STOP questionnaire: a tool to screen patients for obstructive sleep apnea. Anesthesiology. 2008;108(5):812–21. https://pubmed.ncbi.nlm.nih.gov/18431116/.
20. Nagappa M, Liao P, Wong J, Auckley D, Ramachandran SK, Memtsoudis S, et al. Validation of the stop-bang questionnaire as a screening tool for obstructive sleep apnea among different populations: a systematic review and meta-analysis. PLoS One. 2015;10(12):e0143697.
21. Chen L, Pivetta B, Nagappa M, Saripella A, Islam S, Englesakis M, et al. Validation of the STOP-Bang questionnaire for screening of obstructive sleep apnea in the general population and commercial drivers: a systematic review and meta-analysis. Sleep Breath. 2021;25(4):1741. https://pubmed.ncbi.nlm.nih.gov/33507478/.
22. Bonsignore MR, Baiamonte P, Mazzuca E, Castrogiovanni A, Marrone O. Obstructive sleep apnea and comorbidities: a dangerous liaison. Multidiscip Respir Med. 2019 [cited 2021 Nov 14];14(1):8. https://pubmed.ncbi.nlm.nih.gov/30809382/.
23. Garg H. Sleep history taking and examination. Int J Head Neck Surg. 2019;10(1):9–17. https://creativecommons.
24. Young T, Palta M, Dempsey J, Skatrud J, Weber S, Badr S. The occurrence of sleep-disordered breathing among middle-aged adults. N Engl J Med. 1993 [cited 2020 Feb 8];328(17):1230–5. http://www.ncbi.nlm.nih.gov/pubmed/8464434.
25. Phua CQ, Yeo WX, Su C, Mok PKH. Multi-level obstruction in obstructive sleep apnoea: prevalence, severity and predictive factors. J Laryngol Otol. 2017;131(11):982–6.
26. Newman AB, Foster G, Givelber R, Nieto FJ, Redline S, Young T. Progression and regression of sleep-disordered breathing with changes in weight. Arch Intern Med. 2005 [cited 2020 Feb 6];165(20):2408. http://archinte.jamanetwork.com/article.aspx?doi=10.1001/archinte.165.20.2408.
27. Peppard PE, Young T, Palta M, Dempsey J, Skatrud J. Longitudinal study of moderate weight change and sleep-disordered breathing. JAMA. 2000 [cited 2020 Feb 6];284(23):3015. http://www.ncbi.nlm.nih.gov/pubmed/11122588.

28. Nashi N, Kang S, Barkdull GC, Lucas J, Davidson TM. Lingual fat at autopsy. Laryngoscope. 2007;117(8):1467–73.
29. Sung CM, Tan SN, Shin M-H, Lee J, Kim HC, Lim SC, et al. The site of airway collapse in sleep apnea, its associations with disease severity and obesity, and implications for mechanical interventions. Am J Respir Crit Care Med. 2021 [cited 2021 Dec 1];204(1):103–6. http://www.ncbi.nlm.nih.gov/pubmed/33826879.
30. Sung CM, Kim HC, Yang HC. The clinical characteristics of patients with an isolate epiglottic collapse. Auris Nasus Larynx. 2020;47(3):450–7.
31. Kim HY, Sung CM, Bin JH, Kim HC, Lim SC, Yang HC. Patients with epiglottic collapse showed less severe obstructive sleep apnea and good response to treatment other than continuous positive airway pressure: a case-control study of 224 patients. J Clin Sleep Med. 2021;17(3):413–9.
32. Kuo I-C, Hsin L-J, Lee L-A, Fang T-J, Tsai M-S, Lee Y-C, et al. Prediction of epiglottic collapse in obstructive sleep apnea patients: epiglottic length. Nat Sci Sleep. 2021 [cited 2021 Nov 26];13:1985–92. http://www.ncbi.nlm.nih.gov/pubmed/34764713.
33. Franklin KA, Sahlin C, Stenlund H, Lindberg E. Sleep apnoea is a common occurrence in females. Eur Respir J. 2013;41(3):610–5. https://pubmed.ncbi.nlm.nih.gov/22903961/.
34. Young T. The occurrence of sleep disordered brething among middle aged adults. 1993 [cited 2019 March 21]. https://ssl.sb-celje.si/doi/pdf/10.1056/,DanaInfo=www.nejm.org,SSL+NEJM199304293281704.
35. Quintana-Gallego E, Carmona-Bernal C, Capote F, Sánchez-Armengol Á, Botebol-Benhamou G, Polo-Padillo J, et al. Gender differences in obstructive sleep apnea syndrome: a clinical study of 1166 patients. Respir Med. 2004;98(10):984–9. https://pubmed.ncbi.nlm.nih.gov/15481275/.
36. Lin CM, Davidson TM, Ancoli-Israel S. Gender differences in obstructive sleep apnea and treatment implications. Sleep Med Rev. 2008;12(6):481–96. /pmc/articles/PMC2642982/.
37. Ryan CM, Bradley TD. Pathogenesis of obstructive sleep apnea. J Appl Physiol. 2005;99(6):2440–50. https://pubmed.ncbi.nlm.nih.gov/16288102/.
38. Young T, Hutton R, Finn L, Badr S, Palta M. The gender bias in sleep apnea diagnosis. Are women missed because they have different symptoms? Arch Intern Med. 1996;156(21):2445.
39. Whittle AT, Marshall I, Mortimore IL, Wraith PK, Sellar RJ, Douglas NJ. Neck soft tissue and fat distribution: comparison between normal men and women by magnetic resonance imaging. Thorax. 1999 [cited 2020 March 22];54(4):323–8. http://thorax.bmj.com/cgi/doi/10.1136/thx.54.4.323.
40. Ma MA, Kumar R, Macey PM, Yan-Go FL, Harper RM. Epiglottis cross-sectional area and oropharyngeal airway length in male and female obstructive sleep apnea patients. Nat Sci Sleep. 2016 [cited 2021 Aug 9];8:297–304. https://pubmed.ncbi.nlm.nih.gov/27757056/.
41. Sung C-W, Chan W, Chang C-H, Huang P-C, Lien W-C, Chang W-T, et al. Associations between male gender, body size and dimension of the epiglottis. Authorea Prepr; 2020.
42. Zhao C, Viana A, Ma Y, Capasso R. The effect of aging on drug-induced sleep endoscopy findings. Laryngoscope. 2018 [cited 2019 Nov 27];128(11):2644. http://doi.wiley.com/10.1002/lary.27265.
43. Irvine LE, Yang Z, Kezirian EJ, Nimni ME, Han B. Hyoepiglottic ligament collagen and elastin fiber composition and changes associated with aging. Laryngoscope. 2018;128(5):1245–8. https://pubmed.ncbi.nlm.nih.gov/29330863/.
44. Sawatsubashi M, Umezaki T, Kusano K, Tokunaga O, Oda M, Komune S. Age-related changes in the hyoepiglottic ligament: functional implications based on histopathologic study. Am J Otolaryngol Head Neck Med Surg. 2010;31(6):448–52. https://linkinghub.elsevier.com/retrieve/pii/S019607090900163X.
45. Saboisky JP, Stashuk DW, Hamilton-Wright A, Trinder J, Nandedkar S, Malhotra A. Effects of aging on genioglossus motor units in humans. PLoS One. 2014 [cited 2021 Jun 21];9(8):e104572. http://www.ncbi.nlm.nih.gov/pubmed/25111799.
46. Jamieson A, Guilleminault C, Partinen M, Quera-Salva MA. Obstructive sleep apneic patients have craniomandibular abnormalities. Sleep. 1987;9(4):469.

47. Tangugsorn V, Krogstad O, Espeland L, Lyberg T. Obstructive sleep apnoea: multiple comparisons of cephalometric variables of obese and non-obese patients. J Craniomaxillofac Surg. 2000 [cited 2021 Nov 16];28(4):204–12. http://www.ncbi.nlm.nih.gov/pubmed/11110151.
48. Bacon WH, Turlot JC, Krieger J, Stierle JL. Cephalometric evaluation of pharyngeal obstructive factors in patients with sleep apneas syndrome. Angle Orthod. 1990;60(2):115.
49. Cistulli PA. Craniofacial abnormalities in obstructive sleep apnoea: implications for treatment. Respirology. 1996;1(3):167.
50. Lowe AA, Santamaria JD, Fleetham JA, Price C. Facial morphology and obstructive sleep apnea. Am J Orthod Dentofacial Orthop. 1986;90(6):484–91. https://pubmed.ncbi.nlm.nih.gov/3098087/.
51. Neelapu BC, Kharbanda OP, Sardana HK, Balachandran R, Sardana V, Kapoor P, et al. Craniofacial and upper airway morphology in adult obstructive sleep apnea patients: a systematic review and meta-analysis of cephalometric studies. Sleep Med Rev. 2017;31:79.
52. Seto BH, Gotsopoulos H, Sims MR, Cistulli PA. Maxillary morphology in obstructive sleep apnoea syndrome. Eur J Orthod. 2001;23(6):703–14.
53. Aktas O, Erdur O, Cirik AA, Kayhan FT. The role of drug-induced sleep endoscopy in surgical planning for obstructive sleep apnea syndrome. Eur Arch Otorhinolaryngol. 2015 [cited 2019 Feb 14];272(8):2039–43. http://link.springer.com/10.1007/s00405-014-3162-8.
54. Launois SH, Feroah TR, Campbell WN, Issa FG, Morrison D, Whitelaw WA, et al. Site of pharyngeal narrowing predicts outcome of surgery for obstructive sleep apnea. Am Rev Respir Dis. 1993 [cited 2021 Dec 26];147(1):182–9. http://www.ncbi.nlm.nih.gov/pubmed/8420415.
55. Vanderveken OM, Maurer JT, Hohenhorst W, Hamans E, Lin HS, Vroegop AV, et al. Evaluation of drug-induced sleep endoscopy as a patient selection tool for implanted upper airway stimulation for obstructive sleep apnea. J Clin Sleep Med. 2013;9(5):433–8.
56. Ravesloot MJL, de Vries N. One hundred consecutive patients undergoing drug-induced sleep endoscopy: results and evaluation. Laryngoscope. 2011 [cited 2019 Apr 24];121(12):2710–6. http://doi.wiley.com/10.1002/lary.22369.
57. Abdullah VJ, van Hasselt CA. Video sleep nasendoscopy. In: Terris DJGR, editor. Surgical management of sleep apnea and snoring. Boca Raton: Taylor and Francis; 2005. p. 143–54.
58. Riley RW, Powell NB, Guilleminault C. Obstructive sleep apnea syndrome: a review of 306 consecutively treated surgical patients. Otolaryngol Neck Surg. 1993 [cited 2020 March 9];108(2):117–25. http://www.ncbi.nlm.nih.gov/pubmed/8441535.
59. Woodson BT, Wooten MR. Comparison of upper-airway evaluations during wakefulness and sleep. Laryngoscope. 1994 [cited 2020 Feb 6];104(7):821–8. http://www.ncbi.nlm.nih.gov/pubmed/8022243.
60. Campanini A, Canzi P, De Vito A, Dallan I, Montevecchi F, Vicini C. Awake versus sleep endoscopy: personal experience in 250 OSAHS patients. Acta Otorhinolaryngol Ital. 2010 [cited 2020 March 20];30(2):73–7. http://www.ncbi.nlm.nih.gov/pubmed/20559476.
61. Borowiecki BD, Sassin JF. Surgical treatment of sleep apnea. Arch Otolaryngol. 1983;109(8):508–12. http://www.ncbi.nlm.nih.gov/pubmed/6870642.
62. Stuck BA, Maurer J. The Mueller maneuver. In: Friedman M, Jacobowitz O, editors. Sleep apnea and snoring. Amsterdam: Elsevier; 2020. p. 13–22.
63. Soares MCM, Sallum ACR, Gonçalves MTM, Haddad FLM, Gregório LC. Utilização da manobra de Müller na avaliação de pacientes apnéicos: Revisão da literatura. Braz J Otorhinolaryngol. 2009;75(3):463–6.
64. EF Haponik, PL Smith, ME Bohlman, RP Allen, SM Goldman, ER Bleecker. Computerized tomography in obstructive sleep apnea. Correlation of airway size with physiology during sleep and wakefulness. Am Rev Respir Dis. 1983;127(2):221–6. https://doi.org/10.1164/arrd.1983.127.2.221.
65. Genta PR, Sands SA, Butler JP, Loring SH, Katz ES, Demko BG, et al. Airflow shape is associated with the pharyngeal structure causing OSA. Chest. 2017 [cited 2019 March 29];152(3):537–46. http://www.ncbi.nlm.nih.gov/pubmed/28651794.

66. Azarbarzin A, Marques M, Sands SA, Op de Beeck S, Genta PR, Taranto-Montemurro L, et al. Predicting epiglottic collapse in patients with obstructive sleep apnoea. Eur Respir J. 2017 [cited 2021 Jul 13];50(3):1700345. https://doi.org/10.1183/13993003.00345.
67. Isono S. Two valves in the pharynx. Eur Respir J. 2017;50(3):7–9. https://doi.org/10.1183/13993003.01496-2017.
68. Yanagisawa-Minami A, Sugiyama T, Iwasaki T, Yamasaki Y. Primary site identification in children with obstructive sleep apnea by computational fluid dynamics analysis of the upper airway. J Clin Sleep Med. 2020 [cited 2021 Jun 27];16(3):431–439. http://www.ncbi.nlm.nih.gov/pubmed/31992411.
69. Green KK, Kent DT, D'Agostino MA, Hoff PT, Lin HS, Soose RJ, et al. Drug-induced sleep endoscopy and surgical outcomes: a multicenter cohort study. Laryngoscope. 2019;129(3):761.
70. Kwon OE, Jung SY, Al-Dilaijan K, Min JY, Lee KH, Kim SW, et al. Is epiglottis surgery necessary for obstructive sleep apnea patients with epiglottis obstruction? Laryngoscope. 2019 [cited 2019 Nov 20];129(11):2658–62. https://onlinelibrary.wiley.com/doi/abs/10.1002/lary.27808.
71. Steinhart H, Kuhn-Lohmann J, Gewalt K, Constantinidis J, Mertzlufft F, Iro H. Upper airway collapsibility in habitual snorers and sleep apneics: evaluation with drug-induced sleep endoscopy. Acta Otolaryngol. 2000 [cited 2020 Apr 10];120(8):990–4. http://www.tandfonline.com/doi/full/10.1080/00016480050218753.
72. Kellner P, Herzog B, Plößl S, Rohrmeier C, Kühnel T, Wanzek R, et al. Depth-dependent changes of obstruction patterns under increasing sedation during drug-induced sedation endoscopy: results of a German monocentric clinical trial. Sleep Breath. 2016 [cited 2019 Sep 29];20(3):1035–43. https://ssl.sb-celje.si/content/pdf/,DanaInfo=link.springer.com,SSL+10.1007%2Fs11325-016-1348-6.pdf.
73. Fernández-Julián E, García-Pérez MÁ, García-Callejo J, Ferrer F, Martí F, Marco J. Surgical planning after sleep versus awake techniques in patients with obstructive sleep apnea. Laryngoscope. 2014;124(8):1970–4.
74. Eichler C, Sommer JU, Stuck BA, Hörmann K, Maurer JT. Does drug-induced sleep endoscopy change the treatment concept of patients with snoring and obstructive sleep apnea? Sleep Breath. 2013 [cited 2020 Feb 18];17(1):63–8. http://link.springer.com/10.1007/s11325-012-0647-9.
75. Friedman M, Tanyeri H, Lim JW, Landsberg R, Vaidyanathan K, Caldarelli D. Effect of improved nasal breathing on obstructive sleep apnea. Otolaryngol Head Neck Surg. 2000 [cited 2020 March 1];122(1):71–4. http://journals.sagepub.com/doi/10.1016/S0194-5998%2800%2970147-1.
76. Sériès F, St Pierre S, Carrier G. Effects of surgical correction of nasal obstruction in the treatment of obstructive sleep apnea. Am Rev Respir Dis. 1992 [cited 2020 March 15];146(5 Pt 1):1261–5. http://www.atsjournals.org/doi/abs/10.1164/ajrccm/146.5_Pt_1.1261.
77. Victores AJ, Takashima M. Effects of nasal surgery on the upper airway: a drug-induced sleep endoscopy study. Laryngoscope. 2012 [cited 2020 March 15];122(11):2606–10. http://www.ncbi.nlm.nih.gov/pubmed/22886986.
78. Li HY, Wang PC, Chen YP, Lee LA, Fang TJ, Lin HC. Critical appraisal and meta-analysis of nasal surgery for obstructive sleep apnea. Am J Rhinol Allergy. 2011 [cited 2020 March 31];25(1):45–9. http://www.ncbi.nlm.nih.gov/pubmed/21711978.
79. Stewart MG, Witsell DL, Smith TL, Weaver EM, Yueh B, Hannley MT. Development and validation of the Nasal Obstruction Symptom Evaluation (NOSE) scale. Otolaryngol Head Neck Surg. 2004;130(2):157–63. https://pubmed.ncbi.nlm.nih.gov/14990910/.
80. Ishii L, Godoy A, Ishman SL, Gourin CG, Ishii M. The nasal obstruction symptom evaluation survey as a screening tool for obstructive sleep apnea. Arch Otolaryngol Head Neck Surg. 2011;137(2):119–23. https://pubmed.ncbi.nlm.nih.gov/21339396/.
81. Roithmann R, Demeneghi P, Faggiano R, Cury A. Effects of posture change on nasal patency. Braz J Otorhinolaryngol. 2005;71(4):478–84. https://pubmed.ncbi.nlm.nih.gov/16446964/.
82. Miles PG, Vig PS, Weyant RJ, Forrest TD, Rockette HE. Craniofacial structure and obstructive sleep apnea syndrome--a qualitative analysis and meta-analysis of the literature. Am J

Orthod Dentofacial Orthop. 1996 [cited 2021 Nov 16];109(2):163–72. http://www.ncbi.nlm.nih.gov/pubmed/8638562.
83. Martynowicz H, Gac P, Brzecka A, Poreba R, Wojakowska A, Mazur G, et al. The relationship between sleep bruxism and obstructive sleep apnea based on polysomnographic findings. J Clin Med. 2019;8(10):1653. https://pubmed.ncbi.nlm.nih.gov/31614526/.
84. Muto T, Yamazaki A, Takeda S. A cephalometric evaluation of the pharyngeal airway space in patients with mandibular retrognathia and prognathia, and normal subjects. Int J Oral Maxillofac Surg. 2008;37(3):228–31. https://pubmed.ncbi.nlm.nih.gov/18296029/.
85. El H, Palomo JM. Airway volume for different dentofacial skeletal patterns. Am J Orthod Dentofacial Orthop. 2011;139(6):e511. https://pubmed.ncbi.nlm.nih.gov/21640863/.
86. Weiss TM, Atanasov S, Calhoun KH. The association of tongue scalloping with obstructive sleep apnea and related sleep pathology. Otolaryngol Head Neck Surg. 2005;133(6):966–71.
87. Jacobowitz O. Advances in oral appliances for obstructive sleep apnea. Adv Otorhinolaryngol. 2017;80:57–65. https://pubmed.ncbi.nlm.nih.gov/28738372/.
88. Salamanca F, Leone F, Bianchi A, Bellotto RGS, Costantini F, Salvatori P. Surgical treatment of epiglottis collapse in obstructive sleep apnoea syndrome: epiglottis stiffening operation. Acta Otorhinolaryngol Ital 2019 [cited 2020 Feb 12];39(6):404. http://www.ncbi.nlm.nih.gov/pubmed/31950932.
89. Ardran GM, Kemp FH. The mechanism of the larynx. II. The epiglottis and closure of the larynx. Br J Radiol. 1967;40(473):372–89.
90. Tucker WB. A method to describe the pharyngeal airway. Laryngoscope. 2015;125(5):1233–8.
91. Schwab RJ, Remmers JE, Kuna ST, Remmers JE. Anatomy and physiology of upper airway obstruction. In: Kryger MH, Roth TDW, editors. Principles and practice of sleep medicine: fifth edition. 5th ed. Philadelphia: Elsevier Saunders; 2010. p. 983–1000. https://doi.org/10.1016/B978-1-4160-6645-3.00101-8.
92. Isono S, Tanaka A, Tagaito Y, Ishikawa T, Nishino T. Influences of head positions and bite opening on collapsibility of the passive pharynx. J Appl Physiol. 2004 [cited 2021 Aug 3];97(1):339–46. http://www.jap.org.
93. Bonzelaar LB, Salapatas AM, Hwang MS, Andrews CC, Price NY, Friedman M. The effect of oral positioning on the hypopharyngeal airway. Laryngoscope. 2017 [cited 2021 Dec 12];127(6):1471–5. http://www.ncbi.nlm.nih.gov/pubmed/27686476.
94. Fujita S. Pharyngeal surgery for obstructive sleep apnea and snoring. In: Fairbanks DNF, editor. Snoring and obstructive sleep apnea. New York: Raven Press; 1987. p. 101–28.
95. Mallampati SR. Clinical sign to predict difficult tracheal intubation (hypothesis). Can Anaesth Soc J. 1983;30(3 Pt 1):316–7. https://pubmed.ncbi.nlm.nih.gov/6336553/.
96. Friedman M, Salapatas AM, Bonzelaar LB. Updated Friedman Staging System for obstructive sleep apnea. Adv Otorhinolaryngol. 2017 [cited 2020 Feb 22];80:41–8. https://pubmed.ncbi.nlm.nih.gov/28738388/.
97. Sung MW, Lee WH, Wee JH, Lee CH, Kim E, Kim JW. Factors associated with hypertrophy of the lingual tonsils in adults with sleep-disordered breathing. JAMA Otolaryngol Head Neck Surg. 2013;139(6):598–603. https://pubmed.ncbi.nlm.nih.gov/23787418/.
98. Friedman M, Yalamanchali S, Gorelick G, Joseph NJ, Hwang MS. A standardized lingual tonsil grading system: interexaminer agreement. Otolaryngol Head Neck Surg. 2015;152(4):667–72. https://pubmed.ncbi.nlm.nih.gov/25628371/.
99. Friedman M, Tanyeri H, La Rosa M, Landsberg R, Vaidyanathan K, Pieri S, et al. Clinical predictors of obstructive sleep apnea. Laryngoscope. 1999 [cited 2020 Feb 21];109(12):1901–7. http://www.ncbi.nlm.nih.gov/pubmed/10591345.
100. Yahagi N, Kono M, Kitahara M, Watanabe K, Fujiwara Y, Asakawa Y, et al. Causes of airway obstruction during cuffed oropharyngeal airway use. Resuscitation. 2001;48(3):275–8.
101. Shorten GD, Ali HH, Roberts JT. Assessment of patient position for fiberoptic intubation using videolaryngoscopy. J Clin Anesth. 1995;7(1):31–4.
102. Cormack RS, Lehane J. Difficult tracheal intubation in obstetrics. Anaesthesia. 1984 [cited 2020 Feb 22];39(11):1105–11. http://www.ncbi.nlm.nih.gov/pubmed/6507827.

103. Yentis SM, Lee DJ. Evaluation of an improved scoring system for the grading of direct laryngoscopy. Anaesthesia. 1998 [cited 2021 Nov 11];53(11):1041–1044. http://www.ncbi.nlm.nih.gov/pubmed/10023271.
104. Nowakowski M, Williams S, Gallant J, Ruel M, Robitaille A. Predictors of difficult intubation with the Bonfils Rigid Fiberscope. Anesth Analg. 2016 [cited 2021 Nov 2];122(6):1901–6. http://www.ncbi.nlm.nih.gov/pubmed/27028774.
105. Krage R, van Rijn C, Van Groeningen D, Loer SA, Schwarte LA, Schober P. Cormack-Lehane classification revisited. Br J Anaesth. 2010 [cited 2020 Feb 22];105(2):220–7. http://justus.randolph.name/kappa.
106. Ambesh SP, Singh N, Rao PB, Gupta D, Singh PK, Singh U. A combination of the modified Mallampati score, thyromental distance, anatomical abnormality, and cervical mobility (M-TAC) predicts difficult laryngoscopy better than Mallampati classification. Acta Anaesthesiol Taiwan. 2013 [cited 2021 Nov 16];51(2):58–62. http://www.ncbi.nlm.nih.gov/pubmed/23968655.
107. Uzun L, Ugur MB, Altunkaya H, Ozer Y, Ozkocak I, Demirel CB. Effectiveness of the jaw-thrust maneuver in opening the airway: a flexible fiberoptic endoscopic study. ORL Otorhinolarngol Relat Spec. 2005;67(1):39–44.
108. Hiremath AS, Hillman DR, James AL, Noffsinger WJ, Platt PR, Singer SL. Relationship between difficult tracheal intubation and obstructive sleep apnoea. Br J Anaesth. 1998 [cited 2021 Nov 17];80(5):606–11. http://www.ncbi.nlm.nih.gov/pubmed/9691863.
109. Yamashiro Y, Kryger M. Is laryngeal descent associated with increased risk for obstructive sleep apnea? Chest. 2012;141(6):1407–13. https://doi.org/10.1378/chest.10-3238.
110. Bolzer A, Toussaint B, Rumeau C, Gallet P, Jankowski R, Nguyen DT. Can anatomical assessment of hypopharyngolarynx in awake patients predict obstructive sleep apnea? Laryngoscope. 2019;129(12):2782–8.
111. Kezirian EJ, White DP, Malhotra A, Ma W, McCulloch CE, Goldberg AN. Interrater reliability of drug-induced sleep endoscopy. Arch Otolaryngol Head Neck Surg. 2010;136(4):393–7.
112. Moore KE, Phillips C. A practical method for describing patterns of tongue-base narrowing (modification of Fujita) in awake adult patients with obstructive sleep apnea. J Oral Maxillofac Surg. 2002;60(3):252–60.
113. Solomons NB, Prescott CAJ, Laryngomalacia. A review and the surgical management for severe cases. Int J Pediatr Otorhinolaryngol. 1987;13(1):31–9.
114. Janfaza P, Nadol JB, Galla R, Fabian RL, Montgomery WW. Surgical anatomy of the head and neck. Cambridge: Harvard University Press; 2011. p. xi–xii. http://www.jstor.org/stable/10.2307/j.ctvjf9vjb.4.
115. Li S, Wu D, Jie Q, Bao J, Shi H. Lingua-epiglottis position predicts glossopharyngeal obstruction in patients with obstructive sleep apnea hypopnea syndrome. Eur Arch Otorhinolaryngol. 2014;271(10):2737–43.
116. Delakorda M, Ovsenik N. Epiglottis shape as a predictor of obstruction level in patients with sleep apnea. Sleep Breath. 2019;23(1):311–7. http://www.ncbi.nlm.nih.gov/pubmed/30506267.

7 Sleep Studies

Johan Verbraecken

7.1 Introduction

The term "polysomnography" (PSG) was first proposed by Holland, Dement, and Raynal in 1974 [1], and describes the recording, analysis, and interpretation of multiple, simultaneous, physiological parameters that are used in the diagnosis of sleep disorders. Nocturnal PSG can be considered as the gold standard lab technique in the management of sleep-wake disturbances. Respiratory phenomena have to be linked with other sleep features, like sleep stage and leg movements. The following parameters are assessed during sleep by means of PSG:

1. The electroencephalogram (EEG) with different configurations but most often at least C4-M1 and C3-M2. This technique records the electrical activity of the brain from surface electrodes and is mandatory for the identification of sleep and wake. By convention, the EEG electrodes are placed according to the 10–20 electrode placement system [2].
2. The detection of eye movements or electrooculogram (EOG), muscle tone or electromyogram (EMG) of the chin and the lower extremities [3]. The EOG and chin EMG allow the detection of REM sleep, which is characterized by the presence of rapid eye movements and reduced skeletal muscle tone. The EOG electrodes are placed at the right and left outer orbital canthus, one slightly below and the other one slightly above the horizontal axis of the eyes and are refer-

J. Verbraecken (✉)
Department of Pulmonary Medicine and Multidisciplinary Sleep Disorders Center, Antwerp University Hospital, Edegem, Belgium

University of Antwerp, Antwerp, Belgium
e-mail: johan.verbraecken@uza.be

M. Delakorda, N. de Vries (eds.), *The Role of Epiglottis in Obstructive Sleep Apnea*, https://doi.org/10.1007/978-3-031-34992-8_7

enced to the mastoid (M) electrode. The EMG of the submental muscles is recorded from two skin electrodes placed at a location near the chin close to these muscles.

According to international standards, at least four neurophysiological signals are required, one EEG, two EOG, and one chin EMG channel. Consequently, based on the information obtained by EEG, EMG, and EOG, sleep stages can be scored according to the AASM criteria [3]. Ventilation is often measured qualitatively by means of thermistors, but can be assessed more precisely with nasal pressure cannulas, or eventually by means of calibrated respiratory inductance plethysmography [4]. Breathing effort can also be detected by recording movements of chest and abdomen, surface EMG, peripheral artery tonometry (PAT), and changes in pulse transit time (PTT), but most effectively by detection of intrathoracic pressure swings. These swings can be detected invasively by measuring esophageal pressure. Currently, movements of chest and abdomen are most often recorded by respiratory inductance plethysmography (RIP), while few systems still rely on strain gauges, which detect changes in resistance according to length changes. RIP is an evaluation technique which makes use of belts at thorax and abdomen, with an inbuilt electrical wire. This wire behaves as a coil and the features of the coil change when the belt is stretched. The signal is in phase with volume changes of the chest (and abdomen) and changes almost linearly with increasing tidal volume. If respiratory effort is detected during an apnea, this can be explained by obstruction of the upper airway. An overview of the features of these ventilation sensors, with their advantages and disadvantages is shown in Table 7.1. Transcutaneous oxygen saturation is measured by means of pulse oximetry (eventually combined with transcutaneous or end-tidal PCO_2 measures). Sound recording is an indirect method to detect ventilation. Most often, body position (position sensor on the chest) is also registered. Today's sleep laboratories continue to undergo technologic evolution, particularly related to the increased reliance on digital systems, and improved algorithms for automatic analysis based on artificial intelligence [5].

Table 7.1 Physical characteristics of widespread sensors used to assess ventilation during clinical sleep studies

Type	Physical characteristics	Advantages	Disadvantages
Airflow sensors			
Thermistors	Records temperature changes induced by breathing Changes depend on environmental temperature and on mass/inertia of temperature probe Flow/temperature changes are not linear—Extremely difficult to get them linear	Assessment of both nasal and oral airflow Cheap Less effective when breathing through the mouth	Thermistor signal is not well correlated with breath amplitude Consequently, not quantitative, therefore useless in practice Generally resulting in overestimation of the real flow Inadequate to detect flow limitation

Table 7.1 (continued)

Type	Physical characteristics	Advantages	Disadvantages
Nasal cannulas	Detects air pressure changes Flow/pressure changes are nonlinear—Easy to make it linear More sensitive than thermistors for detecting hypopneas and hypoventilation Nasal cannulas have a better negative predictive value and a poorer positive predictive value than RIP	Quantitative Able to detect subtle changes in flow (flow limitation)	No signal when breathing through the mouth Not linear Disposable materials
Effort sensors			
Strain gauges	A strain gauge or load cell is a device used to measure strain on an object. Small voltages are induced in response to movement The sensors are connected with the belts that are placed around chest and abdomen	Cheap	Poorly validated Currently positioned as an obsolete technique, but still used by some systems
Respiratory induction plethysmography (RIP)	Detects changes in volume of chest and abdomen during inspiration and exhalation The RIP belts are embedded with wires, woven in a sinusoidal pattern around the body. An electrical current applied to the wires generates an oscillating signal, in response to variations in resistance associated with changes in body circumference (and behaves like an induction spindle). Analysis of the RIP chest and abdominal channels can indicate a hypopnea	Quantitative Quite linear	Calibration is difficult (especially in obese patients) Costs of belts can rise
Peripheral arterial tone (PAT)	Utilizes the changes in peripheral vascular resistance and oximetry as indirect measures of respiratory signals	Comfortable for subject to wear Few loss of signals	Relatively expensive compared to other respiratory sensors Contraindication when presence of atrial fibrillation and use of alpha blockers Devices utilize two finger probes: a PAT probe and an oximetry probe—Worn on separate digits of the same hand

(continued)

Table 7.1 (continued)

Type	Physical characteristics	Advantages	Disadvantages
Pulse oximetry			
	Two types: – Transmissive pulse oximetry (or transmission pulse oximetry): In this approach, a sensor device is placed on a thin part of the patient's body (fingertip, earlobe, or an infant's foot) – Reflectance pulse oximetry (or reflection pulse oximetry): Does not require a thin section of the person's body (application on the feet, forehead, and chest). The light sources and the photodetector are located on the same surface of the skin Oxygen saturation is estimated by the change in light wavelength between oxygenated and deoxygenated blood in a pulsatile flow. The oximeter probe emits a light that shines through the nail bed and is picked up by a light detector on the opposite side of the finger	Simplicity of use and ability to provide continuous and immediate oxygen saturation values Accurate down to about 70–80% There is good agreement between indices of OSA that require ≥4% oxygen desaturation	Erroneously low reading or false reading may be caused by hypoperfusion of the extremity or from vasoconstriction, incorrect sensor application, highly calloused skin, nail Polish, extraneous light intrusion, misalignment/misplacement, movement Error rates may be higher for adults with dark skin color COPD may cause false readings Pulse oximeters differ in their ability to provide accurate data during conditions of motion or low perfusion In patients with a slow heart rate, a little longer averaging time may be needed (at least a 3-beat average) Nadir in SaO_2 usually follows apnea or hypopnea termination by approximately 6–8 s, secondary to circulation time and instrumental delay Oximeters average over several cycles before producing a reading Oximetry estimate of heart rate may be much lower than the actual rate if the patient has atrial fibrillation or frequent premature beats (only every other beat may provide sufficient signal to oximetry probe for the oximetry software to detect a heartbeat In measuring dynamic events (apneas), different pulse oximeters do not record identical values There is a fluctuation range of up to factor 1.42 between devices

For years, there is also a move to collect data outside of the traditional sleep laboratory setting. Respiratory polygraphy (PG) is performed when one does not include signals such as EEG, EMG, and EOG. This shift is driven by the limited available capacity to perform PSG in the hospital, economical considerations, and the need to assess sleep in the patient's natural sleep environment. To overview this process and direct the patient, sophisticated knowledge of equipment and management procedures is required [6, 7]. This chapter is a review of the clinical aspects of PSG and PG, with some technical aspects in addition. We will also put some emphasis on sleep trackers/wearables and will address new evidence on in-depth flow shape analysis to demonstrate epiglottic collapse.

7.2 In-Lab Attended Polysomnography

In-lab attended PSG is the gold standard technique for assessing sleep-related breathing disorders, including obstructive and central sleep apnea and nocturnal hypoventilation [4]. A sleep study offers in-depth information about both sleep structure and the disturbances in ventilation. Also, data on heart rate, body position, muscle tone, and sleep-related limb movements are obtained. If combined with an audiovisual recording of the sleeping subject, this is called a video PSG. Setting up a PSG requires substantial health care resources, adequate facilities, and experienced medical/paramedical staff. Ideally, the PSG should be performed during the usual sleep period, in order not to interfere with the patient's circadian sleep-wake rhythm. Questionnaires regarding sleep-wake behavior and a sleep diary that solicits information about major sleep-wake periods and naps are useful adjuncts to PSG [8]. Of interest, many patients also report difficulties initiating and/or maintaining sleep and have a subjective total sleep time and quality that is at odds with the objective data assessed in the laboratory (referred to as sleep state misperception). This finding warrants that subjective data be collected systematically, as part of the sleep laboratory evaluation.

PSG is indicated for the diagnosis of sleep-related breathing disorders, including the setup and evaluation of positive airway pressure therapy (PAP), treatment and the evaluation of other treatments (mandibular advancement devices—MAD, surgery); for the evaluation of hypersomnia, including suspected narcolepsy together with a multiple sleep latency test (MSLT), and for the evaluation of sleep-related violent behaviors (or otherwise damaging the patient) [8–10]. More particularly, it can also be indicated for neuromuscular conditions with sleep-related symptoms, and for an assessment of epileptiform sleep interruptions or paroxysmal arousals. Opposite to some current practice, PSG is not a standard indication for chronic pulmonary disorders, epilepsy without sleep-related complaints, typical parasomnia, or for the determination of restless legs, circadian sleep-wake rhythm disorders, depression or first-step assessment of insomnia [8–10].

An in-lab attended PSG fully observed by a sleep technician is the standard technique for assessment of obstructive sleep apnea (OSA). In several guidelines, the following supporting statements have been mentioned [8–10]:

- Up-to-date monitoring with extensive registration of flow, respiratory effort, oxygen saturation, heart activity, sleep position, sound, limb movements, sleep features as well as audiovisual observation, etc.
- A single-night diagnosis performed under attended conditions, so that the test has technical failures (sensor loosening or shifting) by exception.
- Assessment of the effective total sleep time and the simultaneous exact index calculation (including AHI, ODI, sleep efficiency), particularly with comorbid insomnia.
- Sleep disorders can be comorbid; other sleep disorders, especially central sleep apnea syndrome, parasomnia and periodic leg movement disorder can be disentangled with PSG.
- Obtained information is also useful in the presence of clinically relevant comorbidities (chronic obstructive pulmonary disease—COPD, restrictive lung function disorders, systolic or diastolic heart failure and obesity-hypoventilation), since an association can occur during REM sleep or extra sensors can be applied.
- Loss of data rarely occurs, and instantaneous scoring can eventually be done by the attending sleep technician. Optionally, a "split night" approach can be offered when PAP titration is urgently needed.
- PSG can also be considered for medico-legal reasons, such as the workup of patients with cardiorespiratory problems and risk of injury in disabled or disoriented people and in subjects with sleep-related violent behavior.

Generally spoken, in-lab attended PSG is a cost-benefit proof examination.

7.3 Report Format

To take advantage of the results of (video) PSG, the report must meet a number of quality requirements [11]. The PSG report should definitely include information about sleep: sleep times in relation to bedtime, respiratory events like apneas, hypopneas with and without oxygen saturation, its association with body posture and sleep stages, and oxygen saturation (mean, nadir, oxygen desaturation index—ODI, and time <90%) and presence of rhythmic disorders (with or without arousals). An extensive overview of PSG variables and content of an ideal PSG report is shown in Tables 7.2 and 7.3. Critical data must be displayed properly and clearly in tables and graphs. The data must not be amenable to interpretation. Description of the subjective experience of the sleep during the PSG is an integral part of the PSG report. This information allows evaluating whether sleep quality during the analysis was comparable, better or worse than has usually been. Since the results depend on the way in which the sleep and sleep-related events are evaluated, it is necessary to report the scoring method used, which is currently the AASM 2007 (for sleep EEG) and 2012 edition and updates (for respiratory events) [3, 12–14]. It is also common practice to verify and correct any automatic analysis of signals by using visual scoring. Nighttime trends or graphic display of raw data (f.i. O_2 saturation curve),

Table 7.2 Definitions of PSG variables

Sleep	
Lights out (time)	Clock time when the technologist turn the lights out for the patient to go to sleep
Lights on (time)	Clock time when the technologist turns the lights on at the end of the study
Time in bed (TIB) (in minutes)	Time from "lights out" to "lights on"
Total sleep time (TST) (in minutes)	Amount of actual sleep between "lights out" and "lights on"
Sleep (onset) latency (in minutes)	Time from lights out to the first of three continuous epochs of stage N1 or any other sleep stage.
REM sleep latency (in minutes)	Time from lights out to the first epoch of stage REM
Sleep efficiency (percentage)	The amount of time spent sleeping expressed as percentage of TIB
WASO (in minutes)	Wake after sleep onset (the amount of time spent awake after sleep onset)
Arousal index (number/hour)	Amount of arousals per hour of TST
Breathing	
Obstructive apneas (number)	The total number of obstructive sleep apneas during the night
Central apneas (number)	The total number of central sleep apneas during the night
Mixed apneas (number)	The total number of mixed sleep apneas during the night
Hypopneas (number)	The total number of hypopneas during the night
AHI (number/hour)	Apnea-hypopnea index, calculated by adding the apneas and hypopneas during the night and dividing it by TST
AI (number/hour)	Apnea index, calculated by taking the number of apnea events during the night and dividing it by TST
SpO_2	
Mean SpO_2 (%)	The mean oxygen saturation for the entire night
Min SpO_2 (%)	The nadir or lowest oxygen saturation value for the entire night
TimeSpO_2 <90% (or CT90%) (in minutes)	Parameter to express global degree of hypoxemia
ODI (number/hour) ODI3 and ODI4 (number/hour)	Number of oxygen desaturations per hour of TST (≥3% or ≥4%)
Limb movements	
PLMI (number/hour)	Periodic limb movements per hour of TST. Repetitive muscle contractions (0.5–5 s) separated by an interval of 5–90 s
PLMAI (number/hour)	Periodic limb movements associated with microarousal per hour of TST

computer analysis (f.i. EEG power in different spectral bands), and scored events (f.i. hypnogram, arousals, respiratory events) are extremely important (Fig. 7.1):

- To get a general and instant impression on the time course of the studied variables and to demonstrate the interaction with the other parameters.
- To allow quality control: the trend demonstrates at a glance whether the obtained signals are of sufficient quality.

Table 7.3 Overview of the parameters in an ideal PSG report

Administrative data
Recorded parameters
Sleep architecture: • Lights off—Lights on; first and last sleep epoch • TIB—TST—SEI • Sleep latency times (NREM, REM) • Time spent in different sleep stages • WASO, shift in sleep stages, micro- and macroarousals, arousal index, PLM-arousal index (PLMAI)
Respiratory data: • Used scoring method • Number of respiratory events and duration (mean, longest event) • Separation between obstructive, central, and mixed apneas • Respiratory effort-related arousals (RERAs) • Respiratory indices based on body position (AHI supine vs. AHI nonsupine) and sleep stages (AHI-REM vs. AHI-NREM) • Snoring with respect to body position and sleep stage • Data with respect to oxygen saturation (mean, nadir, $SaO_2 < 90\%$, $SaO_2 < 88\%$) • Presence of Cheyne-stokes breathing • Snoring intensity (subjectively, based on video; objectively, based on decibelometry)
Movement activity: • Periodic limb movements (PLMS) • Restless legs (RLS) • Motoric activity during REM sleep • PLMI (periodic limb movement index) • PLMAI (periodic limb movement arousal index)
ECG events
EEG events (sleep fragmentation, alpha-delta pattern, alpha intrusion, influence of drug intake, signal quality)

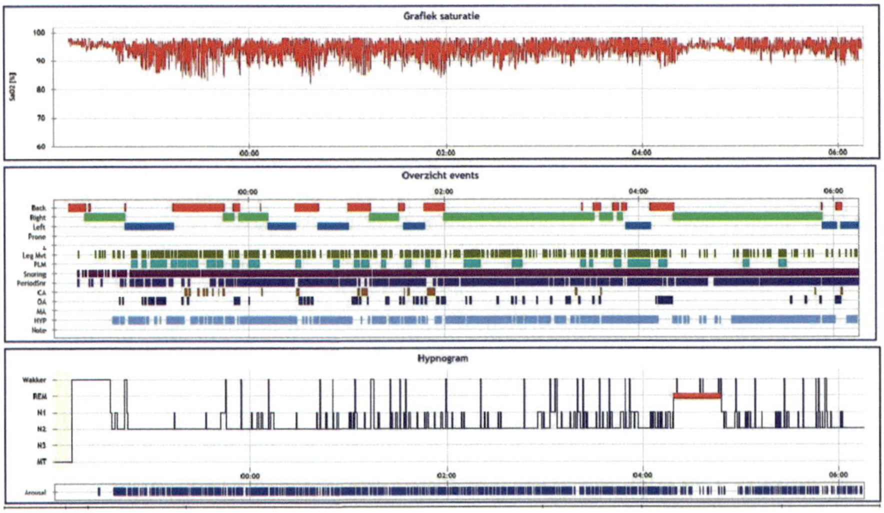

Fig. 7.1 Polysomnographic trend in a patient with severe obstructive sleep apnea

The following parameters and trends can be used:

1. Trends with respect to the neurological activity:
   - Time course of alpha- and delta-power.
   - PLMS, based on low legs EMG or actimetry.
   - Hypnogram.
   - Arousals.
2. Trends with respect to the cardiac and respiratory activity:
   - SaO_2, respiratory event, sound.
   - Heart activity based on RR-interval (brady-tachycardia patterns).
   - Body position.

To evaluate a PSG performed in another sleep lab, it is preferable to have a detailed report with nighttime trends available, or to perform a reanalysis with one's own software. The European Data Format (EDF) allows to exchange raw data between sleep centers which use different software packages [15].

7.4 Ambulatory PSG/PG

Due to the high prevalence of sleep-related breathing disorders in the general public, long waiting lists for diagnostic sleep studies exist in most sleep centers [16]. To tackle this problem, equipment for ambulatory sleep studies has been designed, with a focus on diagnosing OSA. A plethora of studies has been performed to evaluate its reliability and specificity versus the gold standard technique [17, 18]. In the following paragraphs, its use in OSA will be discussed, with emphasis on the indications for diagnosing or ruling out OSA and the strengths and limitations. In real life, each tool has its specific place in the diagnostic area.

7.4.1 Equipment for Ambulatory PSG/PG Versus the Gold Standard Approach

Technically spoken, PSG/PG can be conducted in the patient's natural sleep setting. It facilitates expansion of the measuring capacity, promoting faster access to the test. Plenty of portable systems have been developed meanwhile. The main aim of these systems is to evaluate (obstructive) sleep apnea and have not been extensively evaluated for other indications. Currently, the systems are categorized according to the parameters and sensors used in the presence or absence of a sleep lab technician (Table 7.4) [19]:

- Type 1: PSG fully supervised by a lab technician or by video, conducted at a sleep clinic (sleep staging including EEG, EOG or chin EMG, limb movements, ECG, heart frequency and respiratory measurements with oronasal airflow, thoracoabdominal movements, and pulse oximetry). This is the gold standard.

Table 7.4 Categorization of sleep studies according to the AASM

	Type 1	Type 2	Type 3	Type 4
	Standard supervised PSG	Ambulatory PSG	Ambulatory respiratory polygraphy 4–6 channels	Ambulatory respiratory polygraphy 1–3 channels
Parameters	Minimum of seven, including EEG, chin EMG, EOG, ECG, flow, respiratory effort, SpO_2	Minimum of seven, including EEG, chin EMG, EOG, ECG, flow, respiratory effort, SpO_2	Minimum of four, including ventilation (minimum two channels for respiratory effort, or one for airflow and one for respiratory effort, heart rate or ECG, SpO_2	Minimum of one for SpO_2, flow or thoracic movements
Positional measurement	Present	Optional	Optional	No
EMG OL	Recommended yet optional	Optional	Optional	No
Supervision	Yes	No	No	No
Possibility of interventions	Yes	No	No	No

- Type 2: Unsupervised PSG (at the sleep clinic or at the patient's home).
- Type 3: Patient registration where thoracoabdominal movements and airflow in addition to heart frequency or ECG plus the oximetry are recorded on several channels (4–8).
- Type 4: Ambulatory recording using one to three parameters, usually including pulse oximetry, but not meeting the criteria of type-3 monitors.

At the lower end, devices with even fewer channels, usually 1–3 channels (e.g., RUSleeping, ApneaLink) may record respiratory flow or movement, sometimes even without pulse rate and oximetry. Oximetry is usually part of the methods applied to screen for sleep-disordered breathing. One has to consider false-negative results. Frequent short apneas can occur without significant oxygen saturation dips, f.i. in lean patients with sufficient oxygen reserves [20].

7.4.2 Why/Why Not Ambulatory PG/PSG?

Some of the direct expenses can be lowered or eliminated by sparing on supervision and on the furnishing of the patient rooms. Such an economical approach may sound attractive, but does not necessarily improve cost-effectiveness. Altogether, additional costs are created by repeating sleep studies when ambulatory assessments are technically inadequate, or in negative studies with subjects who have high suspicion of OSA [21]. The sleep comfort of the patient can be a plausible reason for performing sleep testing in the home setting, partly due to the so called "first-night effect" and a familiar environment for the patient. There is scientific evidence for and against this setup. One concern could be that the ecological footprint of sleep studies will increase, due to extra travel time for patient or technician, depending where the hook-up of electrodes will take place.

The drawback is that poorly working electrodes cannot be corrected and the absence of supervision of eventual nocturnal behaviors complicates it interpretation. Failed measurements resulting from technical problems occur in 5–20% of the studies [22]. Such failures can be avoided by proper instructions by skilled and experienced workers, a choice of recorders with robust electrodes and proper sensor hook-up. This could argue for applying a double flow sensor, as recommended by the AASM in 1999 [4].

Lastly, and of major concern, if single polygraphy is performed, patients are likely to have a 30% lower AHI on average, compared to patients investigated by PSG [23]. PGs do not typically include EEG and thus cannot detect hypopneas that lead only to an arousal without significant O_2 desaturation. This is especially important in patients who have a low body mass index (BMI) because they are more likely to have respiratory events that lead to an arousal rather than desaturation [20]. Also, a higher denominator is used in polygraphy to calculate the AHI. Therefore, polygraphy can result in underdiagnosis and misclassification of OSA. Some PGs have an actigraph, which can be used as a surrogate marker for identifying when the patient is awake and asleep [24]. These PGs are not widely available and are more cumbersome and expensive. Moreover, one must remember that this is only a surrogate marker and can give flawed results, particularly in the presence of other causes of sleep fragmentation [24].

Taking all these limitations into account, nowadays ambulatory PSG is considered valid for the evaluation of a wide variety of sleep disorders, as long as video recording or other peripheral equipment is not needed.

7.4.3 Indications for Ambulatory PG: International Guidelines

The guidelines for portable sleep studies are only applicable to PG. PG can be applied when there is a high suspicion of OSA [25], under the prerequisite that some additional conditions are met. Such studies require manual scoring by a skilled sleep lab technician allowing to receive reliable clinically useful data. PG has gained increasing success in the last decade. In 2007, the AASM published a clinical guideline on the implementation of PG for the diagnostic assessment of OSA [6] which forms the starting point for the current indications of PG.

7.4.4 Low or High Pretest Probability of (Obstructive) Sleep Apnea

The use of PG is only recommended in patients with a clinically based low or high suspicion of (obstructive) sleep apnea (low or high pretest probability), whereas it is designated to use PSG to assess patients with an intermediate probability or patients

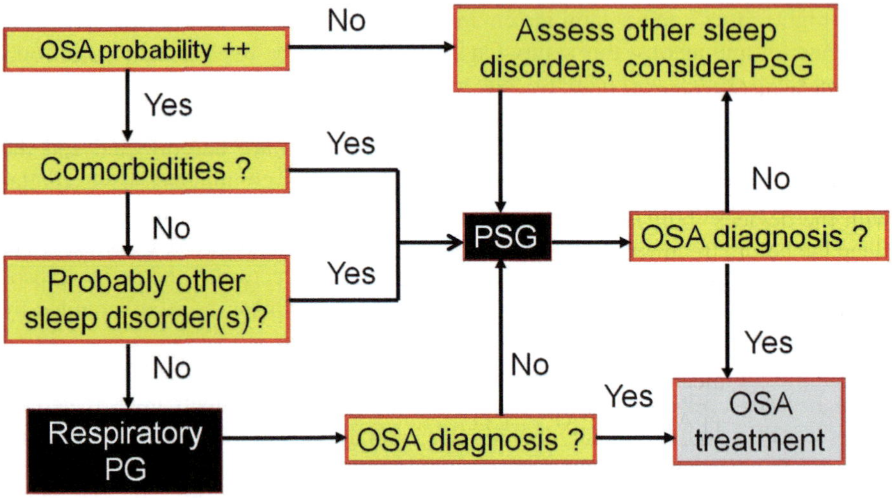

Fig. 7.2 Flowchart to perform polygraphy or polysomnography

with atypical clinical features. A suggested flowchart for using the PG is shown in Fig. 7.2. Obesity by itself is not an indication for obtaining a full PSG. Obese patients who are suspected of having obesity hypoventilation, however, should undergo PSG. Therefore, it is advisable to perform PSG in patients with morbid obesity (BMI $\geq$ 40 kg/m^2). Presence of hypertension or diabetes mellitus are neither a contra-indication to perform PG. On the other hand, in our current health care systems, the majority of patients suspected of having OSA are channeled toward getting the PG, irrespective of their pretest probability. This increases the risk of having false-negative results with the PG. Currently, based on a Spanish network study, long-term effectiveness (6 months) of home respiratory PG protocols is not inferior to PSG management protocols in patients with intermediate-to-high sleep apnea suspicion [26].

7.4.5 Additional Requirements

It is preferable that respiratory PG should only be applied as part of an in-depth sleep assessment performed by a sleep physician. Within this setting, elements of good clinical practice have to be used, summarized in Table 7.5.

7.4.6 Other Indications for OSA

Respiratory PG can also be applied in case of high suspicion for OSA in patients with serious illness, immobility, or safety for whom clinical PSG is not feasible. Finally, PG can be used to assess the efficacy of treatments, such as MAD, surgery, and conservative approaches like weight-reducing measures [6]. The accuracy of this type of assessment can be questioned, given total sleep time is not measured.

Table 7.5 Elements of good clinical practice in sleep assessment

Proper use of healthcare facilities	When an accredited sleep expert-somnologist takes a thorough sleep anamnesis in advance and asks about the sleep pattern, this guarantees a proper sleep diagnosis and excessive use of PG is avoided
Extensive clinical assessment	Comorbidities (both somatic and psychiatric) are common in OSA-referred patients and must be identified and managed. This partly determines what type of registration can be performed
Accurate collection of data	Application of quality criteria, guidelines, recommendations and healthcare programs, plus continued training and schooling of technicians and other staff, contribute to product excellence in terms of quality of the diagnostic data, patient safety and satisfaction, and outcomes
Effective patient management	Optimal treatment results for OSA patients depend on adequate diagnosis as well as effective treatment and follow-up

7.4.7 PG: Limitations of the Current Evidence

PG is predominantly used in patient cohorts with a moderate-to-high suspicion of OSA. However, for the accuracy of a specific test, the test's positive and negative predictive value is largely dependent on the pretest likelihood to have a disease. A clinical assessment conducted by a sleep physician holds promise as the most appropriate manner to estimate the probability of having OSA. The discriminative power of PG, i.e., the capacity to separate mild from severe cases of OSA, has never been thoroughly investigated. Lastly, it has to be emphasized that PG has predominantly been explored in middle-aged patient categories. PG in young or aged people (> 65 years), who often present with multiple ailment or different sleep problems, must be used with the utmost caution [27].

7.4.8 When Not to Perform Respiratory PG

PG is contraindicated for people with high pretest probability for OSA and the presence of important pathologies (heart failure, severe COPD, history of stroke, suspicion of hypoventilation, history of stroke, opiate use, and neuromuscular diseases) that alter the sensitivity and specificity of the sleep study [28]. This statement is based on the rare available data about the accuracy of respiratory PG in subjects presenting with relevant coincident morbidities. In a study with stable COPD (GOLD stage 2 and 3) with high pretest probability of OSA, less than 40% got a respiratory PG of sufficient quality. Compared to full PSG, an intraclass correlation coefficient of 0.47 was present [29]. As a consequence, the AASM stated that the potential drawbacks of applying respiratory PG in these patient categories are not balanced against the anticipated benefits [28]. If suspicion of OSA, together with probable other sleep disorders like insomnia, periodic limb movement disorder (PLMD), central sleep apnea (CSA), parasomnia, narcolepsy or circadian sleep-wake rhythm disorders, respiratory PG is also not indicated. The diagnostic criteria used for other sleep disorders like PLMD, parasomnias, narcolepsy, and circadian rhythm disorders can only be met with PSG.

7.4.9 Methodological Considerations

It is recommended that PG can only be implemented when medical staff and paramedical coworkers meet quality standards. They must be skilled in applying the relevant sensors, instructing and counseling the patient, and analyzing and understanding polygraphic data. The raw signals must be available enabling the sleep evaluators to perform a human analysis of the automated scoring; after that this must be interpreted by an accredited sleep physician. In most studies that concluded that type-3 polygraphs are useful for the assessment of OSA, the scoring was performed either by a technician or both automated and human. A careful analysis of raw data is of utmost importance. When it cannot be come to a diagnosis after ambulatory PG (e.g., loss of electrodes), a clinical PSG (type 1, supervised) must be conducted next if there is a high suspicion of OSA. According to the evidence, a follow-up visit after PG with a certified sleep expert is mandatory. Symptoms can persist despite an accurate diagnosis, which necessitates the expertise and knowledge of a sleep specialist for purposes of reinterpretation and additional treatment. Type-4 devices are not at all advised in the guidelines for the workup of OSA, apart from pulse oximetry in combination with peripheral arterial tonometry (PAT), which is an exception. The AASM considers this type of respiratory PG and the PAT as effective tools for establishing OSA [6, 7, 28, 30]. In PAT, the AHI is derived from heart rate swings in combination with oxygen drops originating from the swings in sympathetic activity induced by repetitive respiratory events. Algorithmic approaches make use of pulse oximetry, PAT, and smartphone applications which allow to transfer the data to the cloud where the data are analyzed automatically with high performance [31]. The use of sophisticated pulse oximeters with short-moving average time, alone or in combination with actimetry, PAT, and questionnaires is promising [32].

7.4.10 Equipment of Choice

One decade ago, a new classification system was introduced to correctly classify the new technologies available for ambulatory PG/PSG [7] (Table 7.6). This equipment is categorized according to measures of sleep, cardiovascular, oximetry, position, effort, and respiration (S.C.O.P.E.R.). Equipment new technology is indicated if a sufficient number of these SCOPER criteria are met and the posttest likelihood of OSA can be raised (positive probability ratio ≥ 5). This indicates that a moderate-to-high pretest likelihood for OSA is anticipated.

Table 7.6 SCOPER classification system

Sleep	Cardiovascular	Oximetry	Position	Effort	Respiratory
S_1—Sleep by three EEG channels × with EOG and EMG	C_1—More than one ECG lead—Can derive events	O_1—Oximetry (finger or ear) with recommended sampling	P_1—Video or visual position measurement	E_1—Two RIP belts	R_1—Nasal pressure and thermal device
S_2—Sleep by less than three EEG with or without EOG or chin EMG	C_2—Peripheral arterial tonometry	O_{1x}—Oximetry (finger or ear) without recommended sampling (per scoring manual) or not described	P_2—Nonvisual position measurement	E_2—One RIP belt	R_2—Nasal pressure
S_3—Sleep surrogate: e.g., actigraphy	C_3—Derived ECG measure (one lead)	O_3—Other oximetry		E_3—Derived effort (e.g., forehead vs. pressure, FVP)	R_3—Thermal device
S_4—Other sleep measure	C_4—Derived pulse (typically from oximetry)			E_4—Other effort measure (including piezo belts)	R_4—Other respiratory measure
	C_5—Other cardiac measure				R_5—Other respiratory measure

7.5 Smart Watches/Wearables and Their Usefulness in Sleep Analysis

Consumer sleep technologies are widespread applications and devices that purport to measure and even improve sleep [33]. Sleep clinicians may frequently encounter these applications in practice and, despite lack of validation against gold standard PSG, familiarity with these devices has become a patient expectation. It is the position of the AASM that these technologies must be FDA cleared and rigorously tested against current gold standards if it is intended to render a diagnosis and/or treatment. Studies focusing on sleep-disordered breathing generally showed that sleep trackers cannot detect, with sufficient accuracy, sleep patterns in this condition [34, 35]. However, these tools may be utilized to enhance the patient-clinician interaction when presented in the context of an appropriate clinical evaluation. Sleep-staging Fitbit models showed most promising performance, especially in differentiating wake from sleep [36]. Fitbit model 5 also offers stress detection via EDA (Electrical Dermal Activity), including a stress management score. It also presents a daily recovery score and a Daily Readiness Score, which indicates whether the user is ready to start the day. However, such features are premium function which is only free for some months. Huawei Band 6 and Xiaomi Mi Band 6 also offer extensive sleep services, but have a privacy concern (links with Chinese government), are energy consuming and are not supported by Google. Moreover, they are also not compatible with third party apps, which is a barrier for connected care. All these devices rely on heart rate activity monitoring and movement detection based on actigraphy. Altogether, although these models are a convenient and economical means for consumers to obtain gross estimates of sleep parameters and time spent in sleep stages, they are of limited specificity and are not a substitute for PSG [37]. However, new versions appear with high speed, and scientific validation is often lacking, or only available with delay. Reviews can be obtained on web platforms from consumers, which are not scientifically sound, but the users' experience can offer useful information. Furthermore, smartphone applications are available, designed for sleep-wake detection through sound and movement sensors [38]. In a study by Fino et al., none of the apps resulted capable of detecting REM sleep, and only one offered significant correlations for sleep efficiency [38]. All apps showed a significant correlation with the PSG-TIB. Each of the studied apps had its limitations, particularly regarding wake and deep sleep detections. So far, smartphone applications for OSA monitoring cannot fulfill the required standards for diagnosis, even in cases where multiple external sensors (e.g., sound, position, and oxygen saturation) are combined [39]. Further technological improvements may, in the near future, allow their use as a supporting tool for assessing sleep conditions and facilitate treatment [39].

7.6 Assessment of Epiglottic Collapse Based on Flow Shape Analysis during PSG/PG

Numerous methods have been developed to aid identification of the site(s) of collapse of the upper airway. Some of them are used in the awake state, while others are used during sleep, which can be either natural, or it can be induced as in the case of drug-induced sleep endoscopy (DISE) [40–42]. Each of these techniques has certain strengths and weaknesses. The disadvantage of most of them is that they are time- and labor-consuming and therefore still not accessible to the majority of the patients. DISE continues to play a dominant role, although some obstruction sites may be overlooked, and a less-than-ideal interobserver agreement has been reported [43]. Recently, new efforts have been made to extract information from the airflow signal monitored by a nasal-pressure cannula. Such methods take full advantage of the sensitivity of this device which, although noncalibrated, provides a respiratory waveform whose morphology approximates that obtained by direct airflow measurements [44]. Diaz et al. developed a new paradigm based on the generation of the respiratory disturbance variable (RDV) that characterizes the breathing signal in a continuous scale of respiratory disturbance, in contrast to the all-or-nothing event detection approach [45]. In the same line, in-depth visual analysis was proposed, given inspiratory flow limitation is a hallmark feature of pharyngeal narrowing. Genta et al. described different airflow shapes observed among OSA patients [46]. Flow shape was classified according to the degree of negative effort dependence (NED), defined as the percent reduction in inspiratory flow from peak to mid-inspiratory flow (the plateau phase) with increasing respiratory effort [(Peak flow-Plateau flow)/Peak flow] × 100 [46]. NED is a reflection of the dynamic compliance of the structure responsible for collapse, with greater NED implying a more compliant airway or structure [46]. Epiglottis collapse was associated with severe NED (89%) and abrupt discontinuities in inspiratory flow, while moderate NED was found among patients with isolated palatal collapse (45%) and lateral wall collapse (50%). Tongue-related obstruction was associated with only a small amount of NED (19%). Moreover, epiglottic collapse often occurred suddenly and produced another flow shape defined as an abrupt discontinuity, characterized by a rapid and severe reduction in airflow (>25% reduction per 50 ms) followed by either constant low or immediate airflow recovery (Fig. 7.3). The epiglottis can be considered as an unstable structure that would sometimes reopen/close repeatedly during inspiration, causing a jagged flow (that can be quantified by the discontinuity and jaggedness indices) [47]. This feature was present among 76% of the flow-limited breaths exhibiting epiglottic collapse [46]. From this it follows that a flat flow limitation pattern (small NED) is indicative of tongue-related obstruction, whereas a scooped-out flow limitation pattern (large NED) suggests that the collapse is due to one of the other pharyngeal structures. Altogether, careful assessment of flow shape may prove to be an inexpensive and noninvasive tool of determining the structure causing upper airway collapse. This approach may be helpful in selecting OSA therapy and allow individualized decision making. In 2019, Mann et al. developed and validated a tool that combines flow shape features across multiple known domains (flattening, scooping, timing, fluttering) to estimate airflow obstruction objectively across a continuum of severities, using the nasal pressure signal as a clinically applicable means to quantify obstruction [48]. The technique is ready for application to routine clinical PSG, given use of nasal pressure did not yield a substantial deterioration in performance compared to pneumotachography as the physiological gold standard.

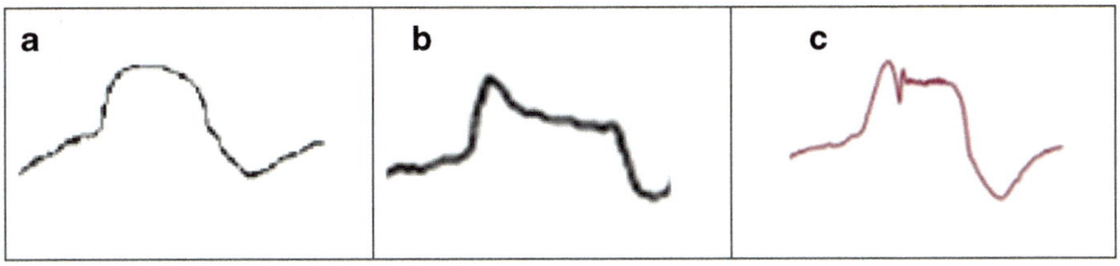

Fig. 7.3 Inspiratory flow curves during sleep in normal and obstructed breathing. (**a**) Unrestricted inspiratory flow during normal conditions. (**b**) Flattened inspiratory flow curve indicating pharyngeal narrowing (flow limitation). (**c**) Flattened inspiratory flow curve with abrupt discontinuity pathognomonic for epiglottic collapse

7.7 Conclusion

PSG is a highly relevant diagnostic tool that should be deployed sparingly due to its relatively high costs and limited availability. Not all sleep disorders deserve to be evaluated with a PSG. PSG is most useful for diagnosing sleep-related breathing disorders, PLMD, narcolepsy as well as some manifestations of parasomnia. There is a rapidly changing landscape and the pace and direction of digital system development will largely depend on cost factors related to clinical PSG. Unsupervised ambulatory PG/PSG can produce usable results as long as certain prerequisites are met. Ideally, PG has to be conducted by sleep experts and with a careful history taking before the decision for sleep testing is made. PG is only indicated with a large pretest likelihood of OSA is present, in patients without clinically relevant comorbidities or possibly coincident sleep pathologies. When it comes to screening, PG is still not indicated due to a lack of profound scientific proof and the lower pretest likelihood. PSG is warranted for a low or moderate risk of OSA, an inconclusive or negative PG, presence of comorbidities, or likelihood of combined sleep problems. It must be remembered, that a patient suspected of having OSA and a negative PG should undergo PSG for further diagnostic evaluation.

References

1. Holland JV, Dement WC, Raynal DM. Polysomnography: a response to a need for improved communication. Presented at the 14th Annual meeting of the Association for the Psychophysiological Study of sleep. Jackson Hole, WY; 1974. p. 121.
2. International Federation of Societies for Electroencephalography and Clinical Neurophysiology. Ten twenty electrode system. EEG Clin Neurophysiol. 1958;10:371–5.
3. Iber C, Ancoli-Israel S, Chesson A, Quan S. The AASM manual for the scoring of sleep and associated events: rules, terminology and technical specifications. 1st ed. Westchester: American Academy of Sleep Medicine; 2007.
4. AASM. Sleep-related breathing disorders in adults: recommendations for syndrome definition and measurement techniques in clinical research. The report of an American Academy of Sleep Medicine Task Force. Sleep. 1999;22:667–89.
5. Van der Plas D, Verbraecken J, Willemen M, Meert W, Davis J. Evaluation of automated hypnogram analysis on multi-scored polysomnographies. Front Digit Health. 2021;3:707589.
6. Collop NA, Anderson WM, Boehlecke B, Claman D, Goldberg R, Gottlieb DJ, et al. Clinical guidelines for the use of unattended portable monitors in the diagnosis of obstructive sleep apnea in adult patients. Portable Monitoring Task Force of the American Academy of Sleep Medicine. J Clin Sleep Med. 2007;3(7):737–47.
7. Collop NA, Tracy SL, Kapur V, Mehra R, Kuhlmann D, Fleishman SA, Ojile JM. Obstructive sleep apnea devices for out-of-center (OOC) testing: technology evaluation. J Clin Sleep Med. 2011;7:531–48.
8. Kushida CA, Littner MR, Morgenthaler T, Alessi CA. Practice parameters for the indication for polysomnography and related procedures: an update for 2005. Sleep. 2005;28:499–521.
9. Standards of Practice Committee Task Force. Practice parameters for the indications of polysomnography and related procedures. Sleep. 1997;20:406–22.
10. Kushida CA, Littner MR, Hirshkowitz M, Morgenthaler TI, Alessi CA, Bailey D, et al. Practice parameters for the use of continuous and bilevel positive airway pressure devices to treat adult patients with sleep-related breathing disorders. Sleep. 2006;29:375–80.

11. Pevernagie D, Verbraecken J. Reporting of videopolysomnography. In: Verbraecken J, Buyse B, Hamburger H, van Kasteel V, van Steenwijk R, editors. Sleep and sleep disorders. A practical handbook. 1st ed. Leuven: Acco; 2019. p. 193–201.
12. Rechtschaffen A, Kales A. Manual of standardized terminology, techniques and scoring system for sleep stage (National Institutes of Health Publication No 204). Washington DC: Public Health Service, U.S. Government Printing Office; 1968.
13. Berry RB, Budhiraja R, Gottlieb DJ, Gozal D, Iber C, Kapur VK, et al. Rules for scoring respiratory events in sleep: update of the 2007 AASM manual for the scoring of sleep and associated events. J Clin Sleep Med. 2012;8(5):597–619.
14. Berry RB, Brooks R, Gamaldo CE, Harding SM, Lloyd RM, Marcus CL, et al. For the American Academy of sleep medicine. The AASM manual for the scoring of sleep and associated events: rules, terminology and technical specifications. Version 2.1. American Academy of Sleep Medicine: Darien, IL; 2014.
15. Kemp B, Olivan J. European data format 'plus' (EDF+), an EDF alike standard format for the exchange of physiological data. Clin Neurophysiol. 2003;114(9):1755–61.
16. Flemons WW, Douglas NJ, Kuna ST, Rodenstein DO, Wheatley J. Access to diagnosis and treatment of patients with suspected sleep apnea. Am J Respir Crit Care Med. 2004;169(6): 668–72.
17. Bruyneel M, Ninane V. Unattended home-based polysomnography for sleep disordered breathing: current concepts and perspectives. Sleep Med Rev. 2014;18:341–7.
18. Mendonça F, Mostafa SS, Ravelo-García AG, Morgado-Dias F, Penzel T. Devices for home detection of obstructive sleep apnea: a review. Sleep Med Rev. 2018;41:149–60.
19. Ferber R, Millman R, Coppola M, Fleetham J, Murray CF, Iber C, et al. ASDA standard of practice: portable recording in the assessment of obstructive sleep apnea. Sleep. 1994;17:378–92.
20. Guilleminault C, Hagen CC, Huynh NT. Comparison of hypopnea definitions in lean patients with known obstructive sleep apnea hypopnea syndrome (OSAHS). Sleep Breath. 2009;13:341–7.
21. Masa JF, Corral J, Pereira R, Duran-Cantolla J, Cabello M, Hernández-Blasco L, et al. Effectiveness of home respiratory polygraphy for the diagnosis of sleep apnoea and hypopnoea syndrome. Thorax. 2011;66(7):567–73.
22. Douglas NJ. Home diagnosis of the obstructive sleep apnoea/hypopnoea syndrome. Sleep Med Rev. 2003;7:53–9.
23. Escourrou P, Grote L, Penzel T, McNicholas WT, Verbraecken J, Tkacova R, et al. The diagnostic method has a strong influence on classification of obstructive sleep apnea. J Sleep Res. 2015;24(6):730–8.
24. Shah P, Gurubhagavatula I. Portable monitoring: practical aspects and case examples. Sleep Med Clin. 2011;6:355–66.
25. McNicholas WT. Diagnosis of obstructive sleep apnea in adults. Proc Am Thorac Soc. 2008;5(2):154–60.
26. Corral J, Sánchez-Quiroga MÁ, Carmona-Bernal C, Sánchez-Armengol Á, de la Torre AS, Durán-Cantolla J, et al. Conventional polysomnography is not necessary for the management of most patients with suspected obstructive sleep apnea. Noninferiority, randomized controlled trial. Am J Respir Crit Care Med. 2017;196(9):1181–90.
27. Tan HL, Gozal D, Ramirez HM, Bandla HP, Kheirandish-Gozal L. Overnight polysomnography versus respiratory polygraphy in the diagnosis of pediatric obstructive sleep apnea. Sleep. 2014;37:255–60.
28. Kapur VK, Auckley DH, Chowdhuri S, Kuhlmann DC, Mehra R, Ramar K, et al. Clinical practice guideline for diagnostic testing for adult obstructive sleep apnea: an American Academy of Sleep Medicine clinical practice guideline. J Clin Sleep Med. 2017;13(3):479–504.
29. Oliveira MG, Nery LE, Santos-Silva R, Sartori DE, Alonso FF, Togeiro SM, et al. Is portable monitoring accurate in the diagnosis of obstructive sleep apnea syndrome in chronic pulmonary obstructive disease? Sleep Med. 2012;13(8):1033–8.
30. Rosen IM, Kirsch DB, Carden KA, Malhotra RK, Ramar K, Aurora RN, et al. American Academy of Sleep Medicine Board of Directors. Clinical use of a home sleep apnea test:

an updated American Academy of Sleep Medicine position statement. J Clin Sleep Med. 2018;14(12):2075–7.
31. Massie F, Mendes de Almeida D, Dreesen P, Thijs I, Vranken J, Klerkx S. An evaluation of the NightOwl home sleep apnea testing system. J Clin Sleep Med. 2018;14(10):1791–6.
32. Fabius TM, Benistant JR, Bekkedam L, van der Palen J, de Jongh FHC, Eijsvogel MMM. Validation of the oxygen desaturation index in the diagnostic workup of obstructive sleep apnea. Sleep Breath. 2019;23(1):57–63.
33. Khosla S, Deak MC, Gault D, Goldstein CA, Hwang D, Kwon Y, et al. American Academy of Sleep Medicine Board of Directors. Consumer sleep technology: an American Academy of Sleep Medicine position statement. J Clin Sleep Med. 2018;14(5):877–80.
34. Gruwez A, Bruyneel AV, Bruyneel M. The validity of two commercially-available sleep trackers and actigraphy for assessment of sleep parameters in obstructive sleep apnea patients. PLoS One. 2019;14(1):e0210569.
35. Moreno-Pino F, Porras-Segovia A, López-Esteban P, Artés A, Baca-García E. Validation of Fitbit Charge 2 and Fitbit Alta HR against polysomnography for assessing sleep in adults with obstructive sleep apnea. J Clin Sleep Med. 2019;15(11):1645–53.
36. Feehan LM, Geldman J, Sayre EC, Park C, Ezzat AM, Yoo JY, et al. Accuracy of fitbit devices: systematic review and narrative syntheses of quantitative data. JMIR Mhealth Uhealth. 2018;6(8):e10527.
37. Haghayegh S, Khoshnevis S, Smolensky MH, Diller KR, Castriotta RJ. Accuracy of wristband Fitbit models in assessing sleep: systematic review and meta-analysis. J Med Internet Res. 2019;21(11):e16273.
38. Fino E, Plazzi G, Filardi M, Marzocchi M, Pizza F, Vandi S, et al. (Not so) Smart sleep tracking through the phone: findings from a polysomnography study testing the reliability of four sleep applications. J Sleep Res. 2020;29(1):e12935.
39. de Zambotti M, Cellini N, Menghini L, Sarlo M, Baker FC. Sensors capabilities, performance, and use of consumer sleep technology. Sleep Med Clin. 2020;15(1):1–30.
40. Van de Perck E, Vroegop AV, Op de Beeck S, Dieltjens M, Verbruggen AE, Van de Heyning PH, et al. Awake endoscopic assessment of the upper airway during tidal breathing: definition of anatomical features and comparison with drug-induced sleep endoscopy. Clin Otolaryngol. 2021;46(1):234–42.
41. Van den Bossche K, Van de Perck E, Wellman A, Kazemeini E, Willemen M, Verbraecken J, et al. Comparison of drug-induced sleep endoscopy and natural sleep endoscopy in the assessment of upper airway pathophysiology during sleep: protocol and study design. Front Neurol. 2021;12:768973.
42. Vroegop AV, Vanderveken OM, Verbraecken JA. Drug-induced sleep endoscopy: evaluation of a selection tool for treatment modalities for obstructive sleep Apnea. Respiration. 2020;99(5):451–7.
43. Carrasco-Llatas M, Zerpa-Zerpa V, Dalmau-Galofre J. Reliability of drug-induced sedation endoscopy: interobserver agreement. Sleep Breath. 2017;21(1):173–9.
44. Hosselet JJ, Norman RG, Ayappa I, Rapoport DM. Detection of flow limitation with a nasal cannula/pressure transducer system. Am J Respir Crit Care Med. 1998;157(5 Pt 1):1461–7.
45. Díaz JA, Arancibia JM, Bassi A, Vivaldi EA. Envelope analysis of the airflow signal to improve polysomnographic assessment of sleep disordered breathing. Sleep. 2014;37(1):199–208.
46. Genta PR, Sands SA, Butler JP, Loring SH, Katz ES, Demko BG, et al. Airflow shape is associated with the pharyngeal structure causing OSA. Chest. 2017;152(3):537–46.
47. Azarbarzin A, Marques M, Sands SA, Op de Beeck S, Genta PR, Taranto-Montemurro L, et al. Predicting epiglottic collapse in patients with obstructive sleep apnoea. Eur Respir J. 2017;50(3):1700345.
48. Mann DL, Terrill PI, Azarbarzin A, Mariani S, Franciosini A, Camassa A, et al. Quantifying the magnitude of pharyngeal obstruction during sleep using airflow shape. Eur Respir J. 2019;54(1):1802262.

Diagnostic Workup by DISE

8

Mickey Leentjens, Patty E. Vonk, and Nico de Vries

8.1 Introduction

Over the past decades, multiple evaluation techniques have been developed to examine the pattern of upper airway (UA) collapse in patients with sleep-disordered breathing, each with important strengths and weaknesses. In the beginning, these techniques were performed in awake patients and included mainly static images rather than dynamic assessments (e.g., Mallampati/Friedman staging, imaging techniques such as computed tomography scanning and magnetic resonance imaging). With growing attention for UA surgery in the treatment of obstructive sleep apnea (OSA), there was a need for a new diagnostic tool to improve patient selection for surgical treatments that are currently available. One of these diagnostic tools is drug-induced sleep endoscopy (DISE).

The introduction of DISE has led to a better understanding of the complexity and multidimensionality of OSA and the key factors involved. DISE allows the physician to assess the pattern of UA narrowing and obstruction during medically induced sleep,

Supplementary Information The online version contains supplementary material available at https://doi.org/10.1007/978-3-031-34992-8_8. The videos can be accessed individually by clicking the DOI link in the accompanying figure caption or by scanning this link with the SN More Media App.

M. Leentjens (✉)
Department of Otorhinolaryngology, OLVG, Location West, Amsterdam, The Netherlands
e-mail: M.Leentjens@olvg.nl

P. E. Vonk
Department of Otorhinolaryngology, Academic Medical Center Amsterdam, Amsterdam, The Netherlands

N. de Vries
Jan Tooropstraat, Onze Lieve Vrouwe Gasthuis, Amsterdam, The Netherlands

M. Delakorda, N. de Vries (eds.), *The Role of Epiglottis in Obstructive Sleep Apnea*, https://doi.org/10.1007/978-3-031-34992-8_8

which as we now know differs from assessment of the UA during awake examination using flexible endoscopy [1]. One of the factors which has been proven to be difficult to assess during awake examination in particular, is a collapse at epiglottis level.

The epiglottis was not typically known for its involvement before the widespread adoption of DISE [2, 3]. The prevalence of epiglottic collapse (EC) was determined to be 11.5% in OSA patients based on awake examinations, which led to an underestimation [4]. Through DISE, it is possible to visualize EC better than by means of the traditional imaging techniques. Several studies have shown that EC can be observed during DISE while it is not detected in awake examination [5–8]. As a result, currently the prevalence of EC is much higher than previously thought [5–8]. DISE has made an important contribution in establishing the diagnosis of EC. However, inconsistent definitions of an EC are reported in literature and different classifications are used to address DISE findings, resulting in a wide variation in the prevalence of EC in OSA patients ranging from 9.7 to 73.5% [8–10].

8.2 DISE Basics

DISE is a dynamic and unique diagnostic tool that provides additional information regarding the degree, level(s), and configuration of obstruction of the collapsible segment of the UA. DISE can be performed in any safe clinical setting, such as an endoscopy suite, an operating theater or a clinical room set up with standard anesthetic equipment. Patients should have basic cardiorespiratory monitoring such as pulse oximetry, blood pressure, and electrocardiogram. Furthermore, it must be possible to administer extra oxygen when necessary. A quiet surrounding with dimmed lights is desirable, since one aims to simulate the situation during natural sleep as close as possible and thus minimize awaking stimuli. Patients should remain nil-per-os for a minimum of 6 h prior to the procedure to avoid regurgitation and aspiration. Atropine or other anticholinergic agents (e.g., glycopyrrolate) can be administered 30 min before DISE to reduce salivation. Although a great variability in drugs used for DISE are reported in the literature, propofol and midazolam are the two drugs most widely used [11]. The use of propofol with target-controlled infusion (TCI), when available, is recommended, as this provides a more stable and reliable sedation in comparison to manual infusion or bolus technique [12]. In addition, it is important to monitor the level of sedation. The bispectral index (BIS) monitoring system is seen as an adequate tool to validate the depth of sedation during DISE [13–15]. Several studies have shown that the collapsibility of structures of the UA increases under DISE in a sedation-dependent manner [16–18]. In particular, an increase in airway obstruction at tongue base level was seen when using propofol or midazolam during deep sedation [18, 19]. As a consequence, a secondary EC could be aggravated according to the sedation depth. Both the TCI technique and BIS monitoring are useful methods for obtaining more clinically relevant DISE results. Once the patient has reached a satisfactory level of sedation, the flexible endoscope is introduced through the nasal cavity.

The levels of snoring and obstruction are assessed observing nasal passage, nasopharynx, velum, oropharynx, tongue base, epiglottis, and larynx consecutively. The role of the epiglottis may be under-recognized as a factor in patients with OSA. A substantial proportion of these patients demonstrate a significant epiglottic involvement to UA collapse during DISE.

8.3 Body Position and Maneuvers

One of the benefits of DISE is that it allows the physician to perform different passive maneuvers with reassessment of UA collapse after each one of them. Historically, DISE was only performed in the supine position. Although it may be technically easier to perform the procedure only in the supine position, various studies have found significant differences when comparing DISE findings in the supine position to nonsupine position [20–22]. In order to mimic the effect of nonsupine sleeping position in nonpositional patients (NPP) during DISE, the head can be rotated to the lateral position [22]. In NPP, findings concerning UA patency during DISE are similar when comparing lateral head rotation and lateral head and trunk rotation. However, in positional patients (PP), this is not the case. In PP, it is recommended to start DISE when the patient is positioned in lateral position, both head and trunk. After adequate observation in this position, the patient can be tilted to the supine position.

Besides body position, two other maneuvers have been described in literature, namely chin-lift and jaw thrust. A chin-lift is a manual closure of the mouth, while jaw thrust (or Esmarch maneuver) is a gentle advancement of the mandible up to approximately 5 mm. By performing jaw thrust, the physician aims to simulate the effect of a mandibular advancement device (MAD) as they both result in protrusion of the mandible. To date, the use of DISE as a selection tool for MAD treatment remains controversial, since the predictive value of DISE for MAD treatment success varies amongst studies. In some studies, better treatment success was found when using a simulation bite during DISE to predict MAD treatment outcome [23–26].

8.4 When to Perform DISE

Prior to DISE, at least a polygraphy (PG) but ideally a polysomnography (PSG) should be performed. The results of this investigation are mandatory for developing customized and effective treatment options. In addition, DISE should only be performed in patients with an acceptable overall anesthetic risk profile. Relative contraindications may include morbid obesity, since UA surgery is generally not indicated in morbidly obese patients. American Society of Anesthesiologists score (ASA) classification 3 and severe cardiovascular comorbidity are other relative contraindications for the outpatient endoscopy setting. Yet, these patients can have their DISE performed in the operating room after approval of an anesthesiologist. Absolute contraindications are ASA classification 4, an allergy to the DISE sedative agents, and pregnancy [12]. Since DISE provides additional information concerning UA collapse, it can be used in patients in whom additional information concerning the dynamics of the UA is considered to be of added value. In general, this is the case when patients have been diagnosed with mild to moderate OSA and surgical intervention is considered as a treatment option by the patient and physician.

Less well researched, and therefore more controversial, is the indication for DISE when MAD or combination of treatments—e.g., MAD + positional therapy (PT), UA surgery + PT—is being considered. DISE is not required if continuous positive airway pressure (CPAP) or PT as monotherapy is being considered, as visualization of the level of obstruction is not mandatory for these treatment modalities.

Although CPAP is the first therapy of choice in patients diagnosed with severe OSA, DISE can be performed when conservative treatment such as CPAP or a MAD fails. In case of treatment failure (e.g., no improvement of respiratory parameters or no improvement of subjective metrics), DISE can be performed with and without the CPAP device in situ to evaluate the remaining cause of UA obstruction leading to treatment failure. Also in case of MAD or CPAP intolerance, DISE can be of additional value to explore other therapeutic options, even in patients with severe OSA.

8.5 Classification Systems for DISE

In literature, several classification systems describe the complex interactions of UA structures during DISE. Some systems do not pay attention to the epiglottis while others try to group multiple structures together in various combinations [27, 28]. For example, Nose Oropharynx Hypopharynx and Larynx (NOHL) classification system, logically, evaluates the following sites: nose, including nasopharynx, oropharynx, hypopharynx, and larynx. A study of da Cunha Viana Jr. et al. showed that VOTE classification system is a more comprehensive classification system in the analysis of the epiglottis during DISE as compared to NOHL classification system [29]. To provide an overview of all classification systems is beyond the scope of this book, as only VOTE describes epiglottic obstruction formats [30].

To date, the most widely used and accepted one is the VOTE classification system (Table 8.1) [30]. It distinguishes between the four different levels and structures that may be involved in UA collapse. VOTE is an acronym for velum (V), oropharynx (O), tongue base (T), and epiglottis (E). The VOTE classification system provides a standardized framework for describing UA collapse in OSA patients enabling an individualized treatment plan.

Table 8.1 The VOTE classification

Structure	Degree of obstruction	Configuration		
		A-P[1]	Lateral	Concentric
Velum				
Oropharynx				
Tongue Base				
Epiglottis				

[a] *A-P* anteroposterior

To assess the degree of airway obstruction, three different categories are used:

1. No obstruction (collapse less than 50% and typically without vibration).
2. A partial obstruction (a collapse between 50 and 75% and typically with vibration).
3. A complete obstruction (a collapse of more than 75% and no airflow).

An X is used when no observation can be made due to poor vision, e.g., hypersecretion.

Depending on the different level(s) involved in UA obstruction, the configuration may be anterior-posterior (A-P), lateral or concentric [30]. Airway obstruction related to the velum can occur in an A-P, concentric, or lateral configuration. The oropharynx collapses in a lateral configuration. As an addendum to the VOTE classification, the obstruction can be distinguished as related solely to the tonsils or including the oropharyngeal lateral walls, with or without a tonsillar component. This is important because this distinction can have implications for treatment selection and outcome. Tongue base obstruction results in A-P narrowing of the UA. Obstruction at epiglottic level occurs in an A-P or lateral collapse, but never concentric. Table 8.1 provides an overview of possible configurations and degree of obstruction at each level.

8.6 Definition of EC

As previously mentioned, an EC can be isolated in A-P configuration, which is also called trapdoor phenomenon or a floppy epiglottis (FE) (Figs. 8.1 and 8.2). This collapse pattern often appears to be related to decreased structural rigidity of the epiglottis. In addition, an EC can be secondary to an A-P collapse of the tongue base, pushing the epiglottis against the posterior pharyngeal wall (Fig. 8.3). Third, a lateral collapse entails lateral folding of the epiglottis during sleep (Fig. 8.4). It can be caused by, for example, an underdevelopment of the epiglottis itself. Most ECs are in A-P configuration, while the lateral type of obstruction is less common [7, 8].

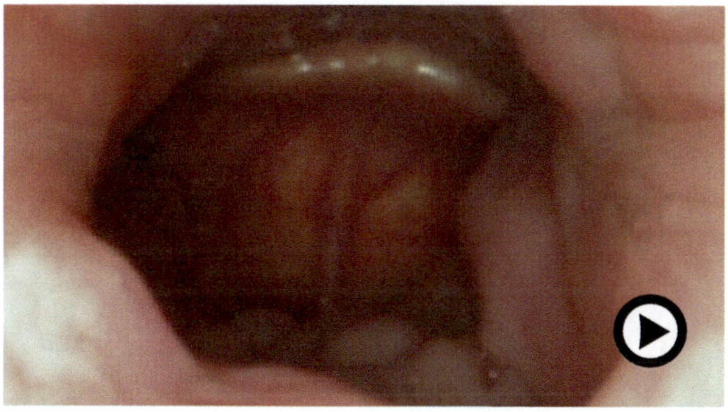

Fig. 8.1 (Video 8.1) Complete anteroposterior obstruction caused by floppy epiglottis and the effect of jaw thrust (courtesy of dr. Matej Delakorda) (▶ https://doi.org/10.1007/000-bf7)

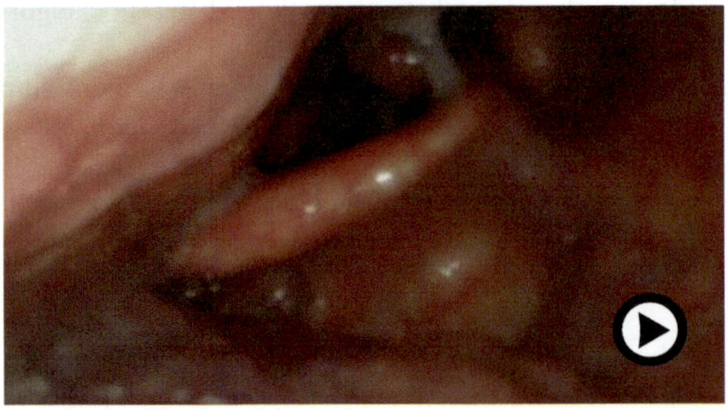

Fig. 8.2 (Video 8.2) Complete anteroposterior obstruction caused by floppy epiglottis and the effect of lateral head rotation (courtesy of dr. Matej Delakorda) (▶ https://doi.org/10.1007/000-bf6)

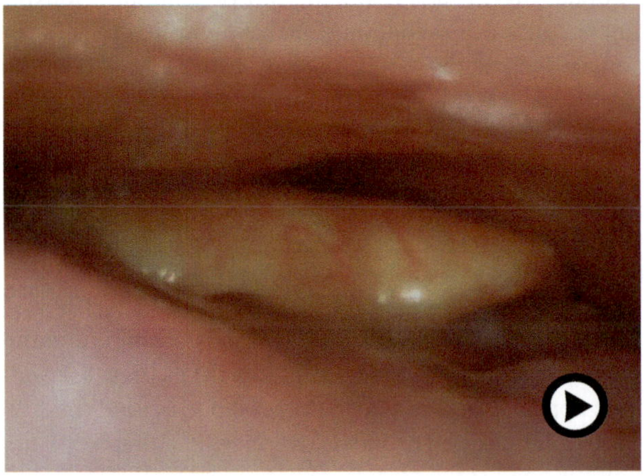

Fig. 8.3 (Video 8.3) Complete anteroposterior epiglottic collapse, secondary to a collapse of the tongue base (courtesy of dr. Matej Delakorda). Video depicting complete anteroposterior obstruction at tongue base and epiglottis level and the effect of jaw thrust and lateral head rotation (Video provided courtesy of dr. Pien Bosschieter) (▶ https://doi.org/10.1007/000-bf5)

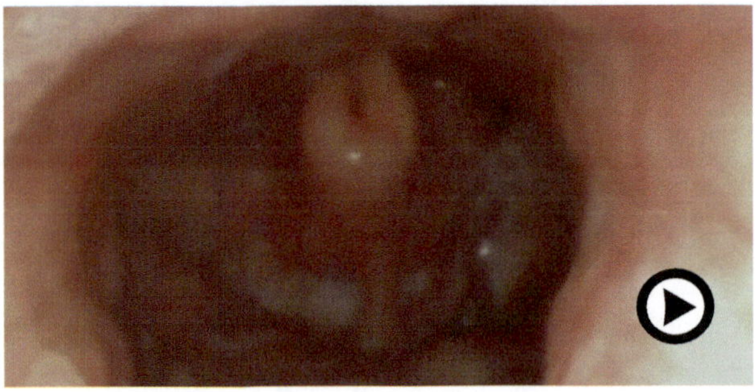

Fig. 8.4 (Video 8.4) Complete lateral, omega-shaped, epiglottic collapse and the effect of jaw thrust (courtesy of dr. Matej Delakorda) (▶ https://doi.org/10.1007/000-bf8)

8.7 FE and Body Position

FE has emerged as a position-dependent phenomenon. A recent study of Vonk et al. indicated that a FE appears almost exclusively in supine body position and to a lesser extent during lateral head (and trunk) rotation [22]. Despite this observation, the prevalence of a FE was similar in NPP and PP. Neither have they found a significant correlation between the presence of FE and positional dependency. This could be explained by the fact that in this study, patients with a FE as part of a multilevel collapse were not excluded. In other studies, evaluating the characteristics of patients with an isolated FE, it was found that, compared to others, they were younger, had lower BMI, and a supine AHI twice as high as the nonsupine AHI. These characteristics are comparable to those of PP [31–34]. Moreover, Marques et al. observed 23 OSA patients who underwent an UA endoscopy during natural sleep to evaluate the effect of sleeping position and the correlation with pharyngeal structures involved in UA collapse. EC was found in six patients who showed substantial improvement in UA patency when turned to lateral body position [35]. In addition, another study showed a positive effect of changing the body position on UA patency in EC [21]. These results were confirmed by a study, in which lateral head rotation was associated with a decrease in EC when compared to supine position [36].

8.8 FE, CPAP Failure, and DISE

In general, CPAP is the treatment of first choice in patients diagnosed with moderate to severe OSA, but some studies indicate that EC might be difficult to treat with conservative treatment option, such as CPAP [37]. CPAP acts as a stent in the UA through the application of continuous positive pressure to avoid mainly pharyngeal collapse during sleep because it widens the UA mostly in lateral dimension [38]. A FE has been linked to CPAP failure, suggesting that the epiglottis is pushed further down into the laryngeal inlet on application of positive pressure [37, 39, 40]. Therefore, recognizing whether a patients' UA collapses at the level of the epiglottis could have important implications for further treatment. In case of suspicion of CPAP failure due to a FE, DISE can be performed with CPAP applied simultaneously. Previously, various studies have shown a benefit of performing DISE for CPAP titration [38, 41, 42]. They evaluated characteristics of airway collapse as possible predictors for CPAP titration level. Shimohata et al. observed 17 patients with multiple system atrophy of which 12 patients showed a FE during DISE [40]. In this study, mild and severe FE were defined as a backward displacement of the epiglottis without and with covering the laryngeal inlet, respectively, during inspiration. They examined the effect of CPAP application on the level of obstruction and the oxygen saturation. Of those with severe FE ($n = 3$), no obvious improvement was observed by using CPAP. In two of the nine patients with mild FE, CPAP application even aggravated the airway obstruction on epiglottic level, which led to a decrease in oxygen saturation. In the remaining seven patients, the degree of obstruction was improved by CPAP. In a study published by Dieleman et al., they observed a FE in 27% of the patients diagnosed with CPAP failure while administering CPAP during DISE [43]. Additionally, they found that some patients who were diagnosed with a FE were previously satisfied with the treatment for many years. This suggests that this phenomenon might be caused by long-term CPAP usage in certain cases.

8.9 Conclusion

DISE is a dynamic and unique diagnostic tool that provides additional information regarding the degree, level(s), and configuration of obstruction of the collapsible segment of the UA. DISE is a valid addition to PG or PSG and clinical assessment of OSA patients. In general, DISE is indicated when UA surgery is being considered as treatment option. In addition, DISE can be performed in case of CPAP or MAD treatment failure to assess the possible reason. The anatomical structures that are involved in narrowing and/or obstruction of the UA are the velum, oropharynx, tongue base, and epiglottis. The degree, configuration, and level(s) of obstruction can be scored by using the VOTE classification system, which is currently the most widely used classification system. By identifying the specific reasons for UA obstruction, the physician can provide a tailor-made treatment plan for each individual patient. Before the widespread adoption of DISE, the role of the epiglottis was under-recognized as a factor in patients with OSA, since it cannot be well assessed during awake examination. A substantial proportion of OSA patients demonstrate a significant epiglottic involvement in UA collapse observed during DISE, which can have implications in possible OSA treatment options. For example, in case of a FE, CPAP may aggravate the degree of obstruction by further pushing the epiglottis down the laryngeal inlet.

References

1. Rabelo FA, Kupper DS, Sander HH, Santos Junior V, Thuler E, Fernandes RM, Valera FC. A comparison of the Fujita classification of awake and drug-induced sleep endoscopy patients. Braz J Otorhinolaryngol. 2013;79(1):100–5. https://doi.org/10.5935/1808-8694.20130017.
2. Vanderveken OM. Drug-induced sleep endoscopy (DISE) as a guide towards upper airway behavior and treatment outcome: the quest for a vigorous standardization of DISE. Sleep Breath. 2018;22(4):897–9. https://doi.org/10.1007/s11325-018-1743-2.
3. Yang HC, Jung EK, Yoon SH, Cho HH. The efficacy of drug induced sleep endoscopy using multimodality monitoring system. PLoS One. 2018;13(12):e0209775. https://doi.org/10.1371/journal.pone.0209775.
4. Catalfumo FJ, Golz A, Westerman ST, Gilbert LM, Joachims HZ, Goldenberg D. The epiglottis and obstructive sleep apnoea syndrome. J Laryngol Otol. 1998;112(10):940–3. https://doi.org/10.1017/s0022215100142136.
5. Cavaliere M, Russo F, Iemma M. Awake versus drug-induced sleep endoscopy: evaluation of airway obstruction in obstructive sleep apnea/hypopnoea syndrome. Laryngoscope. 2013;123(9):2315–8. https://doi.org/10.1002/lary.23881.

6. Fernandez-Julian E, Garcia-Perez MA, Garcia-Callejo J, Ferrer F, Marti F, Marco J. Surgical planning after sleep versus awake techniques in patients with obstructive sleep apnea. Laryngoscope. 2014;124(8):1970–4. https://doi.org/10.1002/lary.24577.
7. Ravesloot MJ, de Vries N. One hundred consecutive patients undergoing drug-induced sleep endoscopy: results and evaluation. Laryngoscope. 2011;121(12):2710–6. https://doi.org/10.1002/lary.22369.
8. Koutsourelakis I, Safiruddin F, Ravesloot M, Zakynthinos S, de Vries N. Surgery for obstructive sleep apnea: sleep endoscopy determinants of outcome. Laryngoscope. 2012;122(11):2587–91. https://doi.org/10.1002/lary.23462.
9. Torre C, Camacho M, Liu SY, Huon LK, Capasso R. Epiglottis collapse in adult obstructive sleep apnea: a systematic review. Laryngoscope. 2016;126(2):515–23. https://doi.org/10.1002/lary.25589.
10. Zhang P, Ye J, Pan C, Xian J, Sun N, Li J, Zhang Y, Kang D. Comparison of drug-induced sleep endoscopy and upper airway computed tomography in obstructive sleep apnea patients. Eur Arch Otorhinolaryngol. 2014;271(10):2751–6. https://doi.org/10.1007/s00405-014-3051-1.
11. Shteamer JW, Dedhia RC. Sedative choice in drug-induced sleep endoscopy: a neuropharmacology-based review. Laryngoscope. 2017;127(1):273–9. https://doi.org/10.1002/lary.26132.
12. De Vito A, Carrasco Llatas M, Ravesloot MJ, Kotecha B, De Vries N, Hamans E, Maurer J, Bosi M, Blumen M, Heiser C, Herzog M, Montevecchi F, Corso RM, Braghiroli A, Gobbi R, Vroegop A, Vonk PE, Hohenhorst W, Piccin O, Sorrenti G, Vanderveken OM, Vicini C. European position paper on drug-induced sleep endoscopy: 2017 update. Clin Otolaryngol. 2018;43(6):1541–52. https://doi.org/10.1111/coa.13213.
13. Babar-Craig H, Rajani NK, Bailey P, Kotecha BT. Validation of sleep nasendoscopy for assessment of snoring with bispectral index monitoring. Eur Arch Otorhinolaryngol. 2012;269(4):1277–9. https://doi.org/10.1007/s00405-011-1798-1.
14. Lo YL, Ni YL, Wang TY, Lin TY, Li HY, White DP, Lin JR, Kuo HP. Bispectral Index in evaluating effects of sedation depth on drug-induced sleep endoscopy. J Clin Sleep Med. 2015;11(9):1011–20. https://doi.org/10.5664/jcsm.5016.
15. Abdullah VJ, Lee DL, Ha SC, van Hasselt CA. Sleep endoscopy with midazolam: sedation level evaluation with bispectral analysis. Otolaryngol Head Neck Surg. 2013;148(2):331–7. https://doi.org/10.1177/0194599812464865.
16. Hong SD, Dhong HJ, Kim HY, Sohn JH, Jung YG, Chung SK, Park JY, Kim JK. Change of obstruction level during drug-induced sleep endoscopy according to sedation depth in obstructive sleep apnea. Laryngoscope. 2013;123(11):2896–9. https://doi.org/10.1002/lary.24045.
17. Kellner P, Herzog B, Plossl S, Rohrmeier C, Kuhnel T, Wanzek R, Plontke S, Herzog M. Depth-dependent changes of obstruction patterns under increasing sedation during drug-induced sedation endoscopy: results of a German monocentric clinical trial. Sleep Breath. 2016;20(3):1035–43. https://doi.org/10.1007/s11325-016-1348-6.
18. Viana A, Zhao C, Rosa T, Couto A, Neves DD, Araujo-Melo MH, Capasso R. The effect of sedating agents on drug-induced sleep endoscopy findings. Laryngoscope. 2019;129(2):506–13. https://doi.org/10.1002/lary.27298.
19. Padiyara TV, Bansal S, Jain D, Arora S, Gandhi K. Dexmedetomidine versus propofol at different sedation depths during drug-induced sleep endoscopy: a randomized trial. Laryngoscope. 2020;130(1):257–62. https://doi.org/10.1002/lary.27903.
20. Lee CH, Kim DK, Kim SY, Rhee CS, Won TB. Changes in site of obstruction in obstructive sleep apnea patients according to sleep position: a DISE study. Laryngoscope. 2015;125(1):248–54. https://doi.org/10.1002/lary.24825.
21. Victores AJ, Hamblin J, Gilbert J, Switzer C, Takashima M. Usefulness of sleep endoscopy in predicting positional obstructive sleep apnea. Otolaryngol Head Neck Surg. 2014;150(3):487–93. https://doi.org/10.1177/0194599813517984.
22. Vonk PE, Ravesloot MJL, Kasius KM, van Maanen JP, de Vries N. Floppy epiglottis during drug-induced sleep endoscopy: an almost complete resolution by adopting the lateral posture. Sleep Breath. 2020;24(1):103–9. https://doi.org/10.1007/s11325-019-01847-x.

23. Eichler C, Sommer JU, Stuck BA, Hormann K, Maurer JT. Does drug-induced sleep endoscopy change the treatment concept of patients with snoring and obstructive sleep apnea? Sleep Breath. 2013;17(1):63–8. https://doi.org/10.1007/s11325-012-0647-9.
24. Johal A, Battagel JM, Kotecha BT. Sleep nasendoscopy: a diagnostic tool for predicting treatment success with mandibular advancement splints in obstructive sleep apnoea. Eur J Orthod. 2005;27(6):607–14. https://doi.org/10.1093/ejo/cji063.
25. Johal A, Hector MP, Battagel JM, Kotecha BT. Impact of sleep nasendoscopy on the outcome of mandibular advancement splint therapy in subjects with sleep-related breathing disorders. J Laryngol Otol. 2007;121(7):668–75. https://doi.org/10.1017/S0022215106003203.
26. Vroegop AV, Vanderveken OM, Dieltjens M, Wouters K, Saldien V, Braem MJ, Van de Heyning PH. Sleep endoscopy with simulation bite for prediction of oral appliance treatment outcome. J Sleep Res. 2013;22(3):348–55. https://doi.org/10.1111/jsr.12008.
27. Kotecha B, Lechner M. Advancing the grading for drug-induced sleep endoscopy—a useful modification of the Croft-Pringle Grading System. Sleep Breath. 2018;22(1):193–4. https://doi.org/10.1007/s11325-017-1611-5.
28. Pringle MB, Croft CB. A grading system for patients with obstructive sleep apnoea—based on sleep nasendoscopy. Clin Otolaryngol Allied Sci. 1993;18(6):480–4. https://doi.org/10.1111/j.1365-2273.1993.tb00618.x.
29. da Cunha Viana A Jr, Mendes DL, de Andrade Lemes LN, Thuler LC, Neves DD, de Araujo-Melo MH. Drug-induced sleep endoscopy in the obstructive sleep apnea: comparison between NOHL and VOTE classifications. Eur Arch Otorhinolaryngol. 2017;274(2):627–35. https://doi.org/10.1007/s00405-016-4081-7.
30. Kezirian EJ, Hohenhorst W, de Vries N. Drug-induced sleep endoscopy: the VOTE classification. Eur Arch Otorhinolaryngol. 2011;268(8):1233–6. https://doi.org/10.1007/s00405-011-1633-8.
31. Ravesloot MJ, Frank MH, van Maanen JP, Verhagen EA, de Lange J, de Vries N. Positional OSA part 2: retrospective cohort analysis with a new classification system (APOC). Sleep Breath. 2016;20(2):881–8. https://doi.org/10.1007/s11325-015-1206-y.
32. Richard W, Kox D, den Herder C, Laman M, van Tinteren H, de Vries N. The role of sleep position in obstructive sleep apnea syndrome. Eur Arch Otorhinolaryngol. 2006;263(10):946–50. https://doi.org/10.1007/s00405-006-0090-2.
33. Oksenberg A, Silverberg DS, Arons E, Radwan H. Positional vs nonpositional obstructive sleep apnea patients: anthropomorphic, nocturnal polysomnographic, and multiple sleep latency test data. Chest. 1997;112(3):629–39. https://doi.org/10.1378/chest.112.3.629.
34. Itasaka Y, Miyazaki S, Ishikawa K, Togawa K. The influence of sleep position and obesity on sleep apnea. Psychiatry Clin Neurosci. 2000;54(3):340–1. https://doi.org/10.1046/j.1440-1819.2000.00705.x.
35. Marques M, Genta PR, Sands SA, Azarbazin A, de Melo C, Taranto-Montemurro L, White DP, Wellman A. Effect of sleeping position on upper airway patency in obstructive sleep apnea is determined by the pharyngeal structure causing collapse. Sleep. 2017;40(3):zsx005. https://doi.org/10.1093/sleep/zsx005.
36. Safiruddin F, Koutsourelakis I, de Vries N. Analysis of the influence of head rotation during drug-induced sleep endoscopy in obstructive sleep apnea. Laryngoscope. 2014;124(9):2195–9. https://doi.org/10.1002/lary.24598.
37. Verse T, Pirsig W. Age-related changes in the epiglottis causing failure of nasal continuous positive airway pressure therapy. J Laryngol Otol. 1999;113(11):1022–5. https://doi.org/10.1017/s0022215100145888.
38. Torre C, Liu SY, Kushida CA, Nekhendzy V, Huon LK, Capasso R. Impact of continuous positive airway pressure in patients with obstructive sleep apnea during drug-induced sleep endoscopy. Clin Otolaryngol. 2017;42(6):1218–23. https://doi.org/10.1111/coa.12851.
39. Dedhia RC, Rosen CA, Soose RJ. What is the role of the larynx in adult obstructive sleep apnea? Laryngoscope. 2014;124(4):1029–34. https://doi.org/10.1002/lary.24494.

40. Shimohata T, Tomita M, Nakayama H, Aizawa N, Ozawa T, Nishizawa M. Floppy epiglottis as a contraindication of CPAP in patients with multiple system atrophy. Neurology. 2011;76(21):1841–2. https://doi.org/10.1212/WNL.0b013e31821ccd07.
41. Lan MC, Hsu YB, Lan MY, Huang YC, Kao MC, Huang TT, Chiu TJ, Yang MC. The predictive value of drug-induced sleep endoscopy for CPAP titration in OSA patients. Sleep Breath. 2018;22(4):949–54. https://doi.org/10.1007/s11325-017-1600-8.
42. Civelek S, Emre IE, Dizdar D, Cuhadaroglu C, Eksioglu BK, Eraslan AK, Turgut S. Comparison of conventional continuous positive airway pressure to continuous positive airway pressure titration performed with sleep endoscopy. Laryngoscope. 2012;122(3):691–5. https://doi.org/10.1002/lary.22494.
43. Dieleman E, Veugen C, Hardeman JA, Copper MP. Drug-induced sleep endoscopy while administering CPAP therapy in patients with CPAP failure. Sleep Breath. 2021;25(1):391–8. https://doi.org/10.1007/s11325-020-02098-x.

Manometry

9

Markus Wirth

9.1 Introduction

Upper airway obstructions can be evaluated with multisensory catheter manometry. Manometry as a method to measure obstructions in both pharynx and larynx was first described in the 80s [1, 2]. The initial purpose using manometry was to determine the level of obstructions within the upper airway in OSA patients and therefore check if surgical treatments needed to be tailored based on it [1]. In an early study by pulmonologist Hudgel, nine OSA patients were measured with an esophageal balloon catheter together with three further catheters that were located in different sites (supralaryngeal airway, oropharynx, and nasopharynx) in the upper airway during sleep [1]. Obstruction sites differed between OSA patients in the study and were not predictable from measurements during wakefulness [1]. The manometry methodology was further developed in particular by two Scandinavian groups which used a single catheter with multiple pressure sensors [2–4]. However, since the length between larynx and nostril differs considerably between individuals [2, 5], it is difficult to assign specific anatomic locations to a pressure sensor [6]. In the clinical setting, it used to be sufficient to separate *upper* obstructions (at the velum) from *lower* obstructions at the level of the tongue base and epiglottis [2].

M. Wirth (✉)
Department of Otolaryngology Head and Neck Surgery, Technical University Munich, Munich, Germany
e-mail: Markus.wirth@tum.de

M. Delakorda, N. de Vries (eds.), *The Role of Epiglottis in Obstructive Sleep Apnea*, https://doi.org/10.1007/978-3-031-34992-8_9

9.2 Overview of Manometry Systems

One frequently used commercially available system (Apneagraph® Spiro, Spiro Medical AS, Bergen, Norway) was developed with only two pressure sensors as depicted in Fig. 9.1. The small catheter (1.3 mm diameter, Fig. 9.2) of the system is deployed transnasally into the pharynx and esophagus. One pressure sensor is located in the esophagus and another just below the soft palate as depicted in Fig. 9.1. Respiratory airflow is measured with thermistors located in the pharynx to detect obstructive events (flow limitations). To determine the obstruction level, the pressure

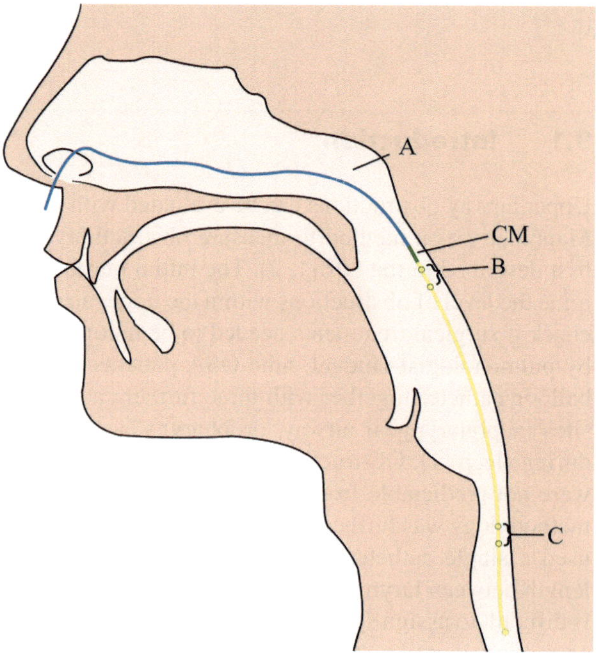

Fig. 9.1 Exemplary depiction of manometry measurements (Apneagraph® Spiro system). *A*—Thermistor recording nasal airflow. *B* and *C*—Sensors measuring local pressure level and airflow. *CM*—Control mark for correct positioning

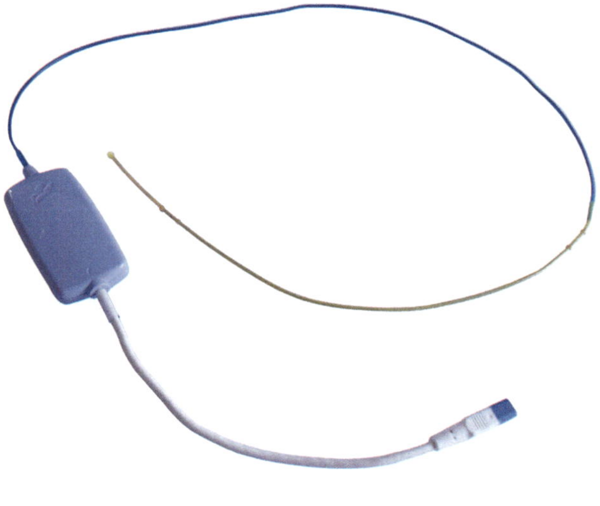

Fig. 9.2 Picture of catheter of Apneagraph® Spiro system (image courtesy Maximilian Bautz). The catheter has a diameter of 1.3 mm

amplitudes between the pressure sensors are compared. The location of partial obstructions can be detected as well, since reduction in airflow is measured with thermistors and the location is determined based on pressure findings. The correct positioning of the catheter is therefore of outmost relevance and controlled with a control mark as shown in Fig. 9.1. Obstructions measured with this system can be differentiated into *upper* (retropalatal), *lower* (retrolingual), and multilevel obstructions. *Lower* obstructions are usually at the level of the tongue base and epiglottis. An example of an upper obstruction analyzed with Apneagraph® Spiro is depicted in

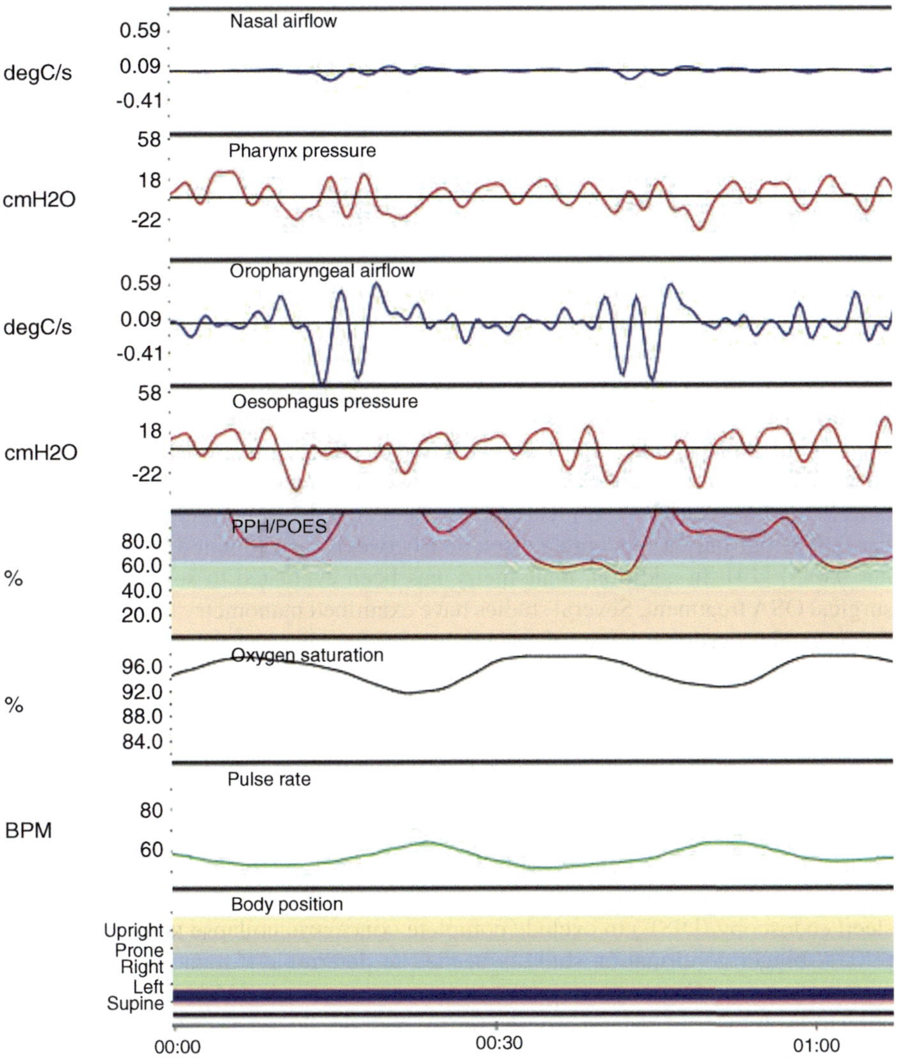

Fig. 9.3 Example of an upper obstruction as displayed in the Apneagraph® Spiro system and the parameters analyzed with the device. As the airflow decreases, the pressure ratio between the pharynx pressure sensor and esophagus pressure sensor displays an upper obstruction. This ratio is depicted in the channel PPH/POES (pressure pharynx/pressure esophagus). The *purple* area denotes upper obstructions, the *green* multilevel obstructions, and the *beige* area lower obstructions

Fig. 9.3. This manometry device provides a good overview of the proportion of obstructions in relevant anatomic locations but does not give a detailed view of the anatomy or the pattern of obstructions [7].

Manometry has been validated in several studies. There was a high correlation between the apnea-hypopnea index (AHI) measured with manometry and polysomnography (PSG) [8–10]. Portable manometry system designed for home sleep studies are not measuring EEG and therefore use, e.g., an actimeter to estimate sleep time. Such a portable manometry system overestimated the sleep time based on actimetry and underestimated the AHI compared to PSG in one study [8]. Another study detected slight changes in sleep architecture with the inserted catheter which were clinically not relevant [11]. The main obstruction sites can also be reliably identified in an ambulatory setting as shown in another study [12]. In the authors' opinion, it is advisable to check for shifting of the catheter after the measurement in the morning.

9.3 Clinical Use

Manometry systems can be used to confirm OSA and determine relevant sleep metrics in patients in an ambulatory setting as outlined above. The esophageal pressure (Pes), the gold standard to determine respiratory effort (RE) according to American Academy of Sleep Medicine (AASM) [13], is also measured with manometry. Respiratory-related arousals (RERA) can be estimated with manometry systems such as the Apneagraph® Spiro device based on flow limitations and respiratory effort (RE) without using EEG signals. However, in a recent study, there was a high correlation between the AHI measured by Apneagraph® Spiro and PSG (Pearson's $r = 0.884$) but only a moderate correlation between the estimated RDI (Pearson's $r = 0.685$) [14]. In addition, manometry has been evaluated to select patients for surgical OSA treatment. Several studies have examined manometry to select patients for surgical procedures at the soft palate. In a prospective case series, selection with manometry for coblation-assisted upper airway procedure (CAUP) resulted in AHI reduction by half in 80% of cases [15]. Hudgel et al. demonstrated that manometry may be beneficial to stratify patients for uvulopalatopharyngoplasty (UPPP) [16]. Nonetheless, another study involving 12 patients who received UPPP showed no benefit of the preoperative use of manometry [17]. A recent small study by the author's research group indicates that a higher percentage of upper (retropalatal) obstructions may be associated with worse treatment outcome after upper airway stimulation (UAS). All patients in this study were preselected with drug-induced sleep endoscopy (DISE) to exclude complete concentric collapse at the soft palate [18]. A bigger confirmation study is needed to determine if manometry could be used as first-line diagnostic to predict treatment success in UAS. In summary, the clinical usefulness of manometry to stratify patients for surgical OSA procedures remains unclear to date.

9.4 Comparison to DISE and Use in Epiglottic Collapse

The current gold standard for the detection of the anatomic location and pattern of obstructions is DISE. DISE is oftentimes used since it is available in many ENT departments and is site-specific, three-dimensional, and safe [19]. Manometry has several advantages but also major drawbacks compared to DISE and can be seen as a complementary screening tool. Manometric examinations are not dependent on the operator's experience as DISE and do not require sedation. In addition, the obstruction levels are continuously recorded throughout a whole night of natural sleep while DISE only reflects a short time frame [20]. A recent study demonstrated the relevance of this finding by comparing manometry with drug-induced sleep fluoroscopy (DISF) in 101 OSA patients [22]. Only seven patients had tongue base obstructions in DISF but the mean percentage of retroglossal obstructive events in the cohort in the manometry examinations was 31.2% [22]. An explanation for this discrepancy could be that DISE with propofol sedation does not simulate REM sleep [21] and it has been demonstrated that *lower* obstructions increase during REM sleep compared to non-REM sleep [9]. Probably one of the most relevant reasons why manometry is not applied more widely in clinical use is the patient's discomfort caused by the inserted catheter. In the author's experience, about 10% of patients do not tolerate the insertion of the catheter. The further development of the catheter has resulted in smaller catheter diameters (<1.5 mm) decreasing patient discomfort. Another relevant disadvantage is the current absence of commercially available manometry systems having the capability to detect the exact anatomic location of obstructions. The development of manometry catheters took place at a time where the role of the epiglottis in OSA was less recognized and the detection of obstructions at this level were therefore probably not a high priority. Hence, manometric systems with only few pressure sensors cannot differentiate between an origin at the epiglottis or at the tongue base and therefore needs to be used in conjunction with DISE in cases with suspicion of collapse of the epiglottis. Manometry could be used as less invasive and cheaper screening tool to identify the main obstruction site. DISE could be used in a separate step, e.g., before a planned surgery to confirm the diagnosis and evaluate the exact anatomic location requiring treatment.

9.5 Outlook

The delineation of pressure changes at the epiglottis is already feasible with high-resolution manometry used to diagnose swallowing disorders [23]. The further development of manometry catheters will presumably enable the differentiation of obstructions at specific anatomic location such as the epiglottis. Already today, whole night manometry measurements provide more information than is currently used for diagnostic purposes and could potentially be used for a more specific topodiagnosis. Recent studies have shown that epiglottic collapse can be predicted based on distinct airflow patterns [24, 25]. The airflow features predictive for epiglottis collapse in the machine learning approach used by Azarbarzin et al. with a pneumotachograph were also highly correlated with nasal pressure signals measured in ten patients [24] which emphasize that manometry could be used to detect epiglottis collapse. The additional application of machine learning could potentially distinguish patterns linked with epiglottic collapse. This would probably require large datasets with patients simultaneously examined with manometry and DISE.

References

1. Hudgel DW. Variable site of airway narrowing among obstructive sleep apnea patients. J Appl Physiol. 1986;61(4):1403–9.
2. Tschopp K. Stellenwert der nächtlichen Manometrie der oberen Luftwege bei Schnarchen und obstruktiver Schlafapnoe. HNO Kompakt. 2009;17(6):1–8.
3. Tvinnereim M, Miljeteig H. Pressure recordings—a method for detecting site of upper airway obstruction in obstructive sleep apnea syndrome. Acta Otolaryngol. 1992;112(sup492):132–40. https://doi.org/10.3109/00016489209136832.
4. Woodson BT, Wooten MR. Manometric and endoscopic localization of airway obstruction after uvulopalatopharyngoplasty. Otolaryngol Head Neck Surg. 1994;111(1):38–43.
5. Han DW, Shim YH, Shin CS, Lee YW, Lee JS, Ahn SW. Estimation of the length of the nares-vocal cord. Anesth Analg. 2005;100(5):1533–5. https://doi.org/10.1213/01.Ane.0000149900.68354.33.
6. Verse T, Pirsig W. Pharyngeal pressure measurements in topodiagnosis of obstructive sleep apnea. HNO. 1997;45(11):898–904. https://doi.org/10.1007/s001060050171.
7. Heo SJ, Park CM, Kim JS. Time-dependent changes in the obstruction pattern during drug-induced sleep endoscopy. Am J Otolaryngol. 2014;35(1):42–7. https://doi.org/10.1016/j.amjoto.2013.08.017.
8. Øverland B, Bruskeland G, Akre H, Skatvedt O. Evaluation of a portable recording device (Reggie) with actimeter and nasopharyngeal/esophagus catheter incorporated. Respiration. 2005;72(6):600–5. https://doi.org/10.1159/000086722.
9. Wirth M, Schramm J, Bautz M, Hofauer B, Edenharter G, Ott A, Heiser C. Reduced upper obstructions in N3 and increased lower obstructions in REM sleep stage detected with manometry. Eur Arch Otorhinolaryngol. 2017;275(1):239–45. https://doi.org/10.1007/s00405-017-4746-x.
10. Reda M, Gibson GJ, Wilson JA. Pharyngoesophageal pressure monitoring in sleep apnea syndrome. Otolaryngol Head Neck Surg. 2001;125(4):324–31. https://doi.org/10.1067/mhn.2001.118076.
11. Chervin RD, Aldrich MS. Effects of esophageal pressure monitoring on sleep architecture. Am J Respir Crit Care Med. 1997;156(3):881–5. https://doi.org/10.1164/ajrccm.156.3.9701021.
12. Rollheim J, Osnes T, Miljeteig H. The sites of obstruction in OSA, identified by continuous measurements of airway pressure and flow during sleep: ambulatory versus in-hospital recordings. Clin Otolaryngol Allied Sci. 1999;24(6):502–6. https://doi.org/10.1046/j.1365-2273.1999.00301.x.
13. Berry RB, Budhiraja R, Gottlieb DJ, Gozal D, Iber C, Kapur VK, Marcus CL, Mehra R, Parthasarathy S, Quan SF, Redline S, Strohl KP, Davidson Ward SL, Tangredi MM. Rules for scoring respiratory events in sleep: update of the 2007 AASM Manual for the Scoring of Sleep and Associated Events. Deliberations of the Sleep Apnea Definitions Task Force of the American Academy of Sleep Medicine. J Clin Sleep Med. 2012;8 (5):597-619:597. https://doi.org/10.5664/jcsm.2172.

14. Olafsson TA, Steinsvik EA, Bachmann-Harildstad G, Hrubos-Strøm H. A validation study of an esophageal probe-based polygraph against polysomnography in obstructive sleep apnea. Sleep Breath. 2021;26(2):575–84. https://doi.org/10.1007/s11325-021-02374-4.
15. Tvinnereim M, Mitic S, Hansen RK. Plasma radiofrequency preceded by pressure recording enhances success for treating sleep-related breathing disorders. Laryngoscope. 2007;117(4):731–6. https://doi.org/10.1097/MLG.0b013e31803250f0.
16. Hudgel DW, Harasick T, Katz RL, Witt WJ, Abelson TI. Uvulopalatopharyngoplasty in obstructive apnea: value of preoperative localization of site of upper airway narrowing during sleep. Am Rev Respir Dis. 1991;143(5_pt_1):942–5. https://doi.org/10.1164/ajrccm/143.5_Pt_1.942.
17. Metes A, Hoffstein V, Mateika S, Cole P, Haight JSJ. Site of airway obstruction in patients with obstructive sleep apnea before and after uvulopalatopharyngoplasty. Laryngoscope. 1991;101(10):1102–8. https://doi.org/10.1288/00005537-199110000-00013.
18. Wirth M, Bautz M, von Meyer F, Hofauer B, Strassen U, Heiser C. Obstruction level associated with outcome in hypoglossal nerve stimulation. Sleep Breath. 2021;26:419. https://doi.org/10.1007/s11325-021-02396-y.
19. Vroegop AV, Vanderveken OM, Verbraecken JA. Drug-induced sleep endoscopy: evaluation of a selection tool for treatment modalities for obstructive sleep apnea. Respiration. 2020;99(5):451–7. https://doi.org/10.1159/000505584.
20. Lee CH, Won TB, Cha W, Yoon IY, Chung S, Kim JW. Obstructive site localization using multisensor manometry versus the Friedman staging system in obstructive sleep apnea. Eur Arch Otorhinolaryngol. 2008;265(2):171–7. https://doi.org/10.1007/s00405-007-0428-4.
21. Rabelo FAW, Küpper DS, Sander HH, Fernandes RMF, Valera FCP. Polysomnographic evaluation of propofol-induced sleep in patients with respiratory sleep disorders and controls. Laryngoscope. 2013;123(9):2300–5. https://doi.org/10.1002/lary.23664.
22. Kim JW, Ahn JC, Choi YS, Rhee CS, Jung HJ. Correlation between short-time and whole-night obstruction level tests for patients with obstructive sleep apnea. Sci Rep. 2021;11(1):1509. https://doi.org/10.1038/s41598-020-80825-w.
23. Silva LC, Herbella FAM, Neves LR, Vicentine FPP, Neto SP, Patti MG. Anatomophysiology of the pharyngo-upper esophageal area in light of high-resolution manometry. J Gastrointest Surg. 2013;17(12):2033–8. https://doi.org/10.1007/s11605-013-2358-3.
24. Azarbarzin A, Marques M, Sands SA, Op de Beeck S, Genta PR, Taranto-Montemurro L, de Melo CM, Messineo L, Vanderveken OM, White DP, Wellman A. Predicting epiglottic collapse in patients with obstructive sleep apnoea. Eur Respir J. 2017;50(3):1700345. https://doi.org/10.1183/13993003.00345-2017.
25. Genta PR, Sands SA, Butler JP, Loring SH, Katz ES, Demko BG, Kezirian EJ, White DP, Wellman A. Airflow shape is associated with the pharyngeal structure causing OSA. Chest. 2017;152(3):537–46. https://doi.org/10.1016/j.chest.2017.06.017.

Acoustic Analysis

10

Zhengfei Huang, Frank Lobbezoo, Ghizlane Aarab,
Nico de Vries, and Antonius A. J. Hilgevoord

10.1 Introduction

Snoring is frequently reported by patients with obstructive sleep apnea (OSA). The reported prevalence rates of snoring in OSA patients range from 50 to 95% [1–3]. According to the definition of the International Classification of Sleep Disorders—Third Edition (ICSD-3), snoring is characterized as "audible vibrations of the upper

Supplementary Information The online version contains supplementary material available at https://doi.org/10.1007/978-3-031-34992-8_10.

Z. Huang (✉)
Department of Clinical Neurophysiology, OLVG, Amsterdam, The Netherlands

Department of Orofacial Pain and Dysfunction, Academic Center for Dentistry Amsterdam (ACTA), University of Amsterdam and Vrije Universiteit Amsterdam, Amsterdam, The Netherlands
e-mail: zf.huang@acta.nl

F. Lobbezoo · G. Aarab
Department of Orofacial Pain and Dysfunction, Academic Center for Dentistry Amsterdam (ACTA), University of Amsterdam and Vrije Universiteit Amsterdam, Amsterdam, The Netherlands

N. de Vries
Department of Orofacial Pain and Dysfunction, Academic Center for Dentistry Amsterdam (ACTA), University of Amsterdam and Vrije Universiteit Amsterdam, Amsterdam, The Netherlands

Department of Otorhinolaryngology–Head and Neck Surgery, OLVG, Amsterdam, The Netherlands

A. A. J. Hilgevoord
Department of Clinical Neurophysiology, OLVG, Amsterdam, The Netherlands

M. Delakorda, N. de Vries (eds.), *The Role of Epiglottis in Obstructive Sleep Apnea*, https://doi.org/10.1007/978-3-031-34992-8_10

airway during respiration in sleep" [4]. In other words, snoring sound can be heard when air passes through the narrowed upper airway and causes vibration or flapping of soft tissues. Due to the noisy nature, snoring sound has always been considered a social nuisance, which is associated with marital disharmony [5]. However, the informative nature of snoring sound has been suggested in the last few years. For example, the peak frequency (Hertz; Hz) of snoring sound was found to increase with the increase of the severity of OSA [6]. Further, a prediction model based on snoring sound parameters (e.g., average power and zero crossing rate) showed an accuracy of 96.4% in distinguishing between OSA snorers and non-OSA snorers [7]. In addition, it was also hypothesized that snoring sound parameters may be potential predictors of the obstruction site in the upper airway [8].

10.2 Clinical Background

Snoring sound parameters were hoped to be useful for the prediction of the obstruction site in the upper airway, because all currently available diagnostic modalities have drawbacks. For example, drug-induced sleep endoscopy (DISE) is a unique and dynamic technique, which enables the observation of the upper airway using a flexible endoscope during drug-induced sleep [9]. In addition to the location of the obstruction site, DISE can also provide information on the level (viz., no obstruction, partial obstruction, and complete obstruction) and configuration (viz., anteroposterior, lateral, and concentric) of the obstruction site [10], which is reported to be essential in the treatment decision-making process [11, 12]. For instance, complete concentric collapse on palatal level (CCCp) is considered an absolute contraindication for upper airway stimulation [11], and prescription of oral appliance therapy makes more sense in case of obstruction at the tongue base than in case of CCCp and complete lateral oropharyngeal collapse [12]. However, both the drug selection and the difference between natural and drug-induced sleep may influence DISE findings [13, 14]. Dynamic magnetic resonance imaging (MRI) is also used to identify the obstruction site in the upper airway, but it is a costly technique, creates noise that may keep patients awake, and may cause claustrophobic effects [15]. Alternatively, both airflow shape and airway pressure measurement can be used to identify the obstruction site during natural sleep, based on the contour of the airflow [16] and the upper airway pressure deflection [17], respectively. However, airflow shape can only be used to identify the obstruction site in patients with single-level obstruction [16], while airway pressure measurement cannot provide information on the abnormal anatomic structures in the upper airway, such as enlarged tonsils [18]. In addition, for patients with multilevel obstruction, only the lowest obstruction site can be identified using airway pressure measurement, while higher obstruction sites are left out [18].

Compared with the abovementioned techniques, snoring sound analysis is a more patient-friendly and feasible method to identify the obstruction site, since

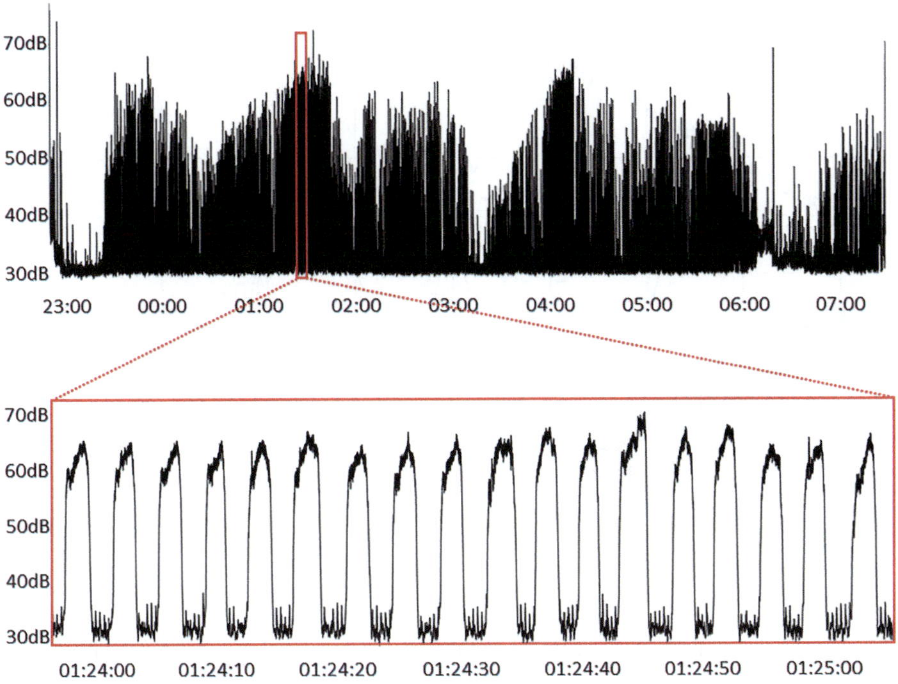

Fig. 10.1 An overnight snoring sound recording. The upper panel is the overview of an overnight snoring sound recording, which started at around 23:00 and ended at around 07:30 the next morning. Each vertical *black line* represents a snoring event. In the temporal domain and the intensity domain, it can be seen that the intensity of the snoring sound varied between 30 dB and 70 dB, and that most high-intensity snoring sounds were generated at around 23:40, 01:30, and 04:10. The *lower panel* is a 1-min snoring epoch (from 01:24:00 to 01:25:00) in the overnight snoring sound recording. This snoring epoch includes 18 snoring events, of which the intensity is higher than 60 dB

snoring sounds can be easily recorded in a patient's bedroom using a noncontact microphone. In addition, snoring sounds during natural sleep can better reflect the dynamic change of the upper airway during natural sleep. Acoustic analysis is mainly performed in three domains, viz., the temporal domain, the intensity domain, and the frequency domain. Analysis in the temporal domain focuses on the variation of sound over time. In intensity domain, sound intensity is commonly expressed as the pressure level of a sound, which is measured in decibel (dB; Fig. 10.1). In frequency domain, mathematical transforms like Fourier transform can transfer an original sound signal into a frequency spectrum, which shows the range of frequencies contained by the sound and the power on these frequencies (Fig. 10.2). The frequency spectrum is therefore considered the "fingerprint" of a sound, which contains the most distinctive information of the sound.

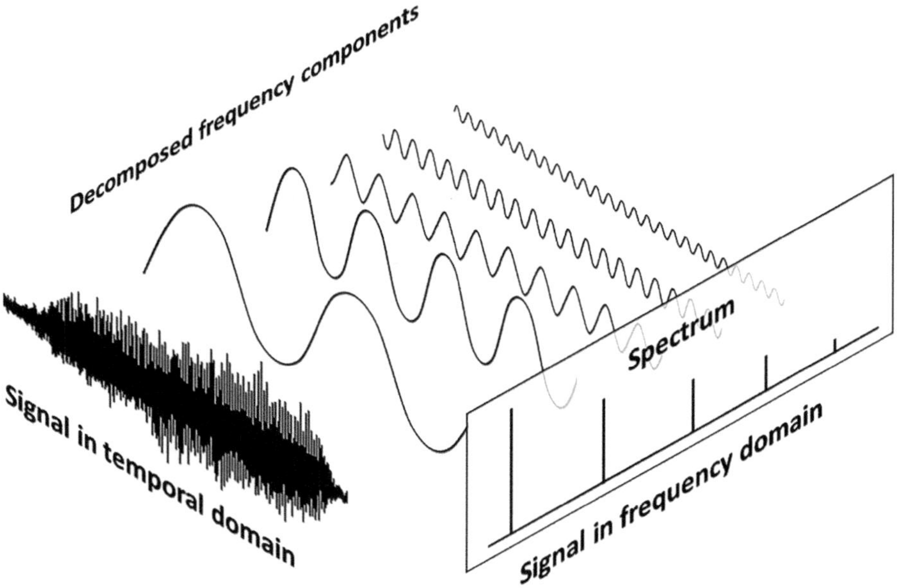

Fig. 10.2 Schematic visualization of Fourier transform. The Fourier transform is a mathematical transform, by which an original sound signal in temporal domain (*left panel*) can be decomposed into sinusoidal oscillations at distinct frequencies ("Decomposed frequency components"), with each sinusoidal oscillation having its own amplitude. A spectrum (*right panel*) is the projection of the amplitudes and frequencies of the sinusoidal oscillations on a plane

10.3 Characteristic Snoring Sound Parameters and Prediction Models

The "source-filter theory" is the theoretical principle of predicting the obstruction site in the upper airway based on snoring sound parameters. This theory was first used to describe speech production [19]. In this theory, the influence of the vocal tract (the acoustic filter) on the sound generated by the vocal cords (the sound source) is emphasized. Similar to speech, the acoustic characteristics of snoring sound depend largely on the anatomy of the upper airway [20]. The chamber-like anatomy makes the upper airway function like a "resonance chamber," in which the original snoring sound waves are either attenuated or amplified. Several characteristic frequency components are considered to reflect the anatomy of the upper airway (Table 10.1). In addition to the acoustic characteristics of epiglottic snoring, previous studies also built prediction models of the obstruction site in the upper airway (viz., velum, oropharynx, tongue base, and epiglottis) based on snoring sound parameters. A summary of studies on epiglottic snoring and epiglottic obstruction is shown in Table 10.2.

Table 10.1 Characteristic frequency components that are considered to reflect the anatomy of the upper airway

Parameter	Explanation
Center frequency [21]	A measure of a central frequency between the upper and lower cutoff frequencies. It is usually defined as the mean of the lower cutoff frequency and the upper cutoff frequency of a band-pass system or a band-stop system $$\text{Center frequency} = \frac{\int_0^{F_s/2} fP(f)\,df}{\int_0^{F_s/2} P(f)\,df}$$ $P(f)$ = spectral power density F_s= sampling frequency df = the standard deviation for the frequency range
Dominant frequency (DF; also known as peak frequency) [22]	The frequency that carries the most energy, i.e., the frequency with the largest amplitude on a spectrum
Formants (F1, F2, F3) [23]	A group of frequencies amplified by a resonator, i.e., three specific frequencies of snoring sound that are amplified by resonating in the upper airway $$H_{(z)} = \frac{1}{1-\sum_{q=i}^{p} a_q z^{-q}}$$ $\alpha_q(q = 1, 2, 3, \ldots, p)$ = the parameters of linear predictive coding (LPC), one of the most powerful speech analysis techniques
Fundamental frequency (F0) [23]	The lowest frequency of a waveform. In mathematics, the F0 of a signal is the greatest common divisor (GCD) of all the frequency components contained in a signal
Mean frequency [22]	The mean frequency of a spectrum is calculated as the sum of the product of the intensity (dB) and the frequency, divided by the sum of the intensity $$\text{Mean frequency} = \frac{\sum_{i-0}^{n} I_i \cdot f_i}{\sum_{i-0}^{n} I_i}$$ n = number of frequency bins in the spectrum f_i = frequency at bin i of n I_i = intensity at bin i of n
Pitch [24]	Pitch is a perceptual property of sounds that allows their ordering on a frequency-related scale

Note: The information in this table is from "Prediction of the obstruction sites in the upper airway in sleep-disordered breathing based on snoring sound parameters: a systematic review" by Huang et al., Sleep Medicine, 2021; 88:116–133. doi: https://doi.org/10.1016/j.sleep.2021.10.015 [25]]

Table 10.2 Summary of studies on epiglottic snoring and epiglottic obstruction

The acoustic characteristics of epiglottic snoring
Agrawal et al. [21] found that the center frequency of epiglottic snoring sound was 442 Hz. Won et al. [26] reported that the mean pitch and first two formants were 447 ± 20.2 Hz, 860.3 ± 141.5 Hz, and 2014.3 ± 175.3 Hz, respectively. The authors also found that the pitch and the first formant of epiglottic snoring were significantly higher than those of soft palatal snoring ($P = 0.001$ and $P = 0.047$, respectively). Consistent with this finding, a systematic review from Huang et al. [25] found that the characteristic frequencies (center frequency, DF, F1, F2, mean frequency, and pitch) of the snoring sound generated from the lower part of the upper airway were higher than those of the snoring sound generated from the upper part of the upper airway.
Prediction models of the obstruction site in the upper airway
Previous studies also built prediction models of obstruction sites (viz., velum, oropharynx, tongue base, and epiglottis) based on snoring sound parameters, especially those in the frequency domain [27]. In these prediction model studies, the reported accuracies ranged from 60.4% [28] to 79.5% [29].
Prediction models of epiglottic obstruction
Specific to epiglottic obstruction, in seven studies that predicted the presence of epiglottic obstruction, the reported accuracies ranged from 53.1% to 96% [27, 29–34]. Of the seven studies, the reported accuracy for epiglottic obstruction was higher than those for velum, oropharynx, and tongue base obstructions in three studies [30–32], higher than those for velum and oropharynx obstructions in two studies [27, 29], and higher than those for oropharynx and tongue base obstructions in two studies [33, 34]. The available evidence suggests that the presence of epiglottic obstruction is relatively more predictable as compared with velum, oropharynx, and tongue base obstructions.

10.4 Limitations of Previous Studies

It needs to be noted that most of the abovementioned prediction model studies only included patients with single-level obstruction, i.e., the obstruction site was also the excitation site of the snoring sound. This means that the association between the acoustic characteristics of snoring sound and the obstruction site was direct. However, it is a clinical reality that a majority of patients with moderate and severe OSA have multilevel obstruction [35]. In such cases, the obstruction site(s) that do(es) not generate a snoring sound also has an impact on snoring sound. As a consequence, the association between the acoustic characteristics of snoring sound and obstruction sites is relatively indirect and complicated. It is therefore more difficult to predict obstruction sites in the upper airway based on snoring sound parameters. Also worth noting is that these prediction model studies were DISE-based studies, which means that the obstruction site was identified using DISE and the snoring sound was also recorded during DISE. Given the difference between natural sleep and drug-induced sleep [36–38], natural sleep-based studies on the association between the obstruction site and snoring sound parameters are needed. In addition, these studies only focused on the location of the obstruction site, while the possibility to predict the level and configuration of epiglottic obstruction and the shape of the epiglottis (viz., flat, concave, and omega-shaped) based on snoring sound parameters have not been explored, even though the influence of these factors on treatment selection is still unclear. Another problem for predicting epiglottic obstruction based on snoring sound parameters is that epiglottic obstruction is often secondary to tongue base obstruction, i.e., a bulky tongue base pushes the epiglottis backwards and causes obstruction [39, 40]. In this case, attention should be paid to tongue base obstruction rather than epiglottic obstruction itself. Hence, it is clinically meaningful to distinguish between primary epiglottic obstruction (e.g., floppy epiglottis) and secondary epiglottic obstruction. However, to the best of the authors' knowledge, no study has investigated the difference between snoring sound generated from primary epiglottic obstruction and that from secondary epiglottic obstruction.

10.5 The Role of the Epiglottis in Snoring

To date, the role of the epiglottis in snoring is still unclear. The reported prevalence rates of the epiglottis being implicated in the generation of snoring sound ranged from 12 to 42.3% [39, 41, 42]. As for isolated epiglottic snoring, Sung et al. [43] identified 11 patients who had an epiglottic anteroposterior obstruction as the only cause of snoring from 334 consecutive DISE examinations, suggesting a prevalence of isolated epiglottic snoring of 3%. Similarly, in another DISE study on 50 snorers, the prevalence of isolated epiglottic snoring was 2% [41]. Two studies [44, 45] reported that no epiglottic snorer was identified in 35 and 23 patients undergoing DISE, respectively. The abovementioned evidence suggests that isolated epiglottic snoring is rare and, compared with the velum and oropharynx, the epiglottis is less commonly implicated in the generation of snoring sound. The authors would like to hypothesize that, as a valve regulating the opening and closing of the trachea, the epiglottis may affect snoring sound by affecting the airflow rather than directly generating snoring sound. Azarbarzin et al. [45] suggested that because the occurrence of epiglottic obstruction is abrupt, due to the immediate cessation of the airflow, the "classical" snoring sound cannot be generated. In addition, it was reported that epiglottic obstruction may generate sounds that are different from the "classical" snoring sound [45]. According to the authors' experience, primary epiglottic obstruction frequently occurs in combination with soft palatal obstruction, generating a different snoring sound than solitary soft palatal snoring sound (Fig. 10.3). In addition, the epiglottis can make other noises during sleep. One such case that the authors have seen in clinic is a patient whose main complaint was "noise during sleep." DISE was prescribed to investigate the patient's upper airway. It was found that the epiglottis flopped into the airway during inspiration. During expiration, the epiglottis straightened up and caused a bubbling sound. This suggests that physicians, especially ENT doctors and sleep clinicians, should keep in mind that epiglottic obstruction may make noises that are different from snoring sound.

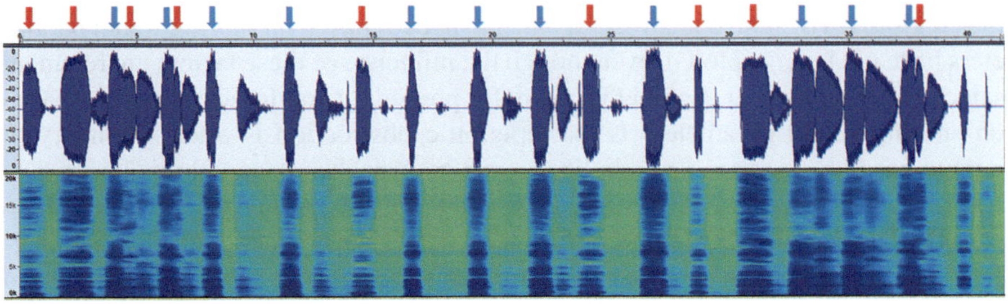

Fig. 10.3 (Audio 10.1) Snoring sounds of epiglottic and soft palatal obstructions. *Red arrows* indicate snoring sounds of primary epiglottic obstruction. *Blue arrows* indicate snoring sounds of soft palatal obstruction. The waveforms of snoring sounds are shown in the upper panels (with *white* background); the amplitudes of waveforms represent the intensities of snoring sounds. In the lower panels (with *green* background), the spectrums show the frequency distribution (0–22 kHz) of the snoring sounds. The *blue* horizontal lines represent the power of the sound, i.e., the more *blue* horizontal lines at certain frequency, the higher power the sound has at this frequency (this sound recording is provided by Dr. Matej Delakorda)

10.6 Conclusion

In summary, using snoring sound parameters to predict the presence of epiglottic obstruction in OSA patients with single-level obstruction can achieve a relatively high accuracy, even though the role of the epiglottis in generating snoring sound is still unclear. Further studies are needed to explore the possibility to predict the presence of epiglottic obstruction in OSA patients with multilevel obstruction based on the acoustic analysis of snoring sound, especially snoring sound during natural sleep. In addition, whether the acoustic analysis of snoring sound can provide information on the level and configuration of epiglottic obstruction and distinguish between primary and secondary epiglottic obstruction need to be studied before using this technique in the clinic. At this stage, snoring sound analysis does not seem to be a viable diagnostic modality for treatment selection.

References

1. Jennum P, Sjøl A. Epidemiology of snoring and obstructive sleep apnoea in a Danish population, age 30-60. J Sleep Res. 1992;1:240–4. https://doi.org/10.1111/j.1365-2869.1992.tb00045.x.
2. Khazaie H, Negahban S, Ghadami MR, Sadeghi Bahmani D, Holsboer-Trachsler E, Brand S. Among middle-aged adults, snoring predicted hypertension independently of sleep apnoea. J Int Med Res. 2018;46:1187–96. https://doi.org/10.1177/0300060517738426.
3. Maimon N, Hanly PJ. Does snoring intensity correlate with the severity of obstructive sleep apnea? J Clin Sleep Med. 2010;6:475–8.
4. American Academy of Sleep Medicine. International classification of sleep disorders. 3rd ed. Darien: American Academy of Sleep Medicine; 2014.
5. Virkkula P, Bachour A, Hytönen M, Malmberg H, Salmi T, Maasilta P. Patient- and bed partner-reported symptoms, smoking, and nasal resistance in sleep-disordered breathing. Chest. 2005;128:2176–82. https://doi.org/10.1378/chest.128.4.2176.

6. Acar M, Yazıcı D, Bayar Muluk N, Hancı D, Seren E, Cingi C. Is there a relationship between snoring sound intensity and frequency and OSAS severity? Ann Otol Rhinol Laryngol. 2016;125:31–6. https://doi.org/10.1177/0003489415595640.
7. Azarbarzin A, Moussavi Z. Snoring sounds variability as a signature of obstructive sleep apnea. Med Eng Phys. 2013;35:479–85. https://doi.org/10.1016/j.medengphy.2012.06.013.
8. Quinn S, Huang L, Ellis P, Williams J. The differentiation of snoring mechanisms using sound analysis. Clin Otolaryngol Allied Sci. 1996;21:119–23. https://doi.org/10.1111/j.1365-2273.1996.tb01313.x.
9. Croft CB, Pringle M. Sleep nasendoscopy: a technique of assessment in snoring and obstructive sleep apnoea. Clin Otolaryngol Allied Sci. 1991;16:504–9. https://doi.org/10.1111/j.1365-2273.1991.tb01050.x.
10. Kezirian E, Hohenhorst W, de Vries N. Drug-induced sleep endoscopy: the VOTE classification. Eur Arch Otorhinolaryngol. 2011;268:1233–6. https://doi.org/10.1007/s00405-011-1633-8.
11. Strollo P, Soose R, Maurer J, de Vries N, Cornelius J, Froymovich O, Hanson R, Padhya T, Steward D, Gillespie B, Woodson T, Van de Heyning P, Goetting M, Vanderveken O, Feldman N, Knaack L, Strohl K, STAR Trial Group. Upper-airway stimulation for obstructive sleep apnea. N Engl J Med. 2014;370:139–49. https://doi.org/10.1056/NEJMoa1308659.
12. Op de Beeck S, Dieltjens M, Verbruggen A, Vroegop A, Wouters K, Hamans E, Willemen M, Verbraecken J, De Backer W, Van de Heyning P, Braem M, Vanderveken O. Phenotypic labelling using drug-induced sleep endoscopy improves patient selection for mandibular advancement device outcome: a prospective study. J Clin Sleep Med. 2019;15:1089–99. https://doi.org/10.5664/jcsm.7796.
13. Chong KB, De Vito A, Vicini C. Drug-induced sleep endoscopy in treatment options selection. Sleep Med Clin. 2019;14:33–40. https://doi.org/10.1016/j.jsmc.2018.11.001.
14. Viana A, Zhao C, Rosa T, Couto A, Neves DD, Araújo-Melo MH, Capasso R. The effect of sedating agents on drug-induced sleep endoscopy findings. Laryngoscope. 2019;129:506–13. https://doi.org/10.1002/lary.27298.
15. Razek A. Diagnostic role of magnetic resonance imaging in obstructive sleep apnea syndrome. J Comput Assist Tomogr. 2015;39:565–71. https://doi.org/10.1097/RCT.0000000000000243.
16. Genta P, Sands S, Butler J, Loring S, Katz E, Demko B, Kezirian E, White D, Wellman A. Airflow shape is associated with the pharyngeal structure causing OSA. Chest. 2017;152:537–46. https://doi.org/10.1016/j.chest.2017.06.017.
17. Hudgel DW. Variable site of airway narrowing among obstructive sleep apnea patients. J Appl Physiol. 1986;61:1403–9. https://doi.org/10.1152/jappl.1986.61.4.1403.
18. Han D, Ye J, Wang J, Yang Q, Lin Y, Wang J. Determining the site of airway obstruction in obstructive sleep apnea with airway pressure measurements during sleep. Laryngoscope. 2002;112:2081–5. https://doi.org/10.1097/00005537-200211000-00032.
19. Titze IR. Principles of vocal production. Englewood Cliffs: Prentice-Hall; 1994.
20. Pevernagie D, Aarts RM, De Meyer M. The acoustics of snoring. Sleep Med Rev. 2010;14:131–44. https://doi.org/10.1016/j.smrv.2009.06.002.
21. Agrawal S, Stone P, McGuinness K, Morris J, Camilleri A. Sound frequency analysis and the site of snoring in natural and induced sleep. Clin Otolaryngol Allied Sci. 2002;27:162–6. https://doi.org/10.1046/j.1365-2273.2002.00554.x.
22. Gürpınar B, Saltürk Z, Kumral T, Civelek S, Izel O, Uyar Y. Analysis of snoring to determine the site of obstruction in obstructive sleep apnea syndrome. Sleep Breath. 2020;25:1427. https://doi.org/10.1007/s11325-020-02252-5.
23. Koo S, Kwon S, Kim Y, Moon J, Kim Y, Jung S. Acoustic analysis of snoring sounds recorded with a smartphone according to obstruction site in OSAS patients. Eur Arch Otorhinolaryngol. 2017;274:1735–40. https://doi.org/10.1007/s00405-016-4335-4.
24. Eberhard Z, Hugo F. Psychoacoustics-facts and models. 2nd ed. Berlin: Springer; 1999.
25. Huang Z, Aarab G, Ravesloot MJL, Zhou N, Bosschieter PFN, van Selms MKA, den Haan C, de Vries N, Lobbezoo F, Hilgevoord AAJ. Prediction of the obstruction sites in the upper airway in sleep-disordered breathing based on snoring sound parameters: a systematic review. Sleep Med. 2021;88:116–33. https://doi.org/10.1016/j.sleep.2021.10.015.

26. Won T, Kim S, Lee W, Han D, Kim D, Kim J, Rhee C, Lee C. Acoustic characteristics of snoring according to obstruction site determined by sleep videofluoroscopy. Acta Otolaryngol. 2012;132(Suppl 1):S13–20. https://doi.org/10.3109/00016489.2012.660733.
27. Qian K, Janott C, Pandit V, Zhang Z, Heiser C, Hohenhorst W, Herzog M, Hemmert W, Schuller B. Classification of the excitation location of snore sounds in the upper airway by acoustic multifeature analysis. IEEE Trans Biomed Eng. 2017;64:1731–41. https://doi.org/10.1109/TBME.2016.2619675.
28. Qian K, Janott C, Deng J, Heiser C, Hohenhorst W, Herzog M, Cummins N, Schuller B. Snore sound recognition: on wavelets and classifiers from deep nets to kernels. Conf Proc IEEE Eng Med Biol Soc. 2017;2017:3737–40. https://doi.org/10.1109/EMBC.2017.8037669.
29. Schmitt M, Janott C, Pandit V, Qian K, Heiser C, Hemmert W, Schuller B. A bag-of-audio-words approach for snore sounds' excitation localisation. Speech Communication; 12. Paderborn: ITG Symposium; 2016.
30. Qian K, Schmitt M, Janott C, Zhang Z, Heiser C, Hohenhorst W, Herzog M, Hemmert W, Schuller B. A bag of wavelet features for snore sound classification. Ann Biomed Eng. 2019;47:1000–11. https://doi.org/10.1007/s10439-019-02217-0.
31. Amiriparian S, Gerczuk M, Ottl S, Cummins N, Freitag M, Pugachevskiy S, Baird A, Schuller B. Snore sound classification using image-based deep Spectrum features. In: Proceedings INTERSPEECH 2017, 18th Annual Conference of the International Speech Communication Association, Stockholm, Sweden, ISCA, August; 2017. p. 3512–6. https://doi.org/10.21437/Interspeech.2017-434.
32. Vesperini F, Galli A, Gabrielli L, Principi E, Squartini S. Snore sounds excitation localization by using scattering transform and deep neural Networks. In: 2018 International Joint Conference on Neural Networks (IJCNN), Rio de Janeiro, Brazil; 2018. https://doi.org/10.1109/IJCNN.2018.8489576.
33. Sun J, Hu X, Chen C, Peng S, Ma Y. Amplitude spectrum trend-based feature for excitation location classification from snore sounds. Physiol Meas. 2020;41:085006. https://doi.org/10.1088/1361-6579/abaa34.
34. Sun J, Hu X, Peng S, Peng C, Ma Y. Automatic classification of excitation location of snoring sounds. J Clin Sleep Med. 2021;17:1031–8. https://doi.org/10.5664/jcsm.9094.
35. Lee E, Cho J. Meta-analysis of obstruction site observed with drug-induced sleep endoscopy in patients with obstructive sleep apnea. Laryngoscope. 2019;129:1235–43. https://doi.org/10.1002/lary.27320.
36. Rabelo F, Kupper D, Sander H, Fernandes R, Valera F. Polysomnographic evaluation of propofol-induced sleep in patients with respiratory sleep disorders and controls. Laryngoscope. 2013;123:2300–5. https://doi.org/10.1002/lary.23664.
37. Murphy M, Bruno M, Riedner B, Boveroux P, Noirhomme Q, Landsness E, Brichant J, Phillips C, Massimini M, Laureys S, Tononi G, Boly M. Propofol anesthesia and sleep: a high-density EEG study. Sleep. 2011;34:283–91A. https://doi.org/10.1093/sleep/34.3.283.
38. Jones T, Ho M, Earis J, Swift A, Charters P. Acoustic parameters of snoring sound to compare natural snores with snores during 'steady-state' propofol sedation. Clin Otolaryngol. 2006;31:46–52. https://doi.org/10.1111/j.1749-4486.2006.01136.x.
39. Salamanca F, Leone F, Bianchi A, Bellotto R, Costantini F, Salvatori P. Surgical treatment of epiglottis collapse in obstructive sleep apnoea syndrome: epiglottis stiffening operation. Acta Otorhinolaryngol Ital. 2019;39:404–8. https://doi.org/10.14639/0392-100X-N0287.
40. Elsobki A, Cahali M, Kahwagi M. LwPTL: a novel classification for upper airway collapse in sleep endoscopies. Braz J Otorhinolaryngol. 2019;85:379–87. https://doi.org/10.1016/j.bjorl.2019.01.010.
41. Quinn SJ, Daly N, Ellis PD. Observation of the mechanism of snoring using sleep nasendoscopy. Clin Otolaryngol Allied Sci. 1995;20:360–4. https://doi.org/10.1111/j.1365-2273.1995.tb00061.x.
42. Xu H, Jia R, Yu H, Gao Z, Huang W, Peng H, Yang Y, Zhang L. Investigation of the source of snoring sound by drug-induced sleep nasendoscopy. ORL J Otorhinolaryngol Relat Spec. 2015;77:359–65. https://doi.org/10.1159/000439597.

43. Sung CM, Kim HC, Yang HC. The clinical characteristics of patients with an isolate epiglottic collapse. Auris Nasus Larynx. 2020;47:450–7. https://doi.org/10.1016/j.anl.2019.10.009.
44. Saunders NA, Vandeleur T, Deves J, Salmon A, Gyulay S, Crocker B, Hensley M. Uvulopalatopharyngoplasty as a treatment for snoring. Med J Aust. 1989;150:177–82. https://doi.org/10.5694/j.1326-5377.1989.tb136420.x.
45. Azarbarzin A, Marques M, Sands SA, Op de Beeck S, Genta PR, Taranto-Montemurro L, de Melo CM, Messineo L, Vanderveken OM, White DP, Wellman A. Predicting epiglottic collapse in patients with obstructive sleep apnoea. Eur Respir J. 2017;50:1700345. https://doi.org/10.1183/13993003.00345-2017.

Part III

Special Section

The Role of the Epiglottis in Pediatric OSA

11

Ashley L. Soaper, Cynthia S. Wang, and Stacey L. Ishman

11.1 Introduction

Obstructive sleep apnea (OSA) is one of the most prevalent health problems in children with an overall prevalence of 1.2–5.7% worldwide [1]. OSA presents differently in children compared to adults (Table 11.1). It can manifest as daytime sleepiness in the adult, while daytime behavioral issues including hyperactivity are more common in children. From a physiologic basis, children are more likely than adults to have long duration partial airway obstruction (hypopneas) rather than discrete apneas. In addition, these hypopneas are more often associated with hypoxemia or hypercapnia in children than in adults. Given that children have lower forced vital capacity and faster respiratory rates than adults, they also tend to desaturate more quickly. Like adults, proper management of OSA in a child is crucial to prevent long-term unfavorable cardiovascular, neurocognitive, and metabolic effects.

The severity of pediatric OSA is based upon normal statistical distribution of polysomnography (PSG) data unlike adult cutoffs which were derived from long-term studies of patient outcomes. For children, mild OSA is defined as an apnea-hypopnea index (AHI) of 1 to <5 events/hour, moderate as an AHI of 5 to <10 events/hour, and severe as an AHI 10 or more events/hour [2]. While adenotonsillar hypertrophy is the most common cause of OSA in children, one-third of children will

Supplementary Information The online version contains supplementary material available at https://doi.org/10.1007/978-3-031-34992-8_11. The videos can be accessed individually by clicking the DOI link in the accompanying figure caption or by scanning this link with the SN More Media App.

A. L. Soaper · C. S. Wang · S. L. Ishman (✉)
Division of Pediatric Otolaryngology-Head and Neck Surgery, Cincinnati Children's Hospital Medical Center, Cincinnati, OH, USA
e-mail: Stacey.Ishman@cchmc.org

M. Delakorda, N. de Vries (eds.), *The Role of Epiglottis in Obstructive Sleep Apnea*, https://doi.org/10.1007/978-3-031-34992-8_11

Table 11.1 Comparison of severity classification, symptoms, and treatment options in pediatric and adult obstructive sleep apnea (OSA)

	Pediatric OSA	Adult OSA
Severity classification	Mild: AHI 1 to <5	Mild: AHI 5 to <15
	Moderate: AHI: 5 to <10	Moderate: AHI 15 to <30
	Severe: AHI 10 or greater	Severe: AHI 30 or greater
Symptoms	• Snoring	• Snoring
	• Discrete apneas less common	• Apnea more commons
	• Daytime sleepiness less common	• Daytime sleepiness very common
	• Hyperactivity	• Headache
	• Aggressive behavior	
Sleep study findings	• Subcortical arousals	• Arousals
First-line treatment	Tonsillectomy and adenoidectomy	CPAP, weight loss

have persistent OSA after adenotonsillectomy. Children with other comorbidities such as Down syndrome, obesity, craniofacial anomalies or neuromuscular disorders have even higher rates of residual OSA [3–5]. Both congenital and sleep-dependent laryngomalacia have been implicated as causes of OSA in infants and in children before and after adenotonsillectomy. In a retrospective study by Verkest et al. of 42 infants, 77% of patients with laryngomalacia who underwent PSG had OSA [6]. While it is likely that this number is overestimated due to the retrospective nature of the study and selection bias, this study suggests that the incidence of OSA is significant in these infants.

Congenital laryngomalacia is the most common cause of stridor in neonates and affects males more than females [7]. It is classically defined as a condition of dynamic collapse of the supraglottic airway based on movement of the arytenoid and epiglottic tissues. This causes symptoms including inspiratory stridor, which is typically worse with feeding and agitation, feeding intolerance, coughing, choking, and regurgitation. Stridor is present at birth in up to 75% of neonates with laryngomalacia and is explained by the Bernoulli effect, in which negative pressure from upper airway obstruction contributes to dynamic collapse of the larynx [7]. In severe cases, which account for 5–10% of all cases, upper airway obstruction can cause failure to thrive, cor pulmonale, pectus excavatum, and even death [8]. Typical endoscopic findings noted in congenital laryngomalacia include redundant or prolapsed arytenoid tissue, shortened aryepiglottic folds, and an omega-shaped, infantile epiglottis (Fig. 11.1).

Most cases present in the first few weeks of life and are self-limited, with symptoms typically resolving by 12–24 months of age (Table 11.2). There is a close association between laryngomalacia and gastroesophageal reflux disease (GERD), with GERD reported in 64% of patients with laryngomalacia [9]. Moreover, several studies have found that infants with laryngomalacia and concomitant GERD have more severe symptoms than those infants with laryngomalacia alone [8, 9].

Sleep-dependent laryngomalacia, also known by multiple monikers including late-onset laryngomalacia, sleep exclusive laryngomalacia, state-dependent

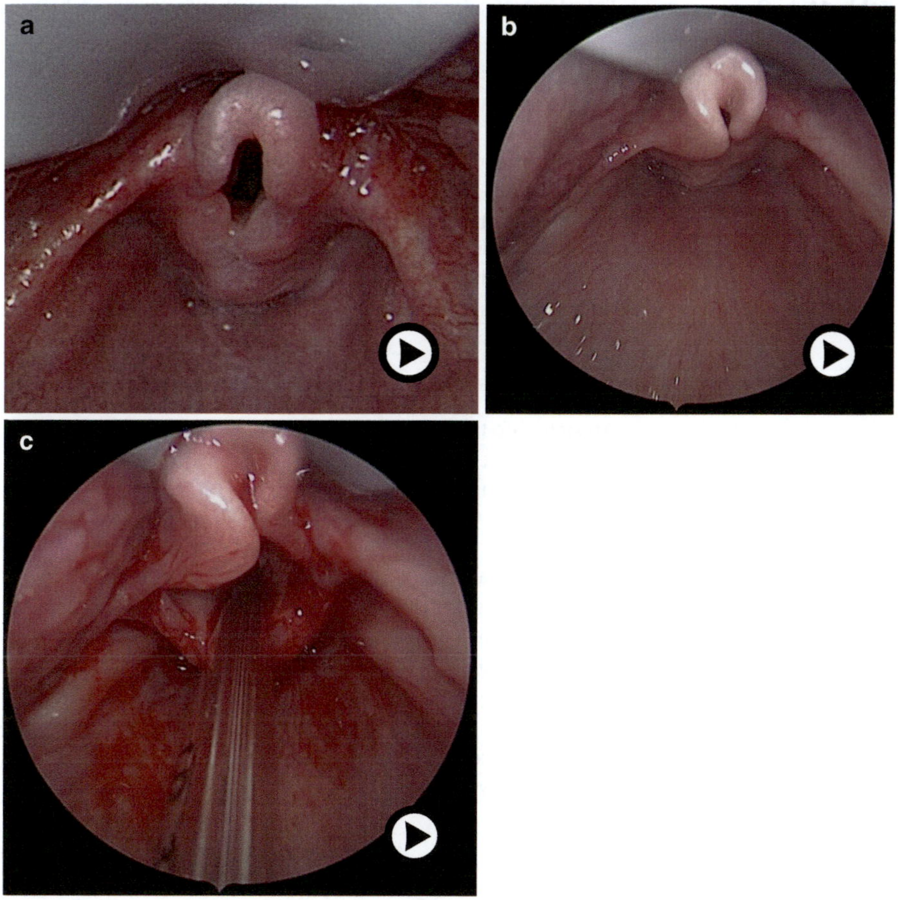

Fig. 11.1 (**a**, **b**) Congenital laryngomalacia on direct laryngoscopy, characterized with shorted aryepiglottic folds and redundant arytenoid tissue, completely obstructing the view of the true vocal folds (**c**) immediately after supraglottoplasty with division of the aryepiglottic folds and removal of redundant arytenoid tissue (► https://doi.org/10.1007/000-bfa)

laryngomalacia, occult laryngomalacia, and sleep-dependent laryngomalacia, was first described by Amin et al. in 1997 [10]. It is characterized by stridor and upper airway obstruction during sleep, without daytime stridor and normal anatomic findings while awake [7]. However, most children determined to have sleep-dependent laryngomalacia present primarily with snoring as reports of stridor during sleep are uncommon. In contrast to congenital laryngomalacia, sleep-dependent laryngomalacia occurs in the absence of the anatomic features seen in children with congenital disease, such as a retroflexed and omega-shaped epiglottis (Fig. 11.2). Sleep-dependent laryngomalacia is also commonly diagnosed in children (2–18 years) and is noted in 3.9% of children who present with sleep-disordered breathing [11] (Table 11.2). Boudewyns et al. noted a 5.4% prevalence of sleep-state laryngomalacia in a group of 37 children who underwent drug-induced sleep endoscopy (DISE) [12].

Table 11.2 Comparison of clinical presentation, diagnosis, and treatment for congenital versus sleep-state laryngomalacia

	Congenital laryngomalacia	Sleep-state laryngomalacia
Age at presentation	Several weeks after birth	> 2 years old
Clinical symptoms	While asleep and awake:	Only while asleep:
	• Mild symptoms	• Snoring
	– Stridor exacerbated by agitation, supine position, feeding	• Stridor (less commonly)
	– Difficulty feeding	• Apneic episodes
	• Severe symptoms	
	– Failure to thrive	
	– Apnea	
	– Cyanosis	
	– Apparent life-threatening event	
	– Cor pulmonale	
	– Pectus excavatum	
Diagnosis	Flexible laryngoscopy	Drug-induced sleep endoscopy
Exam findings	• Supraglottic collapse	• Supraglottic collapse
	• Shortened aryepiglottic folds	• Redundant arytenoid mucosa
	• Redundant arytenoid mucosa	
Nonsurgical management	• Prone positioning	• Supplemental oxygen
	• Supplemental oxygen	• Positive pressure
	• Positive pressure	
	• Antireflux medications	
Surgical management	• Supraglottoplasty	• Supraglottoplasty
	• Epiglottopexy	• Epiglottopexy
	• Tracheostomy	• Tracheostomy

There have been several theories proposed to explain the etiology of laryngomalacia. These include the anatomic or cartilage theory, which suggested that malpositioned or lax laryngeal cartilage was the cause of airway obstruction. In contrast, the neurologic theory of laryngomalacia suggests that reduced tone is the reason for airway collapse and this theory is supported by observations in adults with central nervous system injury who develop laryngomalacia postinjury [10]. More recently, this condition has been hypothesized to be caused by abnormal sensorimotor function which leads to decreased tone, impaired neuromuscular coordination, and flaccidity of the larynx. Based on these last two theories, improvement in congenital laryngomalacia is presumed to occur as the laryngeal reflexes mature [8]. Regardless of mechanism, children with laryngomalacia develop symptoms due to floppiness of the cartilage/soft tissue of the supraglottic larynx with prolapsing of the epiglottis and or the aryepiglottic folds into the airway during inhalation which leads to the symptoms detailed below.

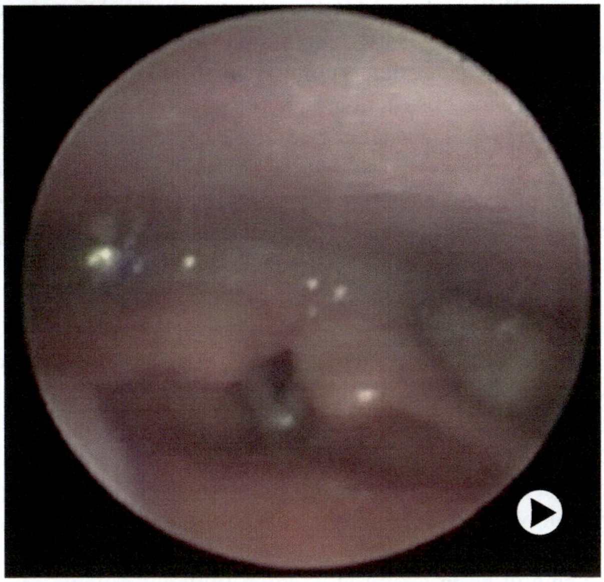

Fig. 11.2 Sleep-state laryngomalacia during a drug-induced sleep endoscopy with demonstration of redundant arytenoid mucosa collapsing into the airway (► https://doi.org/10.1007/000-bf9)

11.2 Evaluation and Diagnosis

Congenital laryngomalacia is a clinical diagnosis often managed with observation by the primary care physician. For children with significant daytime and/or nighttime symptoms who may benefit from further evaluation or management, referral to an otolaryngologist is typically recommended. In the otolaryngology clinic, the diagnosis of congenital laryngomalacia can be confirmed with a flexible fiberoptic laryngoscopy examination. During this assessment, specific attention is placed on the identification of dynamic collapse of the supraglottic structures including findings such as shortened aryepiglottic folds, omega-shaped epiglottis, and prolapse of arytenoid tissue. These findings may be confirmed during laryngoscopy in the operating room when surgical therapy is considered (Fig. 11.1). Congenital laryngomalacia is a major risk factor for OSA in children under one-year of age [13]. Considering this, oximetry and PSG are often used in the workup for those children with laryngomalacia and significant daytime or nighttime signs or symptoms.

Sleep-dependent laryngomalacia is not observed during awake evaluation and typically can only be confirmed during sedated evaluations like DISE. Typical findings on DISE would include redundant arytenoid mucosa with dynamic supraglottic prolapse which obstructs the airway. Experts who created the 2021 expert consensus statement from the American Academy of Otolaryngology—Head and Neck Surgery noted that DISE is useful for assessment of children with OSA after adenotonsillectomy and should be performed prior to additional surgery. Cine magnetic resonance imaging (MRI) may also be a helpful adjunct for diagnosis of patients with this condition. DISE and cine MRI are frequently used to assess patients with persistent OSA. In addition to its use for children with persistent OSA, these assessments are also indicated to evaluate children with small tonsils, those with suspected multilevel airway obstruction, and those unable to tolerate PSG (e.g., developmental delay) [14]. The challenge of these modalities is obtaining the proper level of anesthesia to mimic sleep so that the dynamic movement of the airway can be assessed. While propofol is commonly used to assess adults with OSA, there is currently no consensus regarding the ideal pediatric anesthetic protocol for DISE or cine MRI. We prefer a combination of dexmedetomidine and ketamine. Typically, inhalational agents are used to place an intravenous catheter. They are discontinued once the patient is asleep and a loading dose of dexmedetomidine (2 μg/kg) is given over 10 min, followed by an infusion of 2 μg/kg/h. Once the loading dose of dexmedetomidine is started, ketamine 1 mg/kg is administered. If the patient is inadequately sedated, a second bolus of ketamine 1 mg/kg is administered at the end of the 10-min bolus and the dexmedetomidine is increased to 3 μg/kg/h. If the patient is still moving (e.g., not yet in Ramsay 5 level of sedation) [15], a propofol infusion (50 μg/kg/min) can be started [16]. This must be titrated carefully in order to avoid respiratory depression which may exaggerate airway collapse [14]. During the DISE, the neck should be in a neutral position (without pillows or extension/flexion). We do not typically examine the airway in alternate positions as our sleep lab does not report on positional data. The upper airway should be examined with and without a jaw thrust (at the choana/velum and at base of tongue to assess retroglossal airway), and an oral airway and supplemental oxygen should be removed prior to the evaluation. While children with positional OSA are more likely to demonstrate obstruction at the tongue base or velum, we do not routinely perform DISEs.

11.3 Management of Laryngomalacia

Because most children with congenital laryngomalacia have mild symptoms, they can often be managed conservatively (e.g., with observation) with symptom resolution by 12–24 months of age. Repositioning into a prone position or extending the child's neck during sleep may be used during this period, although caution should be given about prone sleep positioning for infants. In addition, children with signs and symptoms of GERD are treated with either a type 2 histamine antagonist or proton pump inhibitor. It is thought that reflux causes irritation and edema in the airway, worsening the airway obstruction. Treatment of reflux has been associated with improved symptoms and shortened disease course of congenital laryngomalacia [6]. However, evidence supporting causality between GERD and laryngomalacia or benefit from antireflux therapy in patients without GERD symptoms is limited [17].

Nonsurgical treatment for OSA due to congenital or sleep-dependent laryngomalacia can be considered if OSA is mild, if symptoms are mild, or if the patient is not a surgical candidate. For children with congenital laryngomalacia, supplemental oxygen is considered the primary nonsurgical treatment for infants with OSA and has been shown to lower AHI without significant hypoventilation or hypercapnia [18]. Alternatively, for children with sleep-dependent laryngomalacia, continuous positive airway pressure (CPAP) may be considered. Unfortunately, CPAP compliance is low in children (less than 50%) and is not frequently used for children younger than 1 year of age [19]. Common side effects of CPAP include dry mouth, frequent awakening, and poor mask fitting. Mask fitting can be an especially big problem as many masks are too large for young children. Additionally, there is concern that long-term mask use may result in midface flattening in the developing child. For children with mild sleep-dependent laryngomalacia, pharmacologic agents like intranasal steroids and oral montelukast have shown some short-term benefit in children with mild and moderate OSA though evidence is limited.

While most children with congenital laryngomalacia do not require surgical intervention, 5–10% will have severe symptoms (e.g., failure to thrive, feeding difficulties) (Table 11.2) and may benefit from operative intervention [20]. The surgery is typically performed within 1–2 weeks, however occasionally symptoms may be so severe (severe OSA, recurrent acute life-threatening events (ALTEs), inability to coordinate feeding and breathing) that it may be performed urgently [7]. The most common surgery performed to treat laryngomalacia is supraglottoplasty. Epiglottopexy may also be considered for children with independent epiglottic collapse that is severe. Though tracheostomy is rarely performed, it is an option for children with severe disease and comorbid conditions, making resolution of their symptoms unlikely. This may be the case for children with craniofacial abnormalities and those with neurological impairment [7].

Supraglottoplasty involves trimming tight aryepiglottic folds to release the epiglottis and reduce the lateral aryepiglottic fold collapse. It may also include the removal or reduction of redundant arytenoid mucosa. This procedure can be safely performed with the child spontaneously breathing or while intubated. The senior author typically performs this intubated after the administration of an intraoperative dose of intravenous steroid. Intubation puts the aryepiglottic folds on tension, allowing for easier access to trim these tissues. The patient is then placed into suspension with a laryngoscope. This can be performed with several different laryngoscopes (including a Lindholm); however, the senior author prefers a Parsons side-slot laryngoscope and suspension. Using a rigid endoscope, the arytenoid mucosa is grasped, and the tight aryepiglottic folds are trimmed. This can be done with microscissors, although the senior author prefers sharp sinus true cuts [21]. It is important to keep the cut closely associated to the epiglottis. Other techniques include the use of a microscope and alternative methods of tissue removal including the carbon dioxide laser and microdebrider [20]. The redundant arytenoid and aryepiglottic fold mucosa are then trimmed on the lateral side of the arytenoids/folds (using a microdebrider or scissor). Care must be taken to leave a rim of intact mucosa between the aryepiglottic fold cuts and any cut on the arytenoid mucosa to prevent supraglottic scarring. Similarly, it is critical to avoid denuding the interarytenoid mucosa to avoid supraglottic stenosis.

Supraglottoplasty results in improvement in the AHI for children with congenital and sleep-dependent laryngomalacia. A 2016 meta-analysis by Camacho et al. of

138 children with OSA who underwent supraglottoplasty reported that for children with sleep-dependent laryngomalacia, the mean AHI decreased from 14 to 3.3 events/hour and the lowest oxygen saturation increased from 85 to 88%. For those children with congenital laryngomalacia, the mean AHI decreased from 20 to 4.0 events/hour and the lowest oxygen saturation increased from 74 to 88% [22]. A second meta-analysis from 2016 by Lee et al. examined pooled data of 121 patients who underwent a supraglottoplasty, regardless of the type of laryngomalacia, and found a mean decrease in AHI of 8.9 [23].

Epiglottopexy can be considered when addressing OSA-independent epiglottis collapse (epiglottic retroflexion); this is more commonly considered for children with sleep-dependent laryngomalacia [24] (Fig. 11.3). It is performed under general anesthesia with nasotracheal or endotracheal intubation. The lingual surface of the epiglottis, vallecula, and base of tongue are all typically denuded, with either a radiofrequency ablation, electrocautery, or laser, taking care to leave a rim of mucosa along the lateral edges and tip of the lingual epiglottis to prevent swallow dysfunction as recommended by Oomen et al. [25]. The epiglottis may be left to scar to the base of tongue or may be secured to the base of tongue with absorbable interrupted sutures to promote scarring of the epiglottis to the tongue base. The suturing to the tongue base can be technically challenging and it is unclear if outcomes are better than doing it without the suture, so our preference is not to suture. If lingual tonsil hypertrophy is also present, a lingual tonsillectomy can be performed together with the epiglottopexy [25], which we believe can help facilitate scar band formation between the epiglottis and tongue base. Though there are few studies on the effects of epiglottopexy alone on the airway, Zalzal et al. demonstrated a decrease in mean AHI from 5.1 to 1.5 in a cohort of ten patients [24]. The same study also showed similar outcomes in 18 patients who received an epiglottopexy and division of aryepiglottic folds, with an improvement in mean AHI from 5.7 to 3.1. In another series of 19 patients, Baljosevic et al. demonstrated

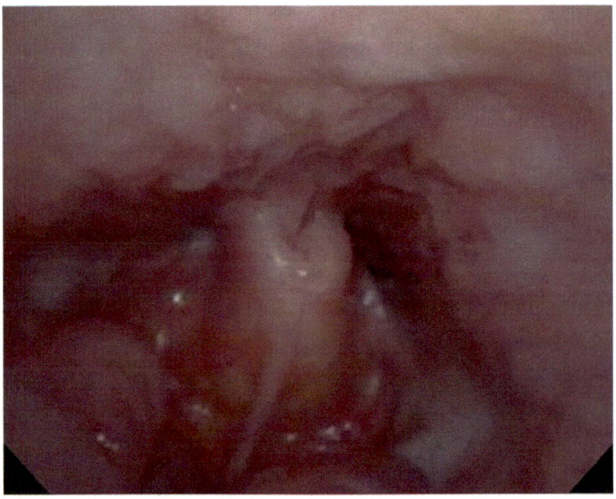

Fig. 11.3 Epiglottic retroflexion on drug-induced sleep endoscopy

improvements in oxygen desaturations and weight gain after both epiglottic suture placement and laser epiglottopexy [26]. The preoperative oxygen desaturation index (ODI) was a mean of 5.8, which improved to 1.2 postoperatively. Preoperative mean oxygen saturation was 89.4 ± 4.3% which improved postoperatively to 96.7 ± 1.1% [26].

Another option for treatment is the epiglottic suture, described in a case series of eight children to specifically address the omega shape of the epiglottis [27]. Under general endotracheal anesthesia, a small strip of mucosa is excised from the lingual surface of the epiglottis and a resorbable suture is placed transversely, bringing together the lateral edges of the cut mucosa, unfurling the epiglottis in the process. Seven of the eight patients demonstrated improved breathing and feeding after the procedure, with one requiring a revision surgery.

Tracheostomy is considered definitive treatment for OSA and laryngomalacia and was previously a mainstay of treatment. Its use has since decreased to avoid the morbidity and mortality associated with tracheostomy. It is most utilized for select patients who have severe laryngomalacia and OSA with significant comorbidities (such as genetic abnormalities, craniofacial syndromes, or neuromuscular disease) [8]. Pediatric tracheostomy is performed in an intubated patient and may be carried out before or after microlaryngoscopy and bronchoscopy. An incision is made either vertically or with a horizontal incision one finger breadth inferior to the cricoid cartilage. The strap muscles are divided in the midline and the thyroid gland is either retracted or divided at the midline. Once the trachea is identified, two stay sutures (we prefer a 4–0 prolene) are placed on either side of midline and spanning 1–2 tracheal rings (often rings 2–3). A midline, vertical incision is made in the trachea spanning two tracheal rings, typically involving tracheal rings 2, 3, or 4. Inferior and superior maturation sutures (we prefer a 4–0 chromic) may be placed in a half horizontal mattress fashion, making a bite into the skin, around a tracheal ring, and back through the skin to mature the skin to the tracheal cartilage. Some providers choose not to use maturation sutures, but they make it easier to replace a tracheostomy tube if it is displaced prior to maturation of the stoma. The endotracheal tube is then pulled back, the tracheostomy tube is placed into the tracheotomy incision with an obturator in place, and tracheostomy ties are placed.

In cases where there is both adenotonsillar hypertrophy and mild laryngomalacia, resolution of the laryngomalacia may occur following adenotonsillectomy alone. In these instances, laryngomalacia is thought to be due to negative inspiratory pressure needed to overcome the upstream obstruction, as explained by the Bernoulli effect [6].

11.4 Postoperative Management

Following supraglottoplasty or epiglottopexy, we recommend overnight admission with continuous pulse oximetry monitoring, which can occur on a hospital floor, stepdown unit, or high-dependency unit (HDU). Once they emerge from anesthesia, the children can resume their normal home diet. An antireflux medication, like a proton pump inhibitor or type 2-histamine blocker, is often given in the postoperative period. No antibiotic therapy is typically given, but a second dose of steroid is frequently given 8 h after surgery. If there are persistent feeding difficulties, a speech language pathology consult may also be requested. For children with OSA, a PSG is recommended at least 1 month after supraglottoplasty or epiglottopexy. Because children at this age typically do not snore, it is important to get objective data to confirm resolution of moderate to severe OSA. In cases of congenital laryngomalacia, a repeat sleep study can be performed as soon as 2–3 weeks after surgery to determine if oxygen or other therapies are needed in these newborns and infants.

Children who undergo tracheostomy are commonly monitored in an intensive care unit (ICU). In our institution, children are in the ICU for at least 5 days while the tracheostomy stoma matures. We also perform the first tracheostomy tie change on postoperative day 3 to minimize skin breakdown and the first tracheostomy tube change on postoperative day 5. The stay sutures are also removed on day 5. If the stoma is healing well and the tracheostomy change is uncomplicated, care of the tracheostomy tube, tracheostomy tube changes, and family education are turned over to the nursing teams.

11.5 Complications

The risk of complications following supraglottoplasty is low, and includes aspiration, supraglottic stenosis, cartilage damage, granuloma formation, and need for revision surgery. Temporary aspiration or dysphagia can occur in 14–25% of patients [6]. A review by Denoyelle et al. (2003) quotes an overall complication rate of 7.4% and major complication rate of 3.7%. Minor complications included granuloma formation, edema, and a posterior fibrous web. Major complications included supraglottic stenosis and need for revision surgery [20]. Another study by Reddy et al. found a 4% rate of supraglottic stenosis following supraglottoplasty [28]. Following supraglottoplasty, children with comorbidities, especially neurologic conditions, tend to have worse feeding and persistent upper airway obstruction than children without comorbidities [8]. For children with multiple comorbidities, one review found that these children had a significantly smaller improvement in their AHI than children without multiple comorbidities [11].

Complications after epiglottopexy are also rare, but because it is less commonly performed, outcomes data are limited. These complications are like those listed above for supraglottoplasty and include aspiration, dysphagia, cartilage damage, granuloma formation, and need for revision surgery. Given the role of the epiglottis in airway protection and swallowing, there is a concern for postoperative dysphagia or aspiration. In a series of five patients, Kanotra et al. studied the swallowing function following an epiglottopexy and found that it did not severely impact swallowing [29]. In a study by Baljosevic et al., 89% of children had preoperative dysphagia and symptoms of GERD ($n = 17$), and postoperatively following epiglottopexy, the dysphagia had resolved in all children and two children had continued GERD symptoms [26].

11.6 Current Gaps in Knowledge

There is much yet to be understood in regard to the impact of laryngomalacia or independent epiglottic collapse on pediatric OSA. Predictors of sleep-dependent laryngomalacia are not yet known. Further investigation is needed into risk factors for sleep-dependent laryngomalacia and whether congenital laryngomalacia carries an increased risk of developing sleep-dependent laryngomalacia in the future. Moreover, little is also known about the efficacy and long-term outcomes of supraglottoplasty or epiglottopexy for the treatment of pediatric sleep apnea and laryngomalacia. Many of the studies evaluating laryngomalacia and OSA are small, single center studies and there is a need for large, multicenter studies to further understand these diagnoses.

11.7 Summary

Overall, congenital laryngomalacia is a common cause of stridor in the neonate and typically presents with stridor with feeding and agitation. This is related to short aryepiglottic folds and an infantile, omega-shaped epiglottis. Sleep-state laryngomalacia is more commonly seen in older children and requires DISE for diagnoses. Both can be important contributors to pediatric OSA and children with persistent OSA following tonsillectomy and adenoidectomy should be evaluated for sleep-dependent laryngomalacia. Most patients with congenital laryngomalacia will improve with conservative measures over time. For those children with sleep-dependent laryngomalacia and children with severe congenital laryngomalacia, surgical management is indicated which can include supraglottoplasty, epiglottopexy, and rarely, tracheostomy.

References

1. Mitchell RB, Archer SM, Ishman SL, Rosenfeld RM, Coles S, Finestone SA, et al. Clinical practice guideline: tonsillectomy in children (update). Otolaryngol Head Neck Surg. 2019;160(1_suppl):S1–S42. https://doi.org/10.1177/0194599818801757.
2. Sterni LM, Tunkel DE. Obstructive sleep apnea in children: an update. Pediatr Clin North Am. 2003;50(2):427–43. https://doi.org/10.1016/s0031-3955(03)00037-3.
3. Friedman M, Wilson M, Lin HC, Chang HW. Updated systematic review of tonsillectomy and adenoidectomy for treatment of pediatric obstructive sleep apnea/hypopnea syndrome. Otolaryngol Head Neck Surg. 2009;140(6):800–8. https://doi.org/10.1016/j.otohns.2009.01.043.
4. Lee CH, Hsu WC, Chang WH, Lin MT, Kang KT. Polysomnographic findings after adenotonsillectomy for obstructive sleep apnoea in obese and non-obese children: a systematic review and meta-analysis. Clin Otolaryngol. 2016;41(5):498–510. https://doi.org/10.1111/coa.12549.
5. Marcus CL, Moore RH, Rosen CL, Giordani B, Garetz SL, Taylor HG, et al. A randomized trial of adenotonsillectomy for childhood sleep apnea. N Engl J Med. 2013;368(25):2366–76. https://doi.org/10.1056/NEJMoa1215881.

6. Verkest V, Verhulst S, Van Hoorenbeeck K, Vanderveken O, Saldien V, Boudewyns A. Prevalence of obstructive sleep apnea in children with laryngomalacia and value of polysomnography in treatment decisions. Int J Pediatr Otorhinolaryngol. 2020;137:110255. https://doi.org/10.1016/j.ijporl.2020.110255.
7. Rutter MJ. Evaluation and management of upper airway disorders in children. Semin Pediatr Surg. 2006;15(2):116–23. https://doi.org/10.1053/j.sempedsurg.2006.02.009.
8. Thompson DM. Abnormal sensorimotor integrative function of the larynx in congenital laryngomalacia: a new theory of etiology. Laryngoscope. 2007;117(6 Pt 2 Suppl 114):1–33. https://doi.org/10.1097/MLG.0b013e31804a5750.
9. Giannoni C, Sulek M, Friedman EM, Duncan NO 3rd. Gastroesophageal reflux association with laryngomalacia: a prospective study. Int J Pediatr Otorhinolaryngol. 1998;43(1):11–20. https://doi.org/10.1016/s0165-5876(97)00151-1.
10. Amin MR, Isaacson G. State-dependent laryngomalacia. Ann Otol Rhinol Laryngol. 1997;106(11):887–90. https://doi.org/10.1177/000348949710601101.
11. Chan DK, Truong MT, Koltai PJ. Supraglottoplasty for occult laryngomalacia to improve obstructive sleep apnea syndrome. Arch Otolaryngol Head Neck Surg. 2012;138(1):50–4. https://doi.org/10.1001/archoto.2011.233.
12. Boudewyns A, Verhulst S, Maris M, Saldien V, Van de Heyning P. Drug-induced sedation endoscopy in pediatric obstructive sleep apnea syndrome. Sleep Med. 2014;15(12):1526–31. https://doi.org/10.1016/j.sleep.2014.06.016.
13. Thevasagayam M, Rodger K, Cave D, Witmans M, El-Hakim H. Prevalence of laryngomalacia in children presenting with sleep-disordered breathing. Laryngoscope. 2010;120(8):1662–6. https://doi.org/10.1002/lary.21025.
14. Wilcox LJ, Bergeron M, Reghunathan S, Ishman SL. An updated review of pediatric drug-induced sleep endoscopy. Laryngoscope Investig Otolaryngol. 2017;2(6):423–31. https://doi.org/10.1002/lio2.118.
15. Sessler CN, Grap MJ, Ramsay MA. Evaluating and monitoring analgesia and sedation in the intensive care unit. Crit Care. 2008;12(Suppl 3):S2. https://doi.org/10.1186/cc6148.
16. Mahmoud M, Radhakrishman R, Gunter J, Sadhasivam S, Schapiro A, McAuliffe J, et al. Effect of increasing depth of dexmedetomidine anesthesia on upper airway morphology in children. Paediatr Anaesth. 2010;20(6):506–15. https://doi.org/10.1111/j.1460-9592.2010.03311.x.
17. Hartl TT, Chadha NK. A systematic review of laryngomalacia and acid reflux. Otolaryngol Head Neck Surg. 2012;147(4):619–26. https://doi.org/10.1177/0194599812452833.
18. Brockbank J, Astudillo CL, Che D, Tanphaichitr A, Huang G, Tomko J, et al. Supplemental oxygen for treatment of infants with obstructive sleep apnea. J Clin Sleep Med. 2019;15(8):1115–23. https://doi.org/10.5664/jcsm.7802.
19. Hawkins SM, Jensen EL, Simon SL, Friedman NR. Correlates of pediatric CPAP adherence. J Clin Sleep Med. 2016;12(6):879–84. https://doi.org/10.5664/jcsm.5892.
20. Denoyelle F, Mondain M, Gresillon N, Roger G, Chaudre F, Garabedian EN. Failures and complications of supraglottoplasty in children. Arch Otolaryngol Head Neck Surg. 2003;129(10):1077–80.; ; discussion 80. https://doi.org/10.1001/archotol.129.10.1077.
21. Tunkel DE, Hotchkiss KS, Ishman S, Brown D. Supraglottoplasty in infants using sinus instruments. Medscape J Med. 2008;10(11):269.
22. Camacho M, Dunn B, Torre C, Sasaki J, Gonzales R, Liu SY, et al. Supraglottoplasty for laryngomalacia with obstructive sleep apnea: a systematic review and meta-analysis. Laryngoscope. 2016;126(5):1246–55. https://doi.org/10.1002/lary.25827.
23. Lee CF, Hsu WC, Lee CH, Lin MT, Kang KT. Treatment outcomes of supraglottoplasty for pediatric obstructive sleep apnea: a meta-analysis. Int J Pediatr Otorhinolaryngol. 2016;87:18–27. https://doi.org/10.1016/j.ijporl.2016.05.015.
24. Zalzal HG, Davis K, Carr MM, Coutras S. Epiglottopexy with or without aryepiglottic fold division: comparing outcomes in the treatment of pediatric obstructive sleep apnea. Am J Otolaryngol. 2020;41(4):102478. https://doi.org/10.1016/j.amjoto.2020.102478.

25. Oomen KP, Modi VK. Epiglottopexy with and without lingual tonsillectomy. Laryngoscope. 2014;124(4):1019–22. https://doi.org/10.1002/lary.24279.
26. Baljosevic I, Minic P, Trajkovic G, Markovic-Sovtic G, Radojicic B, Sovtic A. Surgical treatment of severe laryngomalacia: six month follow-up. Pediatr Int. 2015;57(6):1159–63. https://doi.org/10.1111/ped.12706.
27. Fajdiga I, Beden AB, Krivec U, Iglic C. Epiglottic suture for treatment of laryngomalacia. Int J Pediatr Otorhinolaryngol. 2008;72(9):1345–51. https://doi.org/10.1016/j.ijporl.2008.05.009.
28. Reddy DK, Matt BH. Unilateral vs. bilateral supraglottoplasty for severe laryngomalacia in children. Arch Otolaryngol Head Neck Surg. 2001;127(6):694–9. https://doi.org/10.1001/archotol.127.6.694.
29. Kanotra SP, Givens VB, Keith B. Swallowing outcomes after pediatric epiglottopexy. Eur Arch Otorhinolaryngol. 2020;277(1):285–91. https://doi.org/10.1007/s00405-019-05664-6.

The Role of Obesity in Epiglottis Collapse

12

Christel A. L. de Raaff

12.1 Obesity

Obesity represents a certain amount of excessive adipose tissue, negatively affecting health status, life expectancy, and medical outcomes. The exact definition is formulated with the body mass index (BMI), a ratio of weight in relation to length. It can be calculated by dividing someone's weight in kilograms by his or her height in meters squared (kg/m^2) and enables us to categorize a person as underweight, normal weight, overweight, obese, morbidly obese, or super obese (Table 12.1). Obesity is defined as a BMI $\geq$ 30 kg/m^2. The basis of the BMI was formulated by Adolphe Quetelet between 1830 and 1850 when interest in an index measuring weight came with increasing obesity [1]. Due to its simplicity, the BMI has become a universally used metric for weight.

The overall global population is progressively affected by obesity. Between 1975 and 2016, the prevalence nearly tripled. Worldwide, more than 1.9 billion and over 650 million adults were overweight and obese, respectively. This represents a prevalence of 39% and 13% of the worldwide population [2].

By the year 2030, the number of obese US adults is expected to rise to 40–50% [2]. Knowing that obesity causes multi-organ diseases and decreased life expectancy, this is a threatening perspective for global health.

C. A. L. de Raaff (✉)
Department of Albert Schweitzer Hospital, Dordrecht, The Netherlands

M. Delakorda, N. de Vries (eds.), *The Role of Epiglottis in Obstructive Sleep Apnea*, https://doi.org/10.1007/978-3-031-34992-8_12

Table 12.1 Body Mass Index and weight categories

Body Mass Index (kg/m^2)	Weight category
< 18	Underweight
18–24.9	Normal weight
25–29.9	Overweight
30–34.9	Obesity
35–49.9	Morbid obesity
≥ 50	Super obesity

12.2 Obesity and Obstructive Sleep Apnea (OSA)

Excessive adipose tissue negatively affects the function of organ systems. Anatomical, cardiovascular, metabolic, neuromuscular, and hormonal changes all occur due to obesity. Many of these changes are associated with the presence of obstructive sleep apnea (OSA), being the most prevalent sleep disordered breathing problem and affecting more obese individuals than type II diabetes, hypertension, and dyslipidemia [3].

The pathogenesis of OSA is multifactorial and complex. Local anatomy, obesity, gender, age, sleep position, and sedative drugs are examples of risk factors for OSA and its severity. The prevalence of OSA increases with BMI and age and is more common in men than women. Around 2% and 4% of middle aged women and men, respectively, suffer from OSA in the general population [4]. In morbidly obese individuals, the prevalence increases up to 70% [5]. One of the hypothesis explaining obesity as an important risk factor for OSA is that fat deposition results in diminished pharyngeal airway size, thereby increasing the risk of apneas.

12.3 Fat Tissue in the Pharyngeal Airway

The pharyngeal airway is the upper part of the airway located anteriorly of the cervical spine and between the maxillary and mandibular plane. Besides these bony structures, it is also surrounded by soft tissues including the soft palate, tongue, tonsils, and pharyngeal fat pads. Excessive adipose tissue may be deposited in all parts of these soft tissues, resulting in an increased volume and hence reduced pharyngeal airway or even airway collapse.

Few studies investigating this matter using magnetic resonance imaging (MRI) found a greater amount of fat at several levels surrounding the collapsible segment of the pharynx in patients with OSA.

In 1989, Horner et al. performed MRI in six obese patients with OSA and five weight-matched controls without OSA. Fat deposits were found at all levels of the airway, but were significantly greater posterolateral at the level of the soft palate in OSA patients [6]. In another MRI study of 30 patients with a range of OSA severity and obesity, a significant correlation was found between the AHI as measured with polysomnography and the size of the region enclosed by the mandible [7]. Schwab et al. compared MRI data of 48 OSA patients with data from 48 controls who were matched for gender, age, and ethnicity. Enlargement of the soft tissues at all upper airway levels was observed in OSA patients, yet multivariable analysis identified pharyngeal wall volume and tongue volume as independent risk factors for OSA [8]. A Chinese study group also found a greater thickness of the lateral and posterior pharyngeal wall in the epiglottal region in 18 OSA patients when compared with 19 age-matched controls [9].

The role of obesity and tongue volume was demonstrated by Nashi et al. who assessed fat depositions within the tongue musculature using autopsy specimens from the general population. The amount of fat tissue in the posterior part of the tongue was greater than the anterior part (30% vs. 10%) and was positively correlated with BMI [10].

Although the role of BMI in the development in OSA is well known, excessive fat tissue in the upper airway causing OSA may also be present in normal weight subjects. Mortimore and colleagues compared excess fat deposition between nine obese OSA patients, nine non-obese OSA patients, and nine non-obese non-OSA patients. MRI data showed a 10% and 28% greater neck tissue volume in non-obese OSA and obese-OSA patients, respectively, when compared to control subjects. This excess fat was localized in the anterolateral part of the upper airway [11].

12.4 Role of BMI in Epiglottis Shape

The posterior surface of the epiglottis is slightly concave. It is hypothesized that deformity occurs due to pressure of the excessive fat deposits in the soft tissues surrounding the pharyngeal airway. One study demonstrated the effect of BMI in epiglottis shape changes [12]. Gazayerli and colleagues performed esophagogastroduodenoscopy in more than 50 patients with a varying BMI between 21 and 61 kg/m^2 and noticed a positive correlation between BMI and the extent of epiglottis concavity. Total closure of the epiglottis was observed in extreme cases. The authors evaluated the degree of concavity by drawing lines from the edge points of the epiglottis and measuring the angle between these lines. This angle was 100° in a patient with a BMI of 28 kg/m^2, and 360° in a patient with a BMI of 62 kg/m^2 (Fig. 12.1). This deformity appears to improve after weight loss as a change in epiglottis change was observed in patients who achieved weight loss after laparoscopic gastric banding [12].

However, conclusions on epiglottis convexity should be taken with precautions. This study published an observation rather than a scientific study on the omega shape and the cause of its changes. No scientific background has been published on this matter.

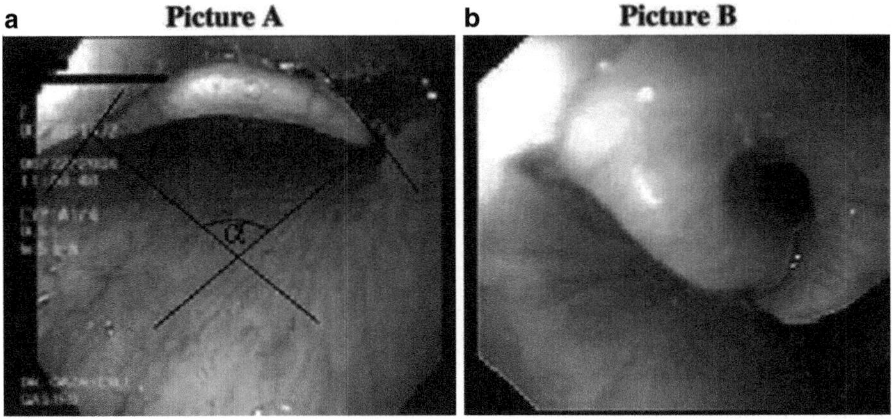

Fig. 12.1 Comparison between the epiglottis of a patient with a BMI of 28 (**a**) and that of a patient with a BMI of 62 (**b**). (Source: Gazayerli et al. Obesity Surgery 2006)

12.5 BMI and Epiglottis Collapse

The gold standard for diagnosing OSA is polysomnography (PSG). Levels of obstruction can be evaluated by MRI, computed tomography (CT), or drug-induced sleep endoscopy (DISE) (Chap. 9). Nowadays, DISE is frequently used in guiding the surgical management of upper airway obstruction and its findings are often graded using VOTE (Velum, Oropharynx, Tongue base and Epiglottis).

Several studies have investigated the role of BMI in epiglottis obstruction. One of the first studies was published by Kuo et al., who performed drug-induced sleep CT in 35 patients with a median AHI of 55.4/h and a median BMI of 26.9 kg/m^2. Epiglottis collapse (EC) was seen in twelve patients (34%). BMI was not different between patients with and without EC [13]. Two studies performed DISE in patients diagnosed with OSA by PSG and evaluated the prevalence and type of EC [14, 15]. Ravesloot and de Vries included 100 consecutive patients with a mean BMI of 27.4 kg/m^2 (SD 4.1). EC was found in 38% of patients; 12% partial anteroposterior (A-P), 16% complete A-P, 2% partial lateral, and 8% complete lateral [14]. In the study of Lan et al. ($N = 64$, mean BMI 27,6 kg/m^2 SD 4.7), EC occurred in 42.2% of patients; 12.5% partial A-P, 26.6% complete A-P, 0% partial lateral, and 3.1% complete lateral [15]. No difference in BMI was found in patients with epiglottis obstruction in both studies. Similar results were published recently in two retrospective studies using DISE after PSG. The first divided patients in to three groups: normal- or underweight ($N = 24$), overweight ($N = 56$), or obese ($N = 31$). Overweight and obese patients showed increasing grades of obstruction at the velum and oropharynx, whereas decreasing grades were noticed at the tongue base and epiglottis [16]. In a large retrospective study of 627 patients, patients were classified in four BMI groups: BMI < 20.75 kg/m^2 (group 1, $n = 45$), BMI 20.75–23 kg/m^2 (group 2, $n = 79$), BMI 23–25 kg/m^2 (group 3, $n = 151$), and BMI >25 kg/m^2 (group 4, $n = 352$). EC occurred in 127 patients (20%). Again, no difference was found between BMI groups [17].

A study that reports other findings was the study by Vroegop et al. who performed DISE after PSG in 1249 patients. Hypopharyngeal collapse including the epiglottis occurred in 38.7% and was more prevalent in the obese population (BMI $\geq$ 30 kg/m^2). BMI was positively correlated with the occurrence of partial lateral, complete concentric, and complete lateral hypopharyngeal collapse. However, the exact role of the epiglottis in these hypopharyngeal collapses was not described [18].

In contrast, Sung et al. retrospectively reviewed 590 patients with complete PSG and DISE data and found a negative correlation of the epiglottis with the BMI ($p < 0.01$), also after adjusting for AHI [19]. This was also shown in the study of Kim and colleagues ($n = 224$), showing a lower BMI in the epiglottic collapse [20].

With these results, it can be concluded that increasing BMI is no risk factor for epiglottis obstruction. Most studies found no role; two found a negative correlation of BMI and EC. As sleep surgery has shown not to be successful in morbidly obese patients, these studies performing DISE prior to sleep surgery included patients with lower BMIs. In order to provide a full overview of the role of obesity in EC, it would be interesting to evaluate the occurrence of EC in the morbidly obese population (BMI > 35 kg/m^2) with OSA.

References

1. Quetelet, Adolphe. Most widely held works by Adolphe Quetelet. 1796–1874. http://www.worldcat.org/identities/lccn-n50050539/.
2. Obesity and overweight. Key facts. Quetelet, Adolphe 1796–1874. Most widely held works by Adolphe Quetelet. http://www.worldcat.org/identities/lccn-n50050539/.
3. White DP. The pathogenesis of obstructive sleep apnea: advances in the past 100 years. Am J Respir Cell Mol Biol. 2006;34(1):1–6.
4. Malhotra A, White DP. Obstructive sleep apnoea. Lancet. 2002;360(9328):237–45.
5. De Raaff CAL, Pierik AS, Coblijn UK, De Vries N, Bonjer HJ, Van Wagensveld BA. Value of routine polysomnography in bariatric surgery. Surg Endosc. 2017;31(1):245–8.
6. Horner RL, Mohiaddin RH, Lowell DG, et al. Sites and sizes of fat deposits around the pharynx in obese patients with obstructive sleep apnea and weight matched controls. Eur Respir J. 1989;2:613–22.
7. Shelton KE, Gay SB, Hollowell DE, et al. Mandible enclosure of upper airway and weight in obstructive sleep apnea. Am Rev Respir Dis. 1993;148:195–200.
8. Schwab RJ, Pasirtstein M, Pierson R, et al. Identificatin of upper airway anatomic risk factors for obstructive sleep apnea with volumetric mangetic resonance imaging. Am J Respir Crit Care Med. 2003;18:522–30.
9. Lin Z, Zhang H, Wang T, Li C, Bai Z. The upper airway MRI of obstructive sleep apnea patients. Zhonghua Er Bi Yan Hou Ke Za Zhi. 2000;35(1):51–4.
10. Nashi N, Kang S, Barkdull GC, et al. Lingual fat at autopsy. Laryngoscopy. 2007;117:1467–73.
11. Mortimore IL, Marshall I, Wraith PK, et al. Neck and total body fat deposition in nonobese and obese patients with sleep apnea compared with that in control subjects. Am J Respir Crit Car Med. 1998;157:280–3.
12. Gazayerli M, Bliebel W, Elhorr A, Elakkary E. The shape of the epiglottis reflects improvement in upper airway obstruction after weight loss. Obes Surg. 2006;16(7):945–7.
13. Kuo I, Hsin L, Lee L, et al. Prediction of epiglottic collapse in obstructive sleep apnea patients: epiglottic length. Nat Sci Sleep. 2021;13:1985–92.

14. Ravesloot MJ, de Vries N. One hundred consecutive patients undergoing drug-induced sleep endoscopy: results and evaluation. Laryngoscope. 2011;121(12):2710–6.
15. Lan MC, Lui SYC, Lan MY, Modi R, Capasso R. Lateral pharyngeal wall collapse associated with hypoxemia in obstructive sleep apnea. Laryngoscope. 2015;125(10):2408–12.
16. Wong SJ, Luitje ME, Karelsky S. Patterns of obstruction on DISE in adults with obstructive sleep apnea change with BMI. Laryngoscope. 2021;131(1):224–9.
17. Woo HJ, Lim JH, Ahn JC, et al. Characteristics of obstructive sleep apnea patients with a low body mass index: emphasis on the obstruction site determined by drug-induced sleep endoscopy. Clin Exp Otorhinolaryngol. 2020;13(4):415–21.
18. Vroegop AV, Vanderveken OM, Boudewyns AN, et al. Drug-induced sleep endoscopy in sleep-disordered breathing: report on 1,249 cases. Laryngoscope. 2014;124:797–802.
19. Sung CM, Tan SH, Shin MH, et al. The site of airway collapse in sleep apnea, its associations with disease severity and obesity, and implications for mechanical interventions. Am J Respir Crit Care Med. 2021;204(1):103–6.
20. Kim HY, Sung CM, Jan HB, Kim HC, Lim SC, Yang HC. Patients with epiglottic collapse showed less severe obstructive sleep apnea and good response to treatment other than continuous positive airway pressure: a case-control study of 224 patients. J Clin Sleep Med. 2021;17(3):413–9.

The Role of the Nose in Pharyngeal Obstructions

13

Thomas Verse

13.1 Introduction

Neither the generation of snoring sounds nor airway obstruction occur in the nose. Nevertheless, the nose is rarely lacking on the agendas of conferences and textbooks about sleep medicine. Already the often-cited Hippokrates (460–370 BC) described a causal connection between nasal polyps and non-restorative sleep. As early as 1581, Levinus Lemnious first mentioned non-restorative sleep caused by oral breathing in supine position [1]. First modern scientific reports date back to the end of the nineteenth century (Table 13.1). In 1898, Wells [2] reported an improvement of vigilance in 8 out of 10 patients following nasal septoplasty.

Looking on modern scientific reports, Stadling et al. [3] investigated 1002 middle aged men, 17% snored. Risk factors for snoring were increased neck circumference, smoking and nasal congestion. Deegan et al. [4] looked for the prevalence of nasal septal deviation in snorers and non-snoring control. Prevalence was found to be 15% in snorers and 13% in non-snorers. Young and colleagues [5] described a three-fold increase of snoring and daytime sleepiness in patients with self-reported nasal congestion. Magliulo et al. [6] examined 50 patients with obstructive sleep apnoea (OSA), only 20% showed no nasal pathology. Nasal obstruction was found in 70% of the patients, allergic and non-allergic rhinitis in 18% and 26%, respectively.

All these data implicate a causal connection of impaired nasal breathing, snoring, daytime fatigue and obstructive sleep apnoea, and thus pharyngeal and maybe laryngeal obstruction.

T. Verse (✉)
Department for Otorhinolaryngology, Head and Neck Surgery, Asklepios Klinikum Hamburg, Asklepios Campus, Hamburg, Germany

Semmelweis University, Budapest, Hungary
e-mail: t.verse@asklepios.com

M. Delakorda, N. de Vries (eds.), *The Role of Epiglottis in Obstructive Sleep Apnea*, https://doi.org/10.1007/978-3-031-34992-8_13

Table 13.1 First reports about the influence of nasal breathing on sleep and well-being

Author	Major Result
Hippocrates 460–370 BC	Nasal polyps are associated with restless sleep
Levinus 1581	Oral breathing in supine position causes unquiet sleep
Catlin 1861	First book: "The breath of life"
Catlin 1890	New edition: "Shut your mouth and save your life"
Guye 1889	Book "Shut your mouth and save your brain"
Cline 1892	Case report: Increase of daytime alertness after septoplasty
Wells 1898	First case series: Alertness increases after septoplasty ($N = 8/10$)

Both, during the awake state and during sleep, the nasal breathing is the physiological route of breathing [7, 8]. Under normal circumstances, less than 10% of human beings breath through their mouths. This makes the nose our major portal for inspired air and hence makes nasal pathology a significant cause for disturbance of the inspirational air flow [9, 10]. With this in mind, many people and physicians likewise assume that nasal pathology also plays a significant role in the pathophysiology of sleep-related breathing disorders (SDB).

In addition, many patients suffering from acute or chronic impairment of nasal breathing report a subjective detoriation of their individual sleep quality with consecutive daytime symptoms like fatigue, sleepiness, lack of concentration, etc. This in turn is leading to many rhinologists having to face expectations of their patients, that improvement of nasal obstruction not only solves daytime symptoms but also reduces the severity of SDB in their daily practice.

This chapter focuses on the relationship between nasal obstruction and sleep quality, as well as on the relationship between nasal obstruction and severity of SDB. As this book deals with the role of the epiglottis in sleep disordered breathing, this chapter tries to find information concerning the influence of nasal breathing on the epiglottis and vice versa.

13.2 Pathophysiology

13.2.1 Nasal Breathing During the Awake State

In the awake state, about 50–60% of the resistance of the complete upper airway is allotted to the nose [11]. This means the biggest part of the entire upper airway resistance is located in the nose. As stated above, the nose can be regarded as the physiological breathing path. In healthy, awake and upright sitting subjects, as much as 92% of the entire airway resistance was found in the nose and only 8% in the oral section of the upper airway [12].

The body position has a considerable influence on nasal resistance. Nasal resistance (Rn) increases if the body position changes from sitting to supine. A shift as little as 10° leads to a significant alteration of Rn. These changes were even more clearly seen in patients with allergic or acute rhinitis as compared to a control group [13].

13.2.2 Nasal Breathing During Sleep

Compared to being awake, Rn does not change if probants fall asleep [14], but the entire upper airway resistance increases distinctively. This implies an increased airway resistance within the pharyngeal and maybe laryngeal sections of the upper airway. In fact, during sleep the biggest part of the entire upper airway resistance is located in the pharyngeal sections. There is no information available that deals with the role of the epiglottis. In other words, relevant changes regarding the entire upper airway resistance while falling asleep occur in the pharynx (and maybe larynx) and not in the nose.

13.2.3 How Can Nasal Obstruction Nonetheless Promote Upper Airway Collapse?

This important question is still open to debate and currently, there are 4 theories being discussed:

13.2.3.1 Starling Resistor

First of all, an increased Rn contributes to the entire resistance of the upper airway (R_{UA}). However, during sleep, Rn only represents a smaller part of $R_{UA.}$ This means that changes in Rn result in relatively slight changes in $R_{UA.}$

In contrast to the nose, the pharynx lacks bony or cartilageous structures to resist the negative pressure on inspiration. Hence, the pharynx is assumed to react like a Starling resistor. A higher preload in terms of an increased Rn is supposed to increase the negative pressure and therefore collapse during inspiration, resulting in an obstruction in the weakest segment of the chain, namely the pharynx. Investigations with unilateral nasal dressings were able to provoke some obstructive apnoea's in non-OSA patients, although the effects were not strong enough to induce a clinically significant obstructive sleep apnoea [15–17]. Another, very interesting study on that matter chose seasonal allergic rhinitis (AR) as a more physiological model for temporary nasal obstruction. Here, polysomnography showed significantly more obstructive breathing events during the season as compared to off-season [18]. Despite the reported result being statistically significant, looking at the absolute values (apnoea index: 0.7/h vs. 1.7/h) shows that this effect is not strong enough to induce clinically significant OSA.

Against the background of the reported data, it can be assumed that a partial nasal obstruction may worsen a preexisting OSA or annoying snoring, but based on the current evidence, it most unlikely represents a major factor in the pathogenesis of OSA.

Increase in Oral Breathing

In case the nose is completely blocked, a switch to oral breathing occurs. By blocking both nares in healthy subjects with a dressing, it could be shown that the critical collapse pressure (Pcrit) during sleep is significantly reduced [19]. A decreased

Pcrit in turn increases the likeliness of airway obstruction. In other words, increased oral breathing destabilises the upper airway. A similar study showed significantly increased upper airway resistance for oral compared with nasal breathing [20]. Two out of 10 healthy subjects developed a clinically significant OSA while their noses were completely occluded, while the other 8 subjects showed little or no changes [21] in their polysomnographies. Apparently, there is a subgroup of patients (20% in the before mentioned study) in which the change from nasal to oral breathing results in clinically notable consequences, while the majority of patients do not show considerable clinical changes. It could be discussed whether the relevant group of patients had either an already existing subclinical SDB or another underlying pathology, even with an open nasal airway.

Loss of Nasal Reflexes

Trigeminally mediated nasal reflexes are crucial to maintaining nasal patency. Several studies could show that local anaesthesia in the nose is able to induce both, central and obstructive, apnoeas [22, 23]. In the first-mentioned study, 3 out of 10 healthy subjects developed transient severe OSA after local anaesthesia in the nose. The other 7 patients did not show any change in their sleep parameters. Using placebo instead of local anaesthesia, no patient developed transient OSA. Additionally, there seems to be a subgroup of patients in which nasal reflexes play an important role in maintaining airway patency.

Nitrogen Monoxide (NO)

Nitric oxide (NO) is produced in significant quantity within the nose and the paranasal sinuses. With the nasal inspiratory airflow, it reaches the lower parts of the airway [24]. NO plays an important role as a bronchial dilator, thereby increasing arterial oxygen saturation [25]. In addition to this important mechanism, NO plays a role in maintaining muscle tone, the neuromuscular control of the pharynx, the respiratory drive, and the regulation of sleep. To our knowledge, a thorough and comprehensive assessment of the role of NO in the pathogenesis of sleep disordered breathing does not exist. To sum it up, nasal obstruction seems to be associated with snoring and apnoeas caused by pharyngeal obstructions. However, a direct correlation between nasal obstruction and the severity of SDB has not been found so far [26]. Currently, this leads to the conclusion that the nose only adds little to the severity of OSA in most patients.

Potential Causal Connection of Nasal Breathing and Epiglottic Obstruction in OSA

The question is, how can impaired nasal breathing lead to a laryngeal airway obstruction caused by the epiglottis? Unfortunately, to date there is almost no data in the literature to answer this question. We know that the epiglottis while asleep may fall back during inspiration causing a complete airway obstruction. We published our first case in a 71-year-old Caucasian male as early as 1999 [27]. This patient had an enlarged and lax epiglottis. This epiglottis appeared unstable in the video endoscopy, was sucked back the posterior wall of the hypopharynx during inspiration and finally obstructed the hypopharynx completely (Fig. 13.1). As a result, the patient was no longer able to accept his CPAP, as with increasing continuous positive airway pressure, the epiglottis was more and more pressed downwards and backwards to the larynx. In other words, the patient developed a secondary CPAP failure with increased AHI-values under PAP-treatment, although he was treated successfully with PAP for a couple of years. So, what changed? Beside the pinna of the ear, the epiglottis is the only organ of the head and neck exclusively consisting of elastic cartilage. Pellnitz 1961 [28] has shown a significant increase in the length, breadth and weight of the epiglottis in males with increasing age, while females show reductions of the same parameters. A histological study of 500 epiglottis specimens obtained at autopsy showed that size increase in male epiglottis is due to the secondary intercellular deposits of by-products of metabolism. This probably reduces the stiffness of the epiglottis in the ageing male, which may increase the risk of airway obstruction during sleep at this level.

Can this context hypothesise a causal connection between impaired nasal breathing and epiglottic obstruction, at least in elder male patients or patients with for other reasons lax epiglottis?

As stated above, impaired nasal breathing implies a higher preload in terms of an increased Rn, and thus is supposed to increase the negative pressure during inspiration within the hypopharynx. The increased negative pressure may result in an epiglottic collapse in patients with a lax epiglottis.

Secondly, mouth breathing narrows the hypopharyngeal section of the upper airway as the tongue moves backwards if the mouth is opened. This means that the upper margin of the epiglottis approximates the posterior pharyngeal wall. This fact again may facilitate epiglottic obstruction.

Thirdly, our case report shows that increasing ventilation pressure may worsen the epiglottic airway collapse. Nasal surgery can help to reduce effective PAP (see below), and might therefore help to avoid airway obstruction caused by the epiglottis.

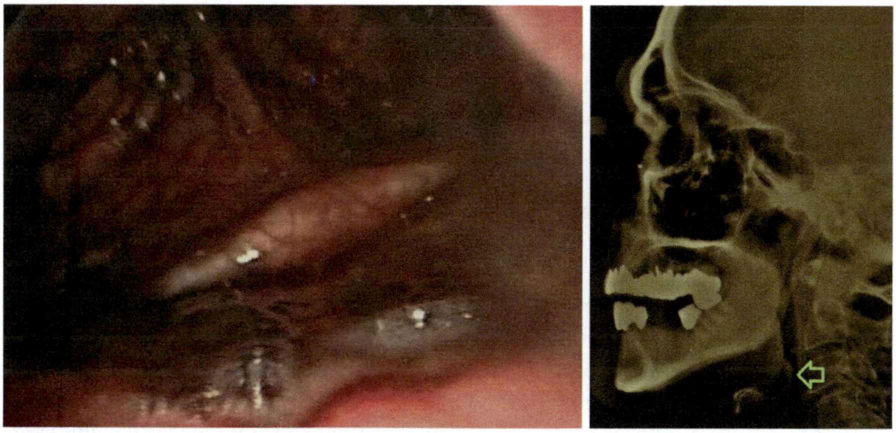

Fig. 13.1 Epiglottic collapse in a 71-year-old male patient. Left side: endoscopic view. Right side: X-ray showing enlarged epiglottis (arrow)

All these theories are speculative. Surprisingly, there is little information about the nose and epiglottis in the literature. Future research seems mandatory.

13.3 Clinical Results

The following data is based on two meta-analyses (published in German and English), which form the basis of the German S2E guideline "ENT-specific therapy of obstructive sleep apnoea in adults" [29] and the German S3 Guideline "The diagnosis and treatment of snoring in adults" [30]. These guidelines only include studies investigating nasal treatments. No other treatments without the nose had been done. Not all references can be mentioned in this book chapter. Please refer to the guidelines. More recent and additional references are given in the reference list below.

13.4 Results of Conservative Treatments

13.4.1 Medication

In a recent metanalysis [31] including 58 RCT, no significant effect of drugs on the severity of OSA in adults could be found. Altogether, a respectable 44 drugs and drug-combinations were investigated. These drugs can be classified into 7 pathomechanism groups. None of these focused on nasal obstruction.

The above-mentioned German guidelines include 2 case-control-series with only 22 patients. These 2 series focused on the effect of nasal decongestion (with xylometazoline) on sleep in patients with OSA. Both did not show any effect on sleep apnoea severity. However, one could report an improvement of sleep quality.

13.4.1.1 Anti-Allergic Treatments

Topical steroids improve both, subjective and objective, quality of sleep in adults with an underlying AR. The amount of improvement significantly correlates with the width of the nasal airway. Two RCT's could show a significant reduction of apnoea-hypopnea-index (AHI) after treatment with several weeks of topical steroids, whilst patients treated with placebo did not show this effect. The effect however was limited to a decrease of 10–20% of the baseline AHI.

In children, a recent Cochrane review [32] detected 5 RCT's (3 using topical steroids and 2 based on Montelucast). All studies could show the superiority of verum versus placebo with regards to objective polysomnographic parameters like AHI, oxygen desaturation index (ODI), respiratory arousal index and nadir oxygen saturation. Again, these effects are highly significant, but in most cases not sufficient to achieve cure of the underlying OSA. Another metanalysis [33], including 5 RCT (Montelucast with or without additional topical steroids), describes the same effects in altogether 166 kids.

Present data prove that anti-allergic treatments may decrease the severity of OSA. One question left unanswered in our knowledge is the duration of these effects after ceasing the anti-allergic treatment.

13.4.2 Nasal Dilators

These can be divided into external (plasters) and internal nasal dilators. The German guideline [29] included data of 194 patients (11 studies) under this category. A recent metanalysis [34] included 147 patients (9 studies). Both metanalysis were not able to find any significant effects of nasal dilators on OSA severity. Two included studies provide additional information on subjective outcome. In both studies, patients significantly benefited from the nasal dilation in terms of reduction of daytime sleepiness although their objective AHI did not change.

Focussing on simple snoring, a number of clinical trials indicate nasal dilators having an effect on snoring [30]. A most recent study [35] including 70 simple snorers did not show any effect of an external nasal dilator on objective snoring parameters. However, as side effects are limited, the German guideline recommends a trial with a nasal dilator for the treatment of simple snoring. There is some trial data indicating that a positive effect of nasal dilators can predict the effect of nasal surgery. In our daily practice, we use nasal dilators in this indication with relatively good results.

13.5 Results of Surgical Treatments

13.5.1 Nasal Surgery for OSA

The metanalysis conducted for the German guideline identified 28 studies including 717 patients having isolated nasal surgery for the treatment of OSA. All studies provided pre- and postoperative polysomnographic data. Since then, a further 4 articles on that topic could be identified [36–39]. All but 5 studies are case-series with a low grade of evidence. An additional most recently published study [40] adds data of 35 patients with and without AR. Table 13.2 summarises the data. Putting all data together, on average the AHI was reduced from 30.4 to 27.5 breathing events per hour of sleep. Only 8 out of 32 studies described a statistically significant decrease of the AHI. This result is in accordance with data that additional nasal surgery does not improve the success rates of multi-level surgery concepts for treating OSA [41]. However, many of the cited studies include individuals that substantially benefited from isolated nasal surgery in terms of their apnoea-hypopnea-index (AHI). The most recent study [40] included 8 patients with and 27 patients without AR. The subgroup of AR-patients profited much more from nasal septoplasty. The surgical success rate was given as 50% (4/8) in patients with AR and only 3.7% (1/27) in patients without AR.

Table 13.2 Effect of isolated nasal surgery on AHI and ESS

Author	*N*	Follow-up	AHI pre	AHI post	P value	ESS pre	ESS post	P value	EBM
Rubin AH et al. 1983	9	1–6	37.8	26.7	< 0.05	No data	No data		4
Dayal VS, Phillipson EA 1985	6	4–44	46.8	28.2	n.s.	No data	No data		4
Caldarelli DD et al. 1985	23	No data	44.2	41.5	n.s.	No data	No data		4
Aubert-Tulkens G et al. 1989	2	2–3	47.5	48.5	–	No data	No data		4
Sériès F et al. 1992	20	2–3	39.8	36.8	n.s.	No data	No data		4
Sériès F et al. 1993	14	2–3	17.8	16	n.s.	No data	No data		4
Utley DS et al. 1997	4	No data	11.9	27	–	7.8	6.8	n.s.	4
Verse T et al. 1998	2	3–4	14	57.7	–	6	12	n.s.	4
Friedman M et al. 2000	22	> 1.5	31.6	39.5	n.s.	No data	No data		4
Kalam I 2002	21	No data	14	11	< 0.05	No data	No data		4
Verse T et al. 2002	26	3–50	31.6	28.9	n.s.	11.9	7.7	< 0.001	4
Kim ST et al. 2004	21	1	39	29	<0.0001	No data	No data		4
Balcerzak J et al. 2004	22	2	48.1	48.8	n.s.	No data	No data		4
Nakata S et al. 2005	12	No data	55.9	47.8	n.s.	11.7	3.3	< 0.045	4
Virkkula P et al. 2006	40	2–6	13.6	14.9	n.s.	No data	No data		4
Koutsourelakis I et al. 2008	27	3–4	31.5	31.5	n.s.	13.4	11.7	< 0.01	2b
Li HY et al. 2008	51	3	37.4	38.1	n.s.	10.0	8.0	< 0.001	4
Nakata S et al. 2008	49	No data	49.6	42.5	n.s.	10.6	4.5		4
Morinaga M et al. 2009	35	No data	43.5	38.6	n.s.	No data	No data		4
Tosun F et al. 2009	27	3	6.7	5.6	n.s.	9.4	4.1	< 0.01	4
Li HY et al. 2009	44	3	36.4	37.5	n.s.	10.6	7.6	< 0.05	3b
Bican A et al. 2010	20	3	43.1	24.6	<0.05	17.1	11.1	< 0.01	4
Choi JH et al. 2011	22	3	28.9	26.1	n.s.	8.8	6.3	< 0.001	4

(continued)

Table 13.2 (continued)

Author	*N*	Follow-up	AHI pre	AHI post	P value	ESS pre	ESS post	P value	EBM
Sufioglu M et al. 2012	28	3	32.5	32.4	n.s.	9.3	5.9	< 0.001	4
Victores AJ + Takashima M 2012	24	3	23.6	20.4	n.s.	12.3	6.6	< 0.05	4
Hu B et al. 2013	79	6	27.7	26.3	n.s.	No data	No data		3b
Poirier J et al. 2014	11	6	33.2	29.4	n.s.	No data	No data		4
Yalamanchali S et al. 2014	56	1.5	33.5	29.4	n.s.	No data	No data		4
Moxness MH et al. 2014	59	3	18.2	16.6	n.s.	10.7	8.9	< 0.001	3b
Park CY et al. 2014	25	2	23.9	12.2	< 0.05	9.7	5.8	< 0.05	4
Shuaib SW et al. 2015	26	4	24.7	16.0	< 0.05	11.5	7.5	= 0.003	4
Xiao Y et al. 2016	30	3	49.7	43.1	< 0.05	No data	No data		3b
Kim SD et al. 2021	35	6	28.5	18.5	< 0.001	7.9	5.3	< 0.001	3b
All	**892**	**1–44**	**30.44**	**27.52**		**10.82**	**6.71**		**B**

Obviously, it is not possible to successfully treat OSA in the vast majority of cases by only performing nasal surgery. Further reviews come to the same conclusion [10, 42, 43].

In contrast, focusing on subjective outcome parameters, nasal surgery has a huge impact on the patient's well-being. Altogether, 17 studies (481 patients) provide data concerning daytime sleepiness as measured with the Epworth Sleepiness Scale, ESS (Table 13.2). Mean ESS values decreased from 10.2 to 6.7. Similar results are shown by a metanalysis from Li and colleagues [42].

Other studies prove significant improvements to other parameters and dimensions of quality of life. Instruments that were used are the "Snore Outcome Survey" [44], the "SF-36" [45], the NOSE-questionnaire [46] and the Pittsburgh Sleep Quality Index [39] amongst other test instruments.

In summary, isolated nasal surgery rarely eliminates OSA completely. More recent studies show at least a limited effect on OSA severity. Maybe patients with AR benefit more. However, nasal surgery has various positive effects on the sleep quality. As patients with OSA often suffer from not-restorative sleep, many patients will benefit from nasal surgery. Another indication for nasal surgery is persisting daytime symptoms after objective relief of OSA (i.e. normalisation of the apnea-hypopnea-index and other polysomnographic parameters). To my personal belief, this fact is too often neglected in our daily practice.

Table 13.3 Effect of isolated nasal surgery on effective PAP (positive airway pressure)

Author	*N*	CPAP pre (cm H_2O)	CPAP post (cm H_2O)	p-Wert	EBM
Mayer-Brix J et al. 1989	3	9.7	6	No data	4
Friedman M et al. 2000	6	9.3	6.7	< 0.05	4
Dorn M et al. 2001	5	11.8	8.6	< 0.05	4
Masdon JL et al. 2004	35	9.7	8.9	n.s.	4
Nakata S et al. 2005	5	16.8	12	< 0.05	4
Zonato AI et al. 2006	17	12.4	10.2	< 0.001	4
Sofioglu M et al. 2012	28	11.2	10.4	n.s.	4
Poirier J et al. 2014	18	11.9	9.2	n.s.	4
All	**117**	**11.2**	**9.4**		**C**

13.5.2 Nasal Surgery and PAP

Nasal surgery proved to facilitate or even enable required PAP-treatments in patients with nasal pathologies [47, 48]. Current data show that the effective positive airway pressure can successfully be reduced by about 2 cm H_2O following nasal surgery (Table 13.3). As results in Table 13.3 show, these data are from non-controlled case series, hence the data need to be regarded as preliminary. Further scientific results may change this assessment.

A recent published series [49] of 14 patients with OSA showed that CPAP can safely be used in the very first night after nasal surgery. Adherence to PAP was reduced in the first week after surgery, but increased to preoperative values in the second week.

13.5.3 Nasal Surgery and Simple Snoring

The work on the German guideline on snoring in adults [30] detected a number of case control series, whereby the follow-up period was generally 6 months. A retrospective study compared the effectiveness of septoplasty and turbinoplasty with other surgical procedures for snoring, and a significant improvement in subjective snoring intensity was seen. Prospective case control series also demonstrated the effect of septoplasty alone on subjective, but not objective, snoring intensity. The results of the above-mentioned studies suggest that a surgical improvement in nasal airflow leads to a subjective reduction in snoring. Not surprisingly, possible side effects and complications of the procedure do not differ from nasal surgery for a primary rhinological indication.

Against the background of these data, the German guideline suggests to offer nasal surgery to patients with objective nasal pathology and a resulting subjective nasal breathing impairment. Due to a lack of evidence, no statement was made on the effectiveness of nasal surgery in snorers with no subjective nasal breathing impairment but objective nasal pathologies. Maybe nasal surgery can help in these cases, too.

13.6 Conclusion

While being awake, the nose contributes up to 60% and therefore plays a great role in the entire resistance of the upper airway; during sleep, the predominant part is contributed by the pharyngeal sections of the upper airway. This is why the nose does not change its resistance during transition from awake to sleep, while the resistance of the pharynx considerably increases. Surprisingly there is little in literature about the nose and epiglottis. Future research is requested.

Against this background it is not surprising that the solvation of nasal obstruction does not significantly affect the severity of OSA in most cases. However, there are exceptions to this rule. Snoring does improve by a certain extent. Patients suffering from allergic or acute rhinitis benefit from anti-allergic treatment.

In contrast to the relatively discrete objective changes in respiratory parameters, the benefit of nasal surgery with regard to the quality of sleep and daytime symptoms and hence quality of life are impressive. This applies to patients with sleep disordered breathing disorders as well for sleep-healthy subjects. In this respect, it should be considered to include sleep disorders caused by impaired nasal breathing into the International Classification of Sleep Disorders (ICSD), where they are not mentioned so far.

In any case, a treatment of nasal obstruction should be considered if a patient is either suffering from subjectively impaired nasal breathing or if his/her relevant daytime fatigue cannot be successfully treated otherwise.

References

1. Lemnious L. The touchstone of complexions. London: Fleetestreete; 1581.
2. Wells WA. Some nervous and mental manifestations occurring in connection with nasal disease. Am J Med Sci. 1898;116:677–92.
3. Stradling JR, Crosby JH, Payne CD. Self reported snoring and daytime sleepiness in men aged 35-65 years. Thorax. 1991;46:807–10.
4. Deegan PC, McNicholas WT. Predictive value of clinical features for the obstructive sleep apnoea syndrome. Eur Respir J. 1996;9:117–24.
5. Young T, Finn L, Palta M. Chronic nasal congestion at night is a risk factor for snoring in a population based cohort study. Arch Intern Med. 2001;161:1514–9.
6. Magliulo G, Iannella G, Ciofalo A, Polimeni A, de Vincentiis M, Pasquariello B, Montevecchi F, Vicini C. Nasal pathologies in patients with obstructive sleep apnoea. Acta Otorhinolaryngol Ital. 2019;39:250–6.
7. Ogura JH. Presidential address. Fundamental understanding of nasal obstruction. Laryngoscope. 1977;87:1225–32.
8. Niinimaa V, Cole P, Mintz S, Shephard RJ. Oronasal distribution of respiratory airflow. Respir Physiol. 1981;43:69–75.
9. Olsen KD, Kern EB, Westbrook PR. Sleep and breathing disturbance secondary to nasal obstruction. Otolaryngol Head Neck Surg. 1981;89:804–10.
10. Georgalas C. The role of the nose in snoring and obstructive sleep apnoea: an update. Eur Arch Otorhinolaryngol. 2011;268:1365–73.
11. Ferris BG Jr, Mead J, Opie LH. Partitioning of respiratory flow resistance in man. J Appl Physiol. 1964;19:653–8.

12. Fitzpatrick MF, Driver HS, Chatha N, Voduc N, Girard AM. Partitioning of inhaled ventilation between the nasal and oral routes during sleep in normal subjects. J Appl Physiol. 2003;94:883–90.
13. Rundcrantz H. Postural variations of nasal patency. Acta Otolaryngol. 1969;68:435–43.
14. Douglas NJ, White DP, Pickett CK, Weil JV, Zwillich CW. Respiration during sleep in normal man. Thorax. 1982;37:840–4.
15. Lavie P, Fischel N, Zomer J, Eliaschar I. The effects of partial and complete mechanical occlusion of the nasal passages on sleep structure and breathing in sleep. Acta Otolaryngol. 1983;95:161–6.
16. Suratt PM, Turner BL, Wilhoit SC. Effect of intranasal obstruction on breathing during sleep. Chest. 1986;90:324–9.
17. Miljeteig H, Hoffstein V, Cole P. The effect of unilateral and bilateral nasal obstruction on snoring and sleep apnea. Laryngoscope. 1992;102:1150–2.
18. McNicholas WT, Tarlo S, Cole P, Zamel N, Rutherford R, Griffin D, Phillipson EA. Obstructive apneas during sleep in patients with seasonal allergic rhinitis. Am Rev Respir Dis. 1982;126:625–8.
19. Meurice JC, Marc I, Carrier G, Sériès F. Effects of mouth opening on upper airway collapsibility in normal sleeping subjects. Am J Respir Crit Care Med. 1996;153:255–9.
20. Fitzpatrick MF, McLean H, Urton AM, Tan A, O'Donnell D, Driver HS. Effect of nasal or oral breathing route on upper airway resistance during sleep. Eur Respir J. 2003;22:827–32.
21. Zwillich CW, Pickett C, Hanson FN, Weil JV. Disturbed sleep and prolonged apnea during nasal obstruction in normal men. Am Rev Respir Dis. 1981;124:158–60.
22. White DP, Cadieux RJ, Lombard RM, Bixler EO, Kales A, Zwillich CW. The effects of nasal anesthesia on breathing during sleep. Am Rev Respir Dis. 1985;132:972–5.
23. McNicholas WT, Coffey M, McDonnell T, O'Regan R, Fitzgerald MX. Upper airway obstruction during sleep in normal subjects after selective topical oropharyngeal anesthesia. Am Rev Respir Dis. 1987;135:1316–9.
24. Djupesland PG, Chatkin JM, Qian W, Cole P, Zamel N, McClean P, Furlott H, Haight JS. Aerodynamic influences on nasal nitric oxide output measurements. Acta Otolaryngol. 1999;119:479–85.
25. Blitzer ML, Lee SD, Creager MA. Endothelium-derived nitric oxide mediates hypoxic vasodilation of resistance vessels in humans. Am J Phys. 1996;271:H1182–5.
26. Leitzen KP, Brietzke SE, Lindsay RW. Correleation between nasal anatomy and objective obstructive sleep apnea severity. Otolaryngol Head Neck Surg. 2014;150:325–31.
27. Verse T, Pirsig W. Age-related changes in the epiglottis causing failure of nasal CPAP therapy. J Laryngol Otol. 1999;113:1022–5.
28. Pellnitz D. Über den durch das Altern bedingten Gestaltswandel der menschlichen epiglottis. Arch Ohren Nasen Kehlkopfheilkd. 1961;178:350–4.
29. Verse T, Dreher A, Heiser C, Herzog M, Maurer JT, Pirsig W, Rohde K, Rothmeier N, Sauter A, Steffen A, Wenzel S, Stuck BA. S2e-guideline: ENT-specific therapy of obstructive sleep apnea in adults. Sleep Breath. 2016;20:1301–11.
30. Stuck BA, Hofauer B. The diagnosis and treatment of snoring in adults. Dtsch Arztebl Int. 2019;116:817–24.
31. Gaisl T, Haile SR, Thiel S, Osswald M, Kohler M. Efficacy of pharmacotherapy for OSA in adults: a systematic review and network meta-analysis. Sleep Med Rev. 2019;46:74–86.
32. Kuhle S, Urschitz MS. Anti-inflammatory medications for obstructive sleep apnea in children. Cochrane Database Syst Rev. 2011;19:CD007074.
33. Liming BJ, Ryan M, Mack D, Ahmad I, Camacho M. Montelukast and nasal corticosteroids to treat pediatric obstructive sleep apnea: a systematic review and meta-analysis. Otolaryngol Head Neck Surg. 2019;160:594–602.
34. Camacho M, Malu OO, Kram YA, Nigam G, Riaz M, Song SA, Tolisano AM, Kushida CA. Nasal dilators (breathe right strips and NoZovent) for snoring and OSA: a systematic review and meta-analysis. Pulm Med. 2016;2016:4841310.

35. Wheatley JR, Amis TC, Lee SA, Ciesla R, Shanga G. Objective and subjective effects of a prototype nasal dilator strip on sleep in subjects with chronic nacturnal congestion. Adv Ther. 2019;36:1657–71.
36. Moxness MH, Nordgard S. An observational cohort study of the effects of septoplasty with or without inferior turbinate reduction in patients with obstructive sleep apnea. BMC Ear Nose Throat Disord. 2014;14:11.
37. Park CY, Hong JH, Lee JH, Lee KE, Cho HS, Lim SJ, Kwak JW, Kim KS, Kim HJ. Clinical effect of surgical correction for nasal pathology on the treatment of obstructive sleep apnea syndrome. PLoS One. 2014;9:e98765.
38. Shuaib SW, Undavia S, Lin J, Johnson CM, Stupak HD. Can functional septothinoplasty independently treat obstructive sleep apnea? Plast Reconstr Surg. 2015;135:1554–65.
39. Xiao Y, Han D, Zang H, Wang D. The effectiveness of nasal surgery on psychological symptoms in patients with obstructive sleep apnea ans nasal obstruction. Acta Otolaryngol. 2016;136:626–32.
40. Kim SD, Jung DW, Lee JW, Park JH, Mun SJ, Cho KS. Relationship between allergic rhinitis and nasal surgery success in patients with obstructive sleep apnea. Am J Otolaryngol Head Neck Surg. 2021;42:103079.
41. Verse T, Baisch A, Maurer JT, Stuck BA, Hörmann K. Multilevel surgery for obstructive sleep apnea: short-term results. Otolaryngol Head Neck Surg. 2006;134:571–7.
42. Li HY, Wang PC, Chen YP, Lee LA, Fang TJ, Lin HC. Critical appraisal and meta-analysis of nasal surgery for obstructive sleep apnea. Am J Rhinol Allergy. 2011;25:45–9.
43. Rombaux P, Liistro G, Hamoir M, Bertrand B, Aubert G, Verse T, Rodenstein D. Nasal obstruction and its impact on sleep-related breathing disorders. Rhinology. 2005;43:242–50.
44. Li HY, Lee LA, Wang PC, Chen NH, Lin Y, Fang TJ. Nasal surgery for snoring in patients with obstructive sleep apnea. Laryngoscope. 2008;118:354–9.
45. Li HY, Lin Y, Chen NH, Lee LA, Fang TJ, Wang PC. Improvement in quality of life after nasal surgery alone for patients with obstructive sleep apnoea and nasal obstruction. Arch Otolaryngol Head Neck Surg. 2008;134:429–33.
46. Stapelton AL, Chang YF, Soose RJ, Gillman GS. The impact of nasal surgery on sleep quality: a prospective outcome study. Otolarynghol Head Neck Surg. 2014;151:868–73.
47. Verse T, Hörmann K. The surgical treatment of sleep-related upper airway obstruction. Dtsch Arztebl Int. 2011;108:216–21.
48. Randerrath WJ, Verbraecken J, Andreas S, Bettega G, Boudewyns A, Hamans E, Jalbert F, Paoli JR, Sanner B, Smith I, Stuck BA, Lacassagne L, Marklund M, Maurer JT, Pepin JL, Valipour A, Verse T, Fietze I. Non-CPAP therapies in obstructive sleep apnoea. Eur Respir J. 2011;37:1000–28.
49. Reilly EK, Boon MS, Vimawala S, Chitguppi C, Patel J, Murphy K, Doghramji K, Nyquist GG, Rosen MR, Rabinowitz MR, Huntley CT. Tolerance of continuous positive airway pressure after sinonasal surgery. Laryngoscope. 2021;131:E1013–8.

Part IV

Conservative Treatment of Epiglottis Collapse

Therapy Decision-Making in Epiglottis Collapse

14

Matej Delakorda and Nico de Vries

14.1 Introduction

The epiglottis has long been a neglected structure in the etiology of obstructive sleep apnea (OSA), and consequently, treating OSA by addressing epiglottic collapse (EC) is relatively new as well. Such neglect of the epiglottis and its role is indeed the main motivation behind this book. In this section of the book, both nonsurgical and surgical treatment modalities are described and discussed. In general, after a careful diagnostic workup (including a meticulous examination of medical history, clinical assessment, a comprehensive sleep study, drug-induced sleep endoscopy (DISE), and imaging when indicated), the doctor and patient should, in a process of shared decision-making, reach a well-balanced choice based on treatment options available in the specific situation. Nonsurgical treatments options include positive airway pressure therapy (CPAP), mandibular advancement devices (MAD), positional therapy, and to a lesser extent myofunctional therapy. On the other hand, a considerable variety of surgical options is available as well.

It is important to realize that in case of EC, treatment might be essentially different from standard OSA therapy. For instance, while CPAP is still the gold standard of therapy for moderate to severe OSA, it can sometimes induce EC that can, in turn, even be an overlooked cause of CPAP failure. In this chapter, we will summarize and comment on these options. We also propose an algorithm for assessment of patients with suspected EC. For further details, we refer to particular chapters in this book.

M. Delakorda (✉)
General Hospital Celje, Celje, Slovenia

N. de Vries
Jan Tooropstraat, Onze Lieve Vrouwe Gasthuis, Amsterdam, The Netherlands
e-mail: n.vries@olvg.nl

M. Delakorda, N. de Vries (eds.), *The Role of Epiglottis in Obstructive Sleep Apnea*, https://doi.org/10.1007/978-3-031-34992-8_14

14.2 CPAP

CPAP is considered the gold standard of therapy for moderate to severe OSA. CPAP has proven to be beneficial and safe, but its efficacy can be limited by poor long-term adherence. Moreover, EC has been linked to (unsuccessful) use of CPAP, suggesting that the epiglottis in some cases is pushed further down into the laryngeal inlet on application of CPAP [1], which aggravates the EC. For further reference, see Chap. 15.

14.3 Mandibular Advancement Devices

A mandibular advancement device (MAD) may also be a treatment option for EC, although there is some controversy regarding its efficacy. In our experience and according to most studies to date, however, MADs are an efficient nonsurgical treatment option for tongue base and/or epiglottis collapse, particularly in patients with mild to moderate OSA. Its effect can be tested with Esmarch repositioning maneuver during DISE. For further reference, see Chap. 17.

14.4 Restoring Nasal Breathing

Mouth breathing during sleep alters the relative positions of the soft structures in the oropharynx. When not in contact with the hard and soft palate, the tongue base moves back, and the epiglottis follows it. This is often seen in DISE when patients open their mouth, and the epiglottis collapses already in the shallow phase of sedation. In this group, it is reasonable to recommend the use of a chin strap to evaluate the effectiveness of nasal breathing restoration. According to patient reports, waking up with a distinctly dry mouth could point to mouth breathing. If the patient cannot breathe satisfactorily through the nose with the chin strap in place, then treatment of nasal obstruction should be considered (surgical or nonsurgical). According to the results of the studies carried out so far, OSA cannot be successfully treated only by restoration of nasal breathing; however, breathing through the mouth can certainly worsen the results of other treatment methods, and this is especially important in cases of obstructions at the level of the tongue base and the epiglottis (for further reference, see Chap. 13).

14.5 Myofunctional Therapy

Myofunctional therapy is interesting and relatively new. The experience with it in general, and in case of epiglottis collapse in particular, is very limited. Further studies are awaited. Since the position of the epiglottis is related to the tongue position, the use of this method should be more sensible in patients with a hypotonic tongue. Newer applications that improve patient participation and progress monitoring can help us with this. Some research already points to the success of such approach (for further reference, see Chap. 16).

14.6 Positional Therapy

The majority of patients with early-stage disease, mild OSA, have a higher frequency and duration of apneic events in the supine position. It has been suggested that epiglottic collapse at this level is affected by sleeping position and seems to occur more often in the supine position compared to non-supine position. The increase in the use of DISE, and performing this procedure in different body positions has given more insight in the involvement of the epiglottis in OSA, particularly with an isolated EC in antero-posterior direction—floppy epiglottis (FE). Vonk et al. showed that a FE is a position-dependent phenomenon. Like a collapse at the level of the tongue base, EC can also be suspected in patients with positional dependence. In case of FE, therefore, positional therapy might be a viable treatment option—proven to be effective [2, 3]. For further reference, see Chap. 18.

14.7 Surgical Treatment

In addition to conventional treatments, several surgical techniques exist. They are described in Part 4 of this book. Several small-scale studies have been published about the techniques, success rates, and complications of epiglottis surgery. Many sleep surgeons are hesitant to opt for epiglottis surgery because of the potential risk of irreversible dysphagia after partial or total epiglottectomy. Fortunately, evidence on and experience with the surgical techniques described in this section do not support the fears of severe irreversible complications. The risk of sequelae must be weighed individually, depending on the severity of the disease, success of conservative treatments, and patient's motivation for such approach. The choice of the described surgical techniques depends on the surgeon's experience, doctor's and patient's preference, severity of the disease, extent, and pattern of the collapse, i.e., isolated epiglottic collapse vs. multilevel obstructions, and availability of, for instance, a laser and robot platform.

In the following section, we will propose an algorithm for assessment of patients with EC as conducted in the authors' institution. It is based on the results of some studies, as well as on the authors' own observations and experience. Before deciding on the surgical treatment of EC, it is necessary to perform follow-up poly(somno) graphy in order to objectify the effect of any previous conservative treatments. The new generation of devices that are being developed for monitoring various OSA-related signs and symptoms can be helpful in evaluating different nonoperative approaches or their combination. Their development has progressed significantly in recent years, and heralds a new era in the field of OSA diagnostics and monitoring.

Assessment of all OSA patients begins with clinical examination. Some studies have shown that patients with EC differ from other patients with OSA in terms of certain poly(somno)graphic and clinical characteristics. EC appears to occur more frequently in men and in patients with a lower average BMI than in other OSA patients [3–8]. The EC group is also characterized by milder degrees of OSA, with less severe desaturations [2]. When dealing with such patients, especially in the initial stage, we must therefore maintain a high level of suspicion for EC. This is especially true for patients in whom CPAP therapy has failed to stabilize the upper airway [1]. If we have a recording of snoring, we can also suspect obstruction at the level of the epiglottis based on the characteristic sound with a higher frequency, usually with occasional complete interruptions [9–11].

EC is confirmed during DISE. We must pay particular attention to the assessment of possible obstructions at the level of the epiglottis in patients who, according to P(S)G and clinical characteristics, correspond to the group of patients with EC. Since the position of the epiglottis is related to the position of the tongue base, the protocol according to which DISE is performed is extremely important. Especially when using propofol, we must be careful not to over-sedate the patient, because the resulting hypotonia of the genioglossus can create "false ECs" [12]. The mentioned effect of the sedation agent can to some extent be avoided by using dexmedetomidine, which has a smaller effect on the tone of upper airway dilators [13]. To assess possible EC, it is necessary to take enough time for DISE and observe as many repetitions of breathing cycles as possible. Therefore, the cooperation between the surgeon and the anesthesiologist is of utmost importance. We should observe and describe the severity and pattern of the EC and check the effects of different maneuvers on EC (mouth closure, jaw thrust, lateral body position). It is important to realize that EC does not behave according to the tube law principle; rather, it is more like a one-way valve with unlimited collapsibility. Once the critical pressure is reached, the epiglottis closes the laryngeal inlet abruptly [14, 15]. As such, EC can be severely influenced by very small changes in UA airflow dynamics.

In the majority of cases, EC is a part of a multilevel obstruction [2]. The prevalence of epiglottis obstructions requiring surgery seems to be lower than that found during DISE, so it is not necessary to perform surgery on all levels/structures causing obstruction or collapses, which are detected during this investigation [16]. In cases of isolated antero-posterior EC, conservative treatment options should be tested first. If the EC is a part of a multilevel obstruction with palatal involvement, we can check the effect of a pharyngeal tube placement during DISE to simulate the palatal surgery (UPPP, or contemporary palatal reconstructive approaches) results. In institutions where this option is available, titration with CPAP can also be performed during DISE to check for the minimal positive pressure needed to stabilize the epiglottis. In cases of secondary EC, it is necessary to evaluate the size of lingual tonsils.

When EC is identified during the DISE, and conservative treatment has failed, then epiglottis surgery should be considered. Epiglottis is located relatively low in the upper respiratory tract and therefore, when assessing its stability, it is also necessary to look for the primary flow-limiting site that may be located at a higher UA level [17]. When there is a significant obstruction at the upper levels of the UA (soft palate, tonsils/lateral pharyngeal walls), it is reasonable to expect that resolving this primary flow-limiting site will also affect the EC. This especially holds true when EC is not complete or when it only occurs intermittently. In such cases, the authors advise a staged approach with palatal surgery (e.g., UPPP with/without tonsillectomy, barbed wired pharyngoplasty) and epiglottis surgery as a secondary intention. Such an approach is also in concordance with the results of some published studies [18]. An exception would be a severe EC in lateral direction (soft, tubular epiglottis type), which usually presents a narrowing with high compliance. In our opinion, this type of obstruction should be addressed with the initial surgical treatment.

The choice of surgical technique in a patient with EC must be adapted to the type of obstruction at this level. EC in anteroposterior direction (floppy epiglottis) is much more common than the lateral type [2]. In the case of EC in the lateral direction with a thin and softened omega-shaped epiglottis, a partial epiglottectomy is probably the most appropriate. Epiglottis stiffening operation or glossoepiglottopexy techniques are the preferred option for EC in the antero-posterior direction, since in the case of lateral EC, in our experience, these techniques most often fail. In cases of secondary EC, tongue base obstruction should be addressed. In patients with severe enlargement of lingual tonsils (Friedman grade 3–4), tongue base reduction either by TORS or coblation should be performed. This procedure can be combined with partial epiglottectomy. When tongue base collapse is a consequence of hypotony, then upper airway stimulation would most probably be the best option.

In Fig. 14.1, we present a proposed algorithm that is used at our institution.

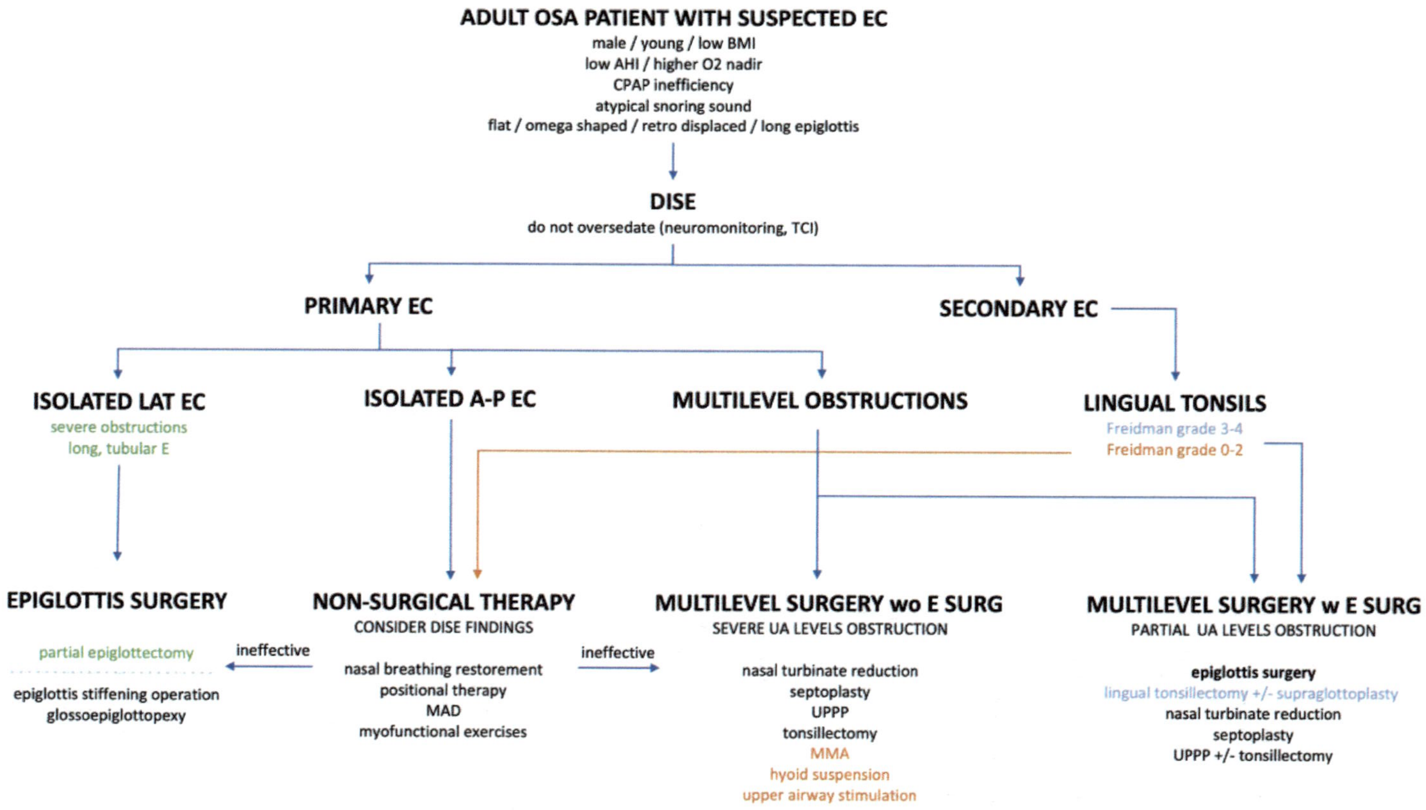

Fig. 14.1 An algorithm for assessment of patients with suspected EC. *TCI* target controlled infusion, *MAD* mandibular advancement device, *UPPP* uvulopalatopharyngoplasty, *MMA* maxillomandibular advancement

14.8 Conclusion

Patients with EC differ from other OSA patients in terms of some demographic and anthropometric characteristics. In most patients, EC is a part of a multilevel obstruction, and the choice of the optimal treatment or combination of different treatment approaches should be carefully selected according to patient's characteristics and preferences. For many patients with EC, positional therapy and MADs may prove very successful. Another important issue is nasal patency that should be resolved when obstructions at the tongue base and/or epiglottis are related to mouth breathing. When those measures fail, surgical treatment should be considered and planned. For this treatment modality, there are many options that should be selected and adapted based on DISE findings.

References

1. Verse T, Pirsig W. Age-related changes in the epiglottis causing failure of nasal continuous positive airway pressure therapy. J Laryngol Otol. 1999;113(11):1022–5; [cited 2020 Mar 21]. https://www.cambridge.org/core/product/identifier/S0022215100145888/type/journal_article.
2. Kim H-Y, Sung C-M, Jang H-B, Kim HC, Lim SC, Yang HC. Patients with epiglottic collapse showed less severe obstructive sleep apnea and good response to treatment other than continuous positive airway pressure: a case-control study of 224 patients. J Clin Sleep Med. 2021;17(3):413–9; [cited 2020 Nov 23]. http://www.ncbi.nlm.nih.gov/pubmed/33094721.
3. Sung CM, Kim HC, Yang HC. The clinical characteristics of patients with an isolate epiglottic collapse. Auris Nasus Larynx. 2020;47(3):450–7.
4. Moore KE, Phillips C. A practical method for describing patterns of tongue-base narrowing (modification of Fujita) in awake adult patients with obstructive sleep apnea. J Oral Maxillofac Surg. 2002;60(3):252–60.
5. Sung C-W, Chan W, Chang C-H, Huang P-C, Lien W-C, Chang W-T, et al. Associations between male gender, body size and dimension of the epiglottis. Authorea Prepr. 2020
6. Ma MA, Kumar R, Macey PM, Yan-Go FL, Harper RM. Epiglottis cross-sectional area and oropharyngeal airway length in male and female obstructive sleep apnea patients. Nat Sci Sleep. 2016;8:297–304; [cited 2021 Aug 9]. https://pubmed.ncbi.nlm.nih.gov/27757056/.
7. Sung CM, Tan SN, Shin M-H, Lee J, Kim HC, Lim SC, et al. The site of airway collapse in sleep apnea, its associations with disease severity and obesity, and implications for mechanical interventions. Am J Respir Crit Care Med. 2021;204(1):103–6; [cited 2021 Dec 1]. http://www.ncbi.nlm.nih.gov/pubmed/33826879.
8. Kim HY, Sung CM, Bin JH, Kim HC, Lim SC, Yang HC. Patients with epiglottic collapse showed less severe obstructive sleep apnea and good response to treatment other than continuous positive airway pressure: a case-control study of 224 patients. J Clin Sleep Med. 2021;17(3):413–9.
9. Agrawal S, Stone P, McGuinness K, Morris J, Camilleri AE. Sound frequency analysis and the site of snoring in natural and induced sleep. Clin Otolaryngol Allied Sci. 2002;27(3):162–6. http://www.ncbi.nlm.nih.gov/pubmed/12071989.
10. Huang Z, Aarab G, Ravesloot MJL, Zhou N, Bosschieter PFN, van Selms MKA, et al. Prediction of the obstruction sites in the upper airway in sleep-disordered breathing based on snoring sound parameters: a systematic review. Sleep Med. 2021;88:116–33. https://doi.org/10.1016/j.sleep.2021.10.015.
11. Lee CH, Bin WT, Kim SY, Lee WH, Han DH, Kim DY, et al. Acoustic characteristics of snoring according to obstruction site determined by sleep videofluoroscopy. Acta Otolaryngol. 2012;132(SUPPL. 1):S13.

12. Hong SD, Dhong HJ, Kim HY, Sohn JH, Jung YG, Chung SK, et al. Change of obstruction level during drug-induced sleep endoscopy according to sedation depth in obstructive sleep apnea. Laryngoscope. 2013;123(11):2896–9.
13. Viana A, Zhao C, Rosa T, Couto A, Neves DD, Araújo-Melo MH, et al. The effect of sedating agents on drug-induced sleep endoscopy findings. Laryngoscope. 2019;129(2):506–13. https://doi.org/10.1002/lary.27298; [cited 2019 Sep 8].
14. Genta PR, Sands SA, Butler JP, Loring SH, Katz ES, Demko BG, et al. Airflow shape is associated with the pharyngeal structure causing OSA. Chest. 2017;152(3):537–46; [cited 2019 mar 29]. http://www.ncbi.nlm.nih.gov/pubmed/28651794.
15. Azarbarzin A, Marques M, Sands SA, Op de Beeck S, Genta PR, Taranto-Montemurro L, et al. Predicting epiglottic collapse in patients with obstructive sleep apnoea. Eur Respir J. 2017;50(3):1700345. https://doi.org/10.1183/13993003.00345; [cited 2021 Jul 13].
16. Blumen MB, Latournerie V, Bequignon E, Guillere L, Chabolle F. Are the obstruction sites visualized on drug-induced sleep endoscopy reliable? Sleep Breath. 2015;19(3):1021–6.
17. Yanagisawa-Minami A, Sugiyama T, Iwasaki T, Yamasaki Y. Primary site identification in children with obstructive sleep apnea by computational fluid dynamics analysis of the upper airway. J Clin Sleep Med. 2020;16(3):431–9; [cited 2021 Jun 27]. http://www.ncbi.nlm.nih.gov/pubmed/31992411.
18. Kwon OE, Jung SY, Al-Dilaijan K, Min JY, Lee KH, Kim SW, et al. Is epiglottis surgery necessary for obstructive sleep apnea patients with epiglottis obstruction? Laryngoscope. 2019;129(11):2658–62. https://doi.org/10.1002/lary.27808; [cited 2019 Nov 20].

Treatment with CPAP 15

Marina Carrasco-Llatas and Joana Vaz de Castro

Abbreviations

AASM	American Academy of Sleep Medicine
AHI	Apnea-hypopnea index
APAP	Auto-adjusting positive airway pressure
BMI	Body mass index
BPAP	Bilevel positive airway pressure
CPAP	Continuous positive airway pressure
CSA	Central sleep apnea
CSR	Cheyne–Stokes respiration
DISE	Drug-induced sleep endoscopy
EF	Ejection fraction
ENT	Ear, nose, and throat
EPAP	Expiratory positive airway pressure
ERS	European Respiratory Society
HF	Heart failure

Supplementary Information The online version contains supplementary material available at https://doi.org/10.1007/978-3-031-34992-8_15. The videos can be accessed individually by clicking the DOI link in the accompanying figure caption or by scanning this link with the SN More Media App.

M. Carrasco-Llatas (✉)
Department of Otorhinolaringology, Hospital Universitario Dr. Peset, Valencia, Spain

Department of Otorhinolaryngology, IMED Hospital, Valencia, Spain

J. Vaz de Castro
ISAMB, Medicine of University of Lisbon, Lisbon, Portugal

Centro de Electroencefalografia e Neurofisiologia Clínica (CENC), Lisbon, Portugal

Comprehensive Health Research Centre - CHRC, Lisbon, Portugal

M. Delakorda, N. de Vries (eds.), *The Role of Epiglottis in Obstructive Sleep Apnea*, https://doi.org/10.1007/978-3-031-34992-8_15

IPAP	Inspiratory positive airway pressure
MAD	Mandibular advancement device
MSA	Multiple system atrophy
OSA	Obstructive sleep apnea
PAP	Positive airway pressure
Pcrit	Critical closing pressure
PS	Pressure support (related to Bilevel PAP)
PSG	Polysomnography
SDB	Sleep disordered breathing
UA	Upper airway

15.1 Introduction to PAP: An Overview

Positive airway pressure (PAP) is the treatment modality in which air is delivered to the lungs through the nasal or oronasal route via a machine, a tube and an interface (mask) (Fig. 15.1) [1]. The interface chosen may be a nasal mask, nasal pillows (nasal cushions) or oronasal (full face) mask (Figs. 15.2, 15.3, 15.4 and 15.5). Air is delivered at a constant pressure (as is the case of continuous PAP - CPAP) or at different pressures, higher during inspiration and lower during expiration (known as bilevel PAP – BPAP) [1]. PAP therapy is the gold standard for treating moderate to severe obstructive sleep apnea (OSA) and other sleep disordered breathing disorders (SDB).

15.1.1 CPAP

Airflow is maintained at a constant pressure throughout the respiratory cycle to splint the airways open, in the presence of spontaneous ventilation. Positive end-expiratory pressure (PEEP) maintains the airway pressure above atmospheric level by exerting pressure that opposes passive emptying of the lungs [2, 3]. This pressure is typically achieved by maintaining a positive pressure flow at the end of expiration [3]. CPAP maintains PEEP, during both inspiration and expiration [2]. Applying PEEP increases the upper airway (UA), alveolar pressure and volume. The latter increases the alveolar surface area by reopening and stabilizing collapsed or

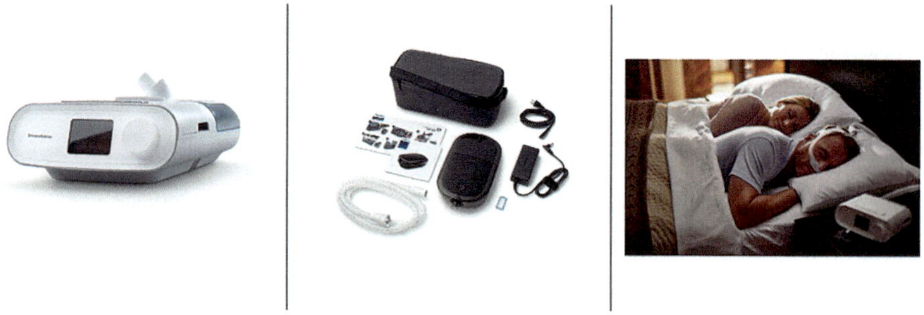

Fig. 15.1 PAP machine and set up. Images courtesy of Philips Iberia

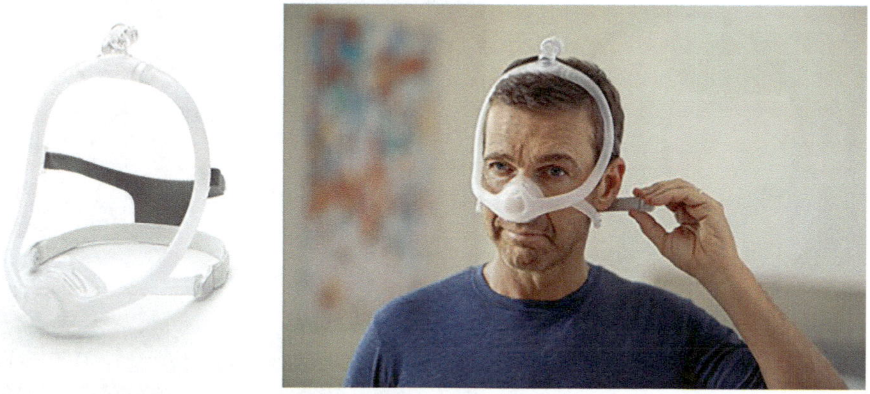

Fig. 15.2 PAP therapy nasal masks. Images courtesy of Philips Iberia

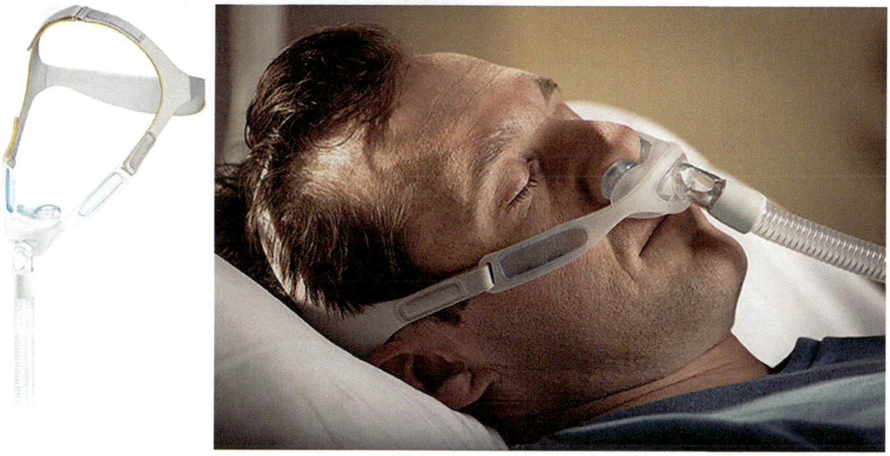

Fig. 15.3 PAP therapy nasal pillows. Images courtesy of Philips Iberia

unstable alveoli [3]. This splinting of the alveoli with positive pressure improves the ventilation–perfusion match, reducing the shunt effect [3].

The optimal pressure level (measured in cm H_2O), may be determined during a night polysomnography (PSG) with CPAP titration or during a CPAP titration night study with standard manual titration. Fixed CPAP pressure derived from prediction formulas are not commonly adopted. With advances in hardware and software, auto-adjusting titrating PAP also known as AutoCPAP (APAP), a continuous pressure is delivered during the night, but at an adjusted pressure depending on events sensed using computer algorithms [4]. For APAP, an upper and lower limit of pressure is established, between the values of 4–20 cm H_2O, usually with intervals no larger than 10 cm H_2O. Currently, the American Academy of Sleep Medicine (AASM) advocates initiating PAP therapy with APAP devices at home or in-laboratory PAP titration, depending on the comorbidities [1, 4].

PAP treatment should provide a low residual apnea-hypopnea index (AHI) and patient tolerance, albeit with an acceptable leakage level (<24 L/min) [1] (Fig. 15.6).

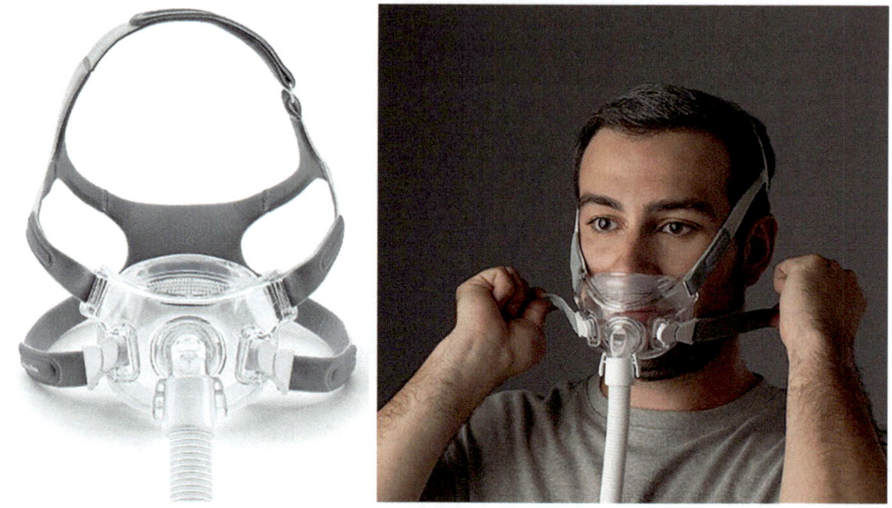

Fig. 15.4 PAP therapy oronasal mask. Images courtesy of Philips Iberia

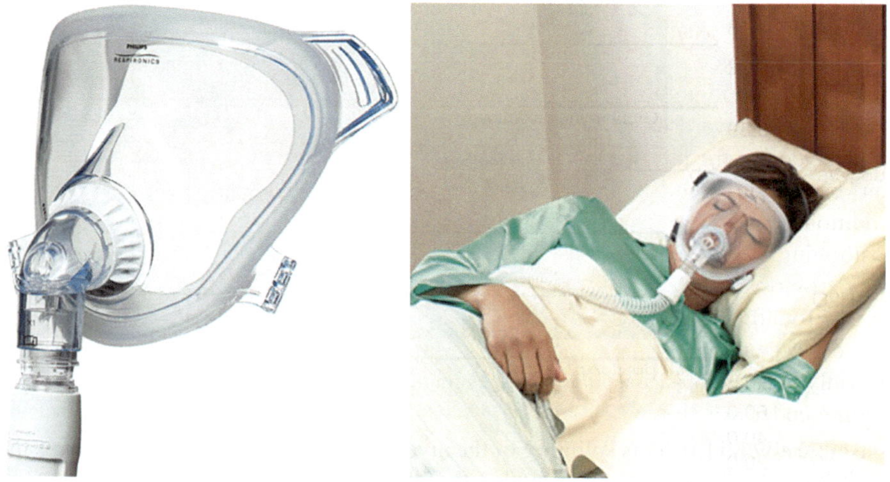

Fig. 15.5 PAP therapy full-face mask. Images courtesy of Philips Iberia

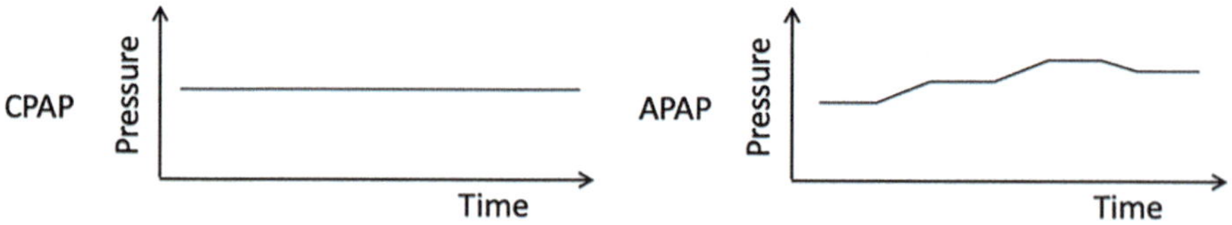

Fig. 15.6 Air pressure delivered with CPAP and with APAP. (Modified from Ref. [5])

15.1.2 Effects of CPAP in the Upper Airway

Increased intraluminal pressure in the upper airway (UA) acts as pneumatic splint. When intraluminal UA pressure exceeds critical closing pressure (Pcrit), passive collapse is prevented [6]. Schwab et al. as well as Torre et al. demonstrated with UA imaging and drug-induced sleep endoscopy (DISE), respectively, that the effect of enlarging the UA is more pronounced in the latero-lateral diameter, compared to the anteroposterior diameter [7, 8]. In 2006, a study by Crawford et al. found that in nine infants (5–12 months old) submitted to an elective brain MRI under anesthesia, with increasing depth of anesthesia cross-sectional area at the tip of the epiglottis decreased by 51% [9]. This resulted from important reductions in antero-posterior diameter but also in the transverse dimensions (38% and 21%, respectively) [9]. Application of CPAP completely reversed the reduction in cross-sectional area primarily by increasing the transverse dimension, by 58% [9]. Therefore, with CPAP, the increase in UA patency is not mediated by its effects on the velopharynx, tongue base, or epiglottis, but on the reduction of thickness of the lateral pharyngeal walls and redistribution of the pharyngeal fat pads [7, 8]. Considering that the antero-posterior diameter is harder to surpass, generally pressures >10 cm H_2O are needed to maintain epiglottic patency in epiglottic obstruction [8]. This pressure may increase further when considering oronasal interfaces, that usually need increased pressures to match the nasal interface. In another study, pressures of >18 cm H_2O were needed to maintain epiglottic patency, meanwhile lesser pressures pushed the epiglottis downwards [10].

Considering the physiological route for breathing begins with the nose, where air can be conditioned, humidified, and filtered, nasal interfaces are preferred. Additionally, promoting nasal breathing stabilizes the velopharynx, promotes correct positioning of the tongue against the hard palate which further increases retropalatal and retroglossal space. Hsu et al. compared oral/oronasal breathers with nasal breathers and found a higher degree and prevalence of lateral pharyngeal wall and tongue base collapse in the former [11]. Therefore, nasal masks should be initially adopted, and only in case of failure, oronasal masks should be provided [1]. Nasal pillows are recommended for those who are claustrophobic, need low-pressure flow, sleep in lateral position, or have a history of skin allergy to silicone [12].

Bear in mind, although in OSA, CPAP therapy is used mainly to increase UA patency, it has benefits elsewhere: (1) increases intrapulmonary pressure and maintains larger end expiratory lung volume, thereby increasing functional residual capacity, (2) decreases breathing effort, (3) improves stability of central respiratory drive, and (4) reduces cardiac preload and afterload with improved cardiac function [1].

15.1.3 Clinical Impact of CPAP

PAP therapy is generally considered the gold-standard for moderate to severe adult OSA (AHI > 15/h). In compliant and tolerant patients, it may be considered superior to other treatment modalities in lowering AHI. CPAP therapy has been shown to be efficacious and indicated in the treatment of excessive sleepiness, impaired quality of life, and comorbid (especially resistant) hypertension [4, 13]. Reflecting how quickly an AHI can be reduced and the UA splinted, CPAP treatment can be used as proof of the causal role of OSA in symptom etiology.

Patients prescribed CPAP should be examined within approximately 2 weeks of starting the treatment and then again between 1 and 2 months later with compliance and efficacy monitored at every visit. Interfaces are replaced every 3–6 months. Patients are followed for as long as they are on CPAP, generally at 6–12 month intervals, depending on treatment success. Repeating polysomnography (PSG) is advocated in case of significant weight change (>10 kg), surgery, or symptom reappearance [14].

According to a statement by the European Respiratory Society (ERS), CPAP is indicated in moderate to severe OSA (AHI > 5/h) for children 1–23 months old, if they are not candidates for, or do not improve after adenotonsillectomy, or other surgical procedures (e.g., supraglottoplasty for severe laryngomalacia) [15]. It may also be applied as a temporary intervention while waiting for the craniofacial surgery, or in cases of hypoventilation with OSA (e.g., spinal muscular atrophy type 1) [15]. In children 1–23 months, CPAP is initiated at 4–6 cm H_2O and titrated up to 10 cm H_2O [15]. After CPAP initiation, PSG is advocated every 2–4 months during the first year of life and every 6 months thereafter to confirm the continued need for treatment and potential need for increased pressure [15].

Children between 2 and 18 years of age with AHI > 5 episodes/hour are at increased risk of sleepiness if they are older but in preschoolers the most common symptom is aggressiveness, attention and cognitive deficits, behavior disorders, elevated blood pressure, primary nocturnal enuresis, decreased quality of life, and respiratory complications post operatively, all conditions which can be reversed with PAP therapy [16]. Usual indications for CPAP for children between 2 and 18 years are: residual OSA after adenotonsillectomy (AHI > 5 episodes/hour), OSA related to obesity, craniofacial abnormalities, or neuromuscular disorders [16]. If nocturnal hypoventilation occurs (e.g., end-tidal carbon dioxide $PCO_2 > 50$ mmHg for 25% of total sleep time or peak end-tidal $PCO_2 > 55$ mmHg), BPAP is preferred [16]. Treatment priority should be given to SDB children with major craniofacial abnormalities, neuromuscular disorders, achondroplasia, Chiari malformation, Down syndrome, mucopolysaccharidoses, and Prader–Willi syndrome [16].

PSG is used to titrate CPAP or BPAP, and is then repeated at least annually (or more often depending on UA growth, changes in percentile, or surgery). There is limited evidence about optimal respiratory supervision for pediatric PAP treatment, but follow-up based on adult CPAP management, with regular and closely scheduled appointments may be warranted [16].

15.1.4 Side Effects, Adherence, and Compliance

Undesired side effects of PAP therapy include: nasal congestion, rhinorrhea, xerostomia, xerophthalmia, epistaxis, skin erythema/eczema, pressure sores, abdominal distention, aerophagia, chest discomfort, difficulty exhaling, and claustrophobia [17, 18]. Other complaints that decrease adherence and compliance related to the device are device loudness, interface leakage, and water condensation in the interface or circuit. In children, a special concern is facial growth, especially in very young children with craniofacial abnormalities. Patient history, physical examination including awake laryngoscopy and DISE may also provide insight to UA obstruction or collapse that once alleviated may also increase CPAP tolerance. The CPAP device can additionally be adjusted to increase compliance with the addition of adequate humidification, temperature setting, interface comfort, and optimized sensor algorithms with modified pressure profiles (e.g., initial pressure relief at expiration) [4, 13].

It is an AASM recommendation that patients should be offered educational interventions prior to PAP therapy initiation, and once treatment is initiated, behavioral, troubleshooting, and telemonitoring-guided interventions [13] (Table 15.1).

Patients most likely to be adherent are either more symptomatic, have higher AHI, or are accompanied with comorbid conditions, such as refractory hypertension. Compliance can be optimized with adequate support systems, be it with family, friends, health practitioners, telemonitoring, educational and psychological support [13]. Adequate CPAP compliance is defined as at least 4 h of use per night during at least 70% of nights, and optimal when used at least 6 h per night [4, 17]. There is a continuous dose–response relationship between hours of use and therapeutic response [4, 13]. Taking into the account that many events occur at the end of the night, which is when patients sometimes take off their interface, this could be an important period of use for CPAP. Ceasing PAP use at the end of the night may be relevant in attenuating PAP therapy benefits.

Table 15.1 PAP therapy side effects and possible solutions. According to Ref. [1, 18]

	Focus	Side effects	Possible solutions
Patient	Nose	Dryness, obstruction Rhinorrhea Epistaxis	Humidifier, nasal gels or vaseline, nasal steroid, anti-histamine, ear, nose and throat (ENT) consultation
	Mouth	Xerostomia	Humidifier
	Eye	Xerophtalmia	Interface adaptation, eye drops
	Skin	Rash, abrasion, erythema, pruritis	Interface adaptation (check mask material, type and untighten)
	UA	Feeling suffocation	ENT consultation (possible anatomical obstruction) Pressure adaptation. Exclusion of acid reflux
CPAP	High pressure	Chest discomfort, abdominal distention, aerophagia, or other ectopic insufflation	Pressure adaptation (reduce pressure), change to APAP from CPAP
	Mask	Claustrophobia	Change to nasal pillows
	Tube	Condensation in tube	Use heated PAP, increase ambient temperature, reduce humidification
	Noise	Airflow leakage	Interface adaptation (change mask or tighten)

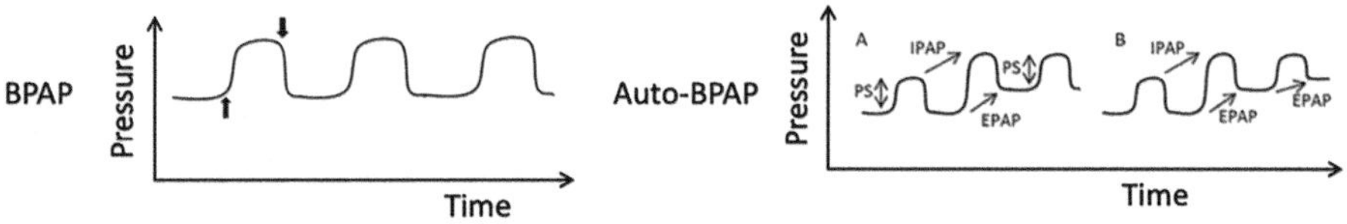

Fig. 15.7 Air pressure delivered with BPAP and AutoBPAP. *IPAP* inspiratory PAP, *EPAP* expiratory PAP, *PS* pressure support, ↑initiation of inspiratory phase, ↓ initiation of expiratory phase. (Modified from Ref. [5])

15.1.5 BiLevel PAP

Bilevel positive airway pressure delivers a higher inspiratory PAP (IPAP) and a lower expiratory PAP (EPAP). There are three different possibilities how BPAP devices interact with the patient's breathing. Respiratory circles can be triggered exclusively by the patients (S modus), be dependent on a minimum breathing frequency or otherwise the device will initiate an inspiration (S/T modus) or are exclusively dependent on the BPAP device (T-modus). Usually, these devices are used in the S/T modus in respiratory failure; however, in SDB patients, they may be used: (1) in concomitant hypoventilation-OSA disorders if hypercapnia does not normalize with CPAP, (2) in patients intolerant to high pressure levels, by encompassing an IPAP, the EPAP may be reduced, (3) in patients needing pressure levels above 20 cm H_2O, (4) to control central sleep apnea (CSA) and Cheyne Stokes respiration (CSR) - there exists very little evidence to justify this indication. Since BPAP might enhance hyperventilation, this therapy, especially in the S modus, is at present not recommended for CSA and CSR [4, 19] (Fig. 15.7).

15.1.6 Adaptive Servo-Ventilation (ASV)

In ASV, positive airway pressure is delivered in an anticyclical manner to the periodic hypo/hyperventilation typical for CSA/CSR [1]. EPAP is either titrated similarly to CPAP or applied by automatic regulation, while pressure support and thus IPAP is adaptive in order to stabilize tidal volume over a device specific time frame [1]. ASV revealed a better control of AHI, excessive daytime sleepiness and biomarkers associated with cardiac heart failure (HF) when compared to oxygen, CPAP, and Bilevel [20]. ASV however is controversial in reducing overall and cardiovascular mortality in CSA with HF and reduced ejection fraction (<45%). In the study on ASV for HF, this therapy reduced the AHI, nevertheless, it was associated with a higher cardiovascular mortality [21]. This applied specially for patients with a severe reduction in the ejection fraction (EF < 30%) and more than 50% central respiratory events [21]. At present, both AASM and ERS do not recommend ASV therapy in heart failure patients with an ejection fraction <45% [21, 22]. While initially developed for CSA with CSR in CHF patients, ASV has been successfully used in patients with idiopathic CSA-CSR, treatment emergent CSA, opioid-associated CSA, and CSA after stroke [1].

15.2 CPAP Diagnostic Possibilities

CPAP might have a role as a tool in patient selection for non-CPAP treatments. It has been shown that the critical closing pressure (Pcrit) has a strong correlation with CPAP pressure. According to Landry et al., lower therapeutic CPAP levels are associated with more negative Pcrit values (less collapsible airway) [23]. Specifically, patients with a CPAP requirement below 6–8 cm H_2O are highly likely to have a mildly collapsible UA (defined by a Pcrit ≤ -2 cm H_2O). Patients who need higher CPAP pressure have more collapsible upper airways and should be more difficult to cure with surgery or mandibular advancement devices (MADs) [23]. The CPAP pressure needed to open the airway may offer a hint on the structure responsible for the collapse. Torres et al. demonstrated with nasal CPAP and DISE that a pressure of 15 cm H_2O was enough to splint collapses in all their patients (n = 15), while values at 5 cm H_2O did not make much of a difference. Nasal CPAP pressures of 10 cm H_2O were sufficient to surpass velopharyngeal and oropharyngeal obstructions, but 15 cm H_2O was necessary for tongue base and epiglottic obstruction [8]. Similarly, Sung et al., using simultaneous PAP-DISE, demonstrated that most patients with isolated epiglottic collapse needed pressures >12 cm H_2O [24]. Likewise, Kim et al. showed that patients with epiglottic collapse had relatively low body mass index (BMI) and less severe OSA [25]. Additionally, they were unlikely to respond to CPAP therapy; therefore, it is possible that patients with mild OSA that are intolerant to CPAP at low pressures (due to a sense of suffocation), may have predominantly epiglottic collapse, and this could be solved with higher pressures. Nevertheless, this idea needs to be proven in prospective studies and with larger populations.

Although it is not directly the focus of this chapter, the authors found it pertinent to report that CPAP may also be used to diagnose laryngeal clefts using flexible endoscopy. Laryngeal clefts are uncommon but important causes of stridor in infants, for which direct laryngoscopy is the recommended method, as flexible endoscopy is not sensitive enough [26]. CPAP-flexible laryngoscopy applied via an endoscopy mask can be titrated to open the upper esophageal sphincter and spread the inter-arytenoid folds at 10–15 cm H_2O unmasking obscured laryngeal clefts [26].

On the other hand, CPAP can be used during DISE to demonstrate the etiology of patient intolerance [27]. Ideally, the same mask that the patient is using at home should be employed; however, testing other types of masks during DISE could reveal the impact of UA collapse with different masks maintaining the same pressure levels [28]. Fig. 15.8 (Video 15.1) shows DISE-CPAP performed to evaluate the best mask to be attached to CPAP. The exam was performed with the same

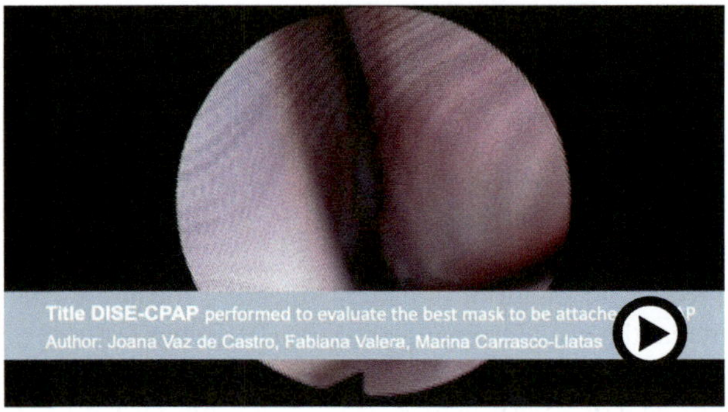

Fig. 15.8 (Video 15.1) DISE-CPAP performed to evaluate the best mask to be attached to CPAP (► https://doi.org/10.1007/000-bfc)

pressure and three different masks (nasal, oronasal, and prong), showing a better airway area with nasal mask when compared to the other two. As epiglottis continued to eventually collapse even with nasal mask, chin strap was added. This maneuver juxtaposed to nasal mask prevented the epiglottic collapse.

15.3 CPAP Treatment in Certain Epiglottic Pathologies

Epiglottic obstruction is associated with certain states, such as, multiple system atrophy (MSA) and laryngomalacia, both of which are frequently associated with OSA. In MSA, UA obstruction occurs not only at the level of vocal cords, but also at the tongue base, velopharynx, and laryngeal inlet. Obstruction of the laryngeal inlet is provoked by a floppy epiglottis that is sucked in during inspiration, by an unknown mechanism [29]. Although awake laryngoscopy did not reveal floppy epiglottis in any of the patients included in the study conducted by Shimohata et al. (n = 17), DISE revealed a floppy epiglottis in 71% (12/17) with 5 patients worsening with CPAP >8 cm H_2O. Of these 5 cases, 3 had severe floppy epiglottis (downward displacement of the epiglottis with covering of the laryngeal inlet during inspiration), but two had mild laryngomalacia (no covering of the laryngeal inlet). One-year follow-up revealed another mild patient developing severe floppy epiglottis over the time. In patients with MSA, a laryngeal motor tone abnormality associated with neurodegeneration and Bernoulli effect may influence the development of floppy epiglottis [29]. This suggests that in MSA there might be a disease progression of epiglottic obstruction with CPAP.

As many as 77–93% of children with laryngomalacia may have OSA [30, 31]. Infants with laryngomalacia can achieve improved ventilatory pattern and unloaded respiratory muscle effort (decreased respiratory rate and esophageal pressure swings) with CPAP (pressures between 8 and 10 cm H_2O) which is preferred compared to BPAP [15, 32].

15.4 Epiglottis Collapse as Cause of CPAP Failure and how to Diagnose it

It has been previously stated that epiglottic collapse can be a cause of CPAP low adherence. In fact, according to the European position paper, one of the indications for DISE are patients who do not tolerate CPAP [33]. Most of the times, DISE will show the epiglottic collapse and it is assumed that this structure is implicated, especially when the patients report that they feel suffocated during the night. Fig. 15.9 (Video 15.2) shows DISE-CPAP titration, with different pressures and jaw thrust maneuver, in a patient intolerant to CPAP use. Epiglottic collapse occurred despite high pressure and was even worse with the increase of CPAP level from 13 to 14 cm H_2O. Jaw thrust maneuver prevented the hypopharyngeal and epiglottic collapse. This patient was then indicated to MMA, with success.

The fact that many CPAP intolerant patients undergo DISE might be the cause of the high rates of epiglottic collapse reported in the literature. In the systematic review performed by Torre et al. in 2015, the incidence of epiglottic collapse ranged from 9.6% to 73.5% [34]. This enormous difference in the series published is probably caused by the heterogeneity of the studies (differences in OSA severity, BMI, anatomy, etc.) but there might also be differences in the terminology used by the different authors. Some authors may include only primary epiglottic collapse while others, both primary and secondary epiglottic collapse. Primary collapse is caused by a floppy epiglottis collapsing in the anteroposterior direction or, even more rarely, folding laterally, as for example in laryngomalacia. Secondary epiglottic collapse is an anteroposterior collapse due to posterior displacement of the tongue base, and is more frequent than primary collapse.

In some patients performing DISE and CPAP simultaneously will show the cause of the intolerance. The case series articles published performing CPAP-DISE showed that epiglottic collapse was the cause of intolerance in 27–61% of the patients [10, 27, 35]. The differences in reported numbers is probably caused by the

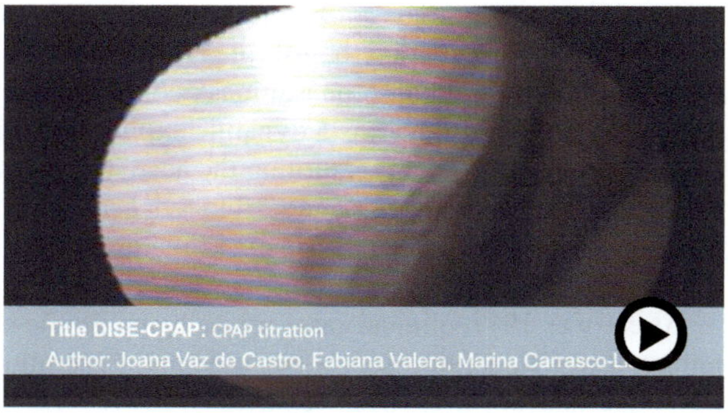

Fig. 15.9 (Video 15.2) DISE-CPAP titration with different pressures and jaw thrust maneuvers (► https://doi.org/10.1007/000-bfb)

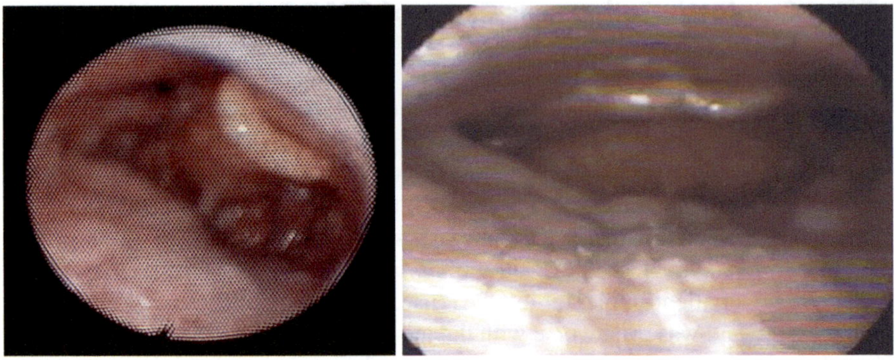

Fig. 15.10 DISE-CPAP showing epiglottic collapse in a child 10 years old with persistent OSA after adenotonsillectomy (left) and in an adult (right)

small sample size in each study and heterogeneity, as in the study by Yui et al., where partial epiglottic collapse was also included [35]. Nevertheless, in all these series there was also persistent collapse in all the UA areas except in the lateral pharyngeal walls, which caused the CPAP intolerance in other patients. Dieleman et al. also reported that in 10% of cases in their series, no UA collapse was observed during CPAP-DISE [27] (Fig. 15.10).

When performing CPAP-DISE, it is of the upmost importance to use the same mask as the patient is using every night, as this may influence the tolerance. If the patient usually uses a nasal mask, the fiberscope can be inserted through the inferior part of the sealing silicone. In case of an oronasal mask, a flexible fiberscope may be inserted through side holes, under the mask, or with an adapted mask [27]. Alternatively, a fiberscope can be passed through a bronchoscopy swivel adapter with a self-sealing diaphragm between the mask and CPAP circuit [8] (Fig. 15.11).

Some patients with severe OSA and CPAP intolerance might have a high surgical risk and UA surgery may not be the first option. Nevertheless, performing CPAP-DISE in these patients may be useful. Yui et al. showed that the same pressure of CPAP applied through an oronasal mask could not open the UA as well as a nasal mask [36]. As CPAP-DISE is a dynamic exploration where maneuvers can be performed, changing mask type, turning the head, advancing the mandible, or adding a MAD, ameliorate conditions and lead to reduced pressure and increased adherence. Videos 15.1 and 15.2 show the image of the pharynx with different maneuvers and PAP pressures.

As early as 1987, clinical cases reporting epiglottic collapse as a cause for CPAP failure, using videofluoroscopy, emerged in the literature. and at that time the DISE technique had not even been reported yet [37, 38]. However, DISE offers many advantages over videofluoroscopy; therefore, it should remain the preferred diagnostic tool. During awake fiberoptic examination, the collapse of a floppy epiglottis

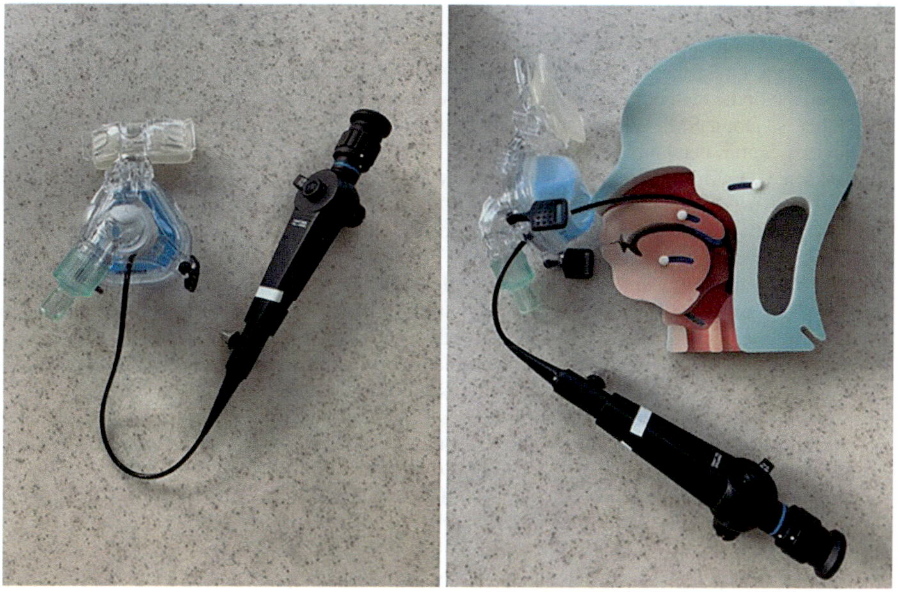

Fig. 15.11 Insertion of the fiberscope through the adapted hole of the mask. Adopted from Dieleman [27]

observed during inspiration can also raise suspicion for epiglottic collapse associated with CPAP intolerance [39].

The shape of the flow signal during conventional PSG is related to the structure causing the collapse. It has been reported that the epiglottic collapse causes a specific curve, with features of discontinuity and jaggedness in nasal cannula or pneumotachograph. Meanwhile, non-epiglottic collapse often produces a "flat-top" flow shape [40]. Therefore, exploring the flow curve under CPAP titration might be another method to discover whether the epiglottis is the cause of intolerance, but as far as we know, there are no publications on this subject so far. In fact, this noninvasive method could answer the question if some types of epiglottic collapse could be solved with CPAP. Intuitively, anteroposterior epiglottic collapse due to a floppy epiglottis may worsen with the increased pressure, but it could happen that lateral collapse of the epiglottis could be relieved. We could not find any publications exploring this idea either.

In conclusion, the studies performed with CPAP-DISE show that the epiglottis is the structure responsible for CPAP intolerance in an important number of patients. The easiest way to diagnose epiglottic collapse is DISE and it is performed in a high proportion of patients with CPAP intolerance and less frequently on those with optimal CPAP adaptation. To elucidate which epiglottic characteristics could predict CPAP (in)tolerance, it would be interesting to perform DISE-CPAP on all patients before CPAP therapy initialization.

References

1. Pevernagie D, Sastry M, van Maanen JP. D. Sleep related breathing disorders: treatment. In: Sleep medicine textbook. Regensburg: European Sleep Research Society; 2021. p. 357–77.
2. Gupta S, Donn SM. Continuous positive airway pressure: physiology and comparison of devices. Semin Fetal Neonatal Med. 2016;21:204–11.
3. Jackson CD, Mosenifar Z What is positive end-expiratory pressure (PEEP) therapy and how is it used with mechanical ventilation? Medscape. 2020. https://www.medscape.com/answers/304068–104,783/what-is-positive-end-expiratory-pressure-peep-therapy-and-how-is-it-used-with-mechanical-ventilation.
4. Patil SP, Ayappa IA, Caples SM, Kimoff RJ, Patel SR, Harrod CG. Treatment of adult obstructive sleep apnea with positive airway pressure: an American Academy of Sleep Medicine Clinical Practice Guideline. J Clin Sleep Med. 2019;15:335–43.
5. Basner RC, Parthasarathy S, editors. Nocturnal non-invasive ventilation: theory, evidence, and clinical practice. Cham: Springer; 2015. https://doi.org/10.1007/978-1-4899-7624-6.
6. Sullivan CE, Berthon-Jones M, Issa FG, Eves L. Reversal of obstructive sleep apnoea by continuous positive airway pressure applied through the nares. Lancet. 1981;317:862–5.
7. Schwab RJ, Pack AI, Gupta KB, Metzger LJ, Oh E, Getsy JE, Hoffman EA, Gefter WB. Upper airway and soft tissue structural changes induced by CPAP in normal subjects. Am J Respir Crit Care Med. 1996;154:1106–16.
8. Torre C, Liu SY, Kushida CA, Nekhendzy V, Huon LK, Capasso R. Impact of continuous positive airway pressure in patients with obstructive sleep apnea during drug-induced sleep endoscopy. Clin Otolaryngol. 2017;42:1218–23.
9. Crawford MW, Rohan D, Macgowan CK, Yoo S-J, Macpherson BA. Effect of propofol anesthesia and continuous positive airway pressure on upper airway size and configuration in infants. Anesthesiology. 2006;105:45–50.
10. Hybášková J, Jor O, Novák V, Zeleník K, Matoušek P, Komínek P. Drug-induced sleep endoscopy changes the treatment concept in patients with obstructive sleep apnoea. Biomed Res Int. 2016;2016:6583216.
11. Hsu Y, Lan M, Huang Y, Kao M, Lan M. Association between breathing route, oxygen desaturation, and upper airway morphology. Laryngoscope. 2021;131(2):E659. https://doi.org/10.1002/lary.28774.
12. Lin H-C, Weaver EM, Lin H-S, Friedman M. Multilevel obstructive sleep apnea surgery. Adv Otorhinolaryngol. 2017;80:109–15.
13. Patil SP, Ayappa IA, Caples SM, Kimoff RJ, Patel SR, Harrod CG. Treatment of adult obstructive sleep apnea with positive airway pressure: An American Academy of sleep medicine systematic review, meta-analysis, and GRADE assessment. J Clin Sleep Med. 2019;15:301–34.
14. Pagel JF, Pandi-Perumal SR. Primary care sleep medicine. Cham: Springer; 2014. https://doi.org/10.1007/978-1-4939-1185-1.
15. Kaditis AG, Alonso Alvarez ML, Boudewyns A, et al. ERS statement on obstructive sleep disordered breathing in 1- to 23-month-old children. Eur Respir J. 2017;50:1700985.
16. Kaditis AG, Alonso Alvarez ML, Boudewyns A, et al. Obstructive sleep disordered breathing in 2- to 18-year-old children: diagnosis and management. Eur Respir J. 2016;47:69–94.
17. Sawyer AM, Gooneratne NS, Marcus CL, Ofer D, Richards KC, Weaver TE. A systematic review of CPAP adherence across age groups: clinical and empiric insights for developing CPAP adherence interventions. Sleep Med Rev. 2011;15:343–56.
18. Li H-Y, Lee L-A, Tsai M-S, Chen N-H, Chuang L-P, Fang T-J, Shen S-C, Cheng W-N. How to manage continuous positive airway pressure (CPAP) failure—hybrid surgery and integrated treatment. Auris Nasus Larynx. 2020;47:335–42.
19. Johnson KG, Johnson DC. Bilevel positive airway pressure worsens central apneas during sleep. Chest. 2005;128:2141–50.
20. Teschler H, Döhring J, Wang Y-M, Berthon-Jones M. Adaptive pressure support servo-ventilation: a novel treatment for Cheyne-stokes respiration in heart failure. Am J Respir Crit Care Med. 2001;164:614–9.

21. Cowie MR, Woehrle H, Wegscheider K, et al. Adaptive servo-ventilation for central sleep apnea in systolic heart failure. N Engl J Med. 2015;373:1095–105.
22. Aurora RN, Bista SR, Casey KR, Chowdhuri S, Kristo DA, Mallea JM, Ramar K, Rowley JA, Zak RS, Heald JL. Updated adaptive servo-ventilation recommendations for the 2012 AASM guideline: the treatment of central sleep apnea syndromes in adults: practice parameters with an evidence-based literature review and meta-analyses. J Clin Sleep Med. 2016;12:757–61.
23. Landry SA, Joosten SA, Eckert DJ, Jordan AS, Sands SA, White DP, Malhotra A, Wellman A, Hamilton GS, Edwards BA. Therapeutic CPAP level predicts upper airway collapsibility in patients with obstructive sleep apnea. Sleep. 2017;40(6):zsx056. https://doi.org/10.1093/sleep/zsx056.
24. Sung CM, Kim HC, Yang HC. The clinical characteristics of patients with an isolate epiglottic collapse. Auris Nasus Larynx. 2020;47:450–7.
25. Kim HCH-Y, Sung C-M, Jang H-B, Kim HCH-Y, Lim SC, Yang HC. Patients with epiglottic collapse showed less severe obstructive sleep apnea and good response to treatment other than continuous positive airway pressure: a case-control study of 224 patients. J Clin Sleep Med. 2020;17(3):413. https://doi.org/10.5664/jcsm.8904.
26. Trachsel D, Hammer J. CPAP to diagnose laryngeal clefts by flexible endoscopy in infants. Pediatr Pulmonol. 2018;53:1284–7.
27. Dieleman E, Veugen CCAFM, Hardeman JA, Copper MP. Drug-induced sleep endoscopy while administering CPAP therapy in patients with CPAP failure. Sleep Breath. 2020;25(1):391. https://doi.org/10.1007/s11325-020-02098-x.
28. Andrade RGS, Madeiro F, Piccin VS, Moriya HT, Schorr F, Sardinha PS, Gregório MG, Genta PR, Lorenzi-Filho G. Impact of acute changes in CPAP flow route in sleep apnea treatment. Chest. 2016;150:1194–201.
29. Shimohata T, Tomita M, Nakayama H, Aizawa N, Ozawa T, Nishizawa M. Floppy epiglottis as a contraindication of CPAP in patients with multiple system atrophy. Neurology. 2011;76:1841–2.
30. Tanphaichitr A, Tanphaichitr P, Apiwattanasawee P, Brockbank J, Rutter MJ, Simakajornboon N. Prevalence and risk factors for central sleep apnea in infants with laryngomalacia. Otolaryngol Head Neck Surg. 2014;150:677–83.
31. Verkest V, Verhulst S, Van Hoorenbeeck K, Vanderveken O, Saldien V, Boudewyns A. Prevalence of obstructive sleep apnea in children with laryngomalacia and value of polysomnography in treatment decisions. Int J Pediatr Otorhinolaryngol. 2020;137:110255.
32. Essouri S, Nicot F, Clément A, Garabedian E-N, Roger G, Lofaso F, Fauroux B. Noninvasive positive pressure ventilation in infants with upper airway obstruction: comparison of continuous and bilevel positive pressure. Intensive Care Med. 2005;31:574–80.
33. De Vito A, Carrasco Llatas M, Ravesloot MJ, et al. European position paper on drug-induced sleep endoscopy: 2017 update. Clin Otolaryngol. 2018;43:1541–52.
34. Torre C, Camacho M, Liu SY-C, Huon L-K, Capasso R. Epiglottis collapse in adult obstructive sleep apnea: a systematic review. Laryngoscope. 2016;126:515–23.
35. Yui MS, Tominaga Q, Lopes BCP, Eckeli AL, de Almeida LA, Rabelo FAW, Küpper DS, Valera FCP. Can drug-induced sleep endoscopy (DISE) predict compliance with positive airway pressure therapy? A pilot study. Sleep Breath; 2021. https://doi.org/10.1007/s11325-021-02360-w.
36. Yui MS, Tominaga Q, Lopes BCP, Eckeli AL, Rabelo FAW, Küpper DS, Valera FCP. Nasal vs. oronasal mask during PAP treatment: a comparative DISE study. Sleep Breath. 2020;24:1129–36.
37. Andersen APD, Alving J, Lildholdt T, Wulff CH. Obstructive sleep apnea initiated by a lax epiglottis: a contraindication for continuous positive airway pressure. Chest. 1987;91:621–3.
38. Croft CB, Pringle M. Sleep nasendoscopy: a technique of assessment in snoring and obstructive sleep apnoea. Clin Otolaryngol Allied Sci. 1991;16:504–9.
39. Verse T, Pirsig W. Age-related changes in the epiglottis causing failure of nasal continuous positive airway pressure therapy. J Laryngol Otol. 1999;113:1022–5.
40. Azarbarzin A, Marques M, Sands SA, et al. Predicting epiglottic collapse in patients with obstructive sleep apnoea. Eur Respir J. 2017;50:1700345.

Orofacial Myofunctional Therapy 16

Carlos O'Connor-Reina and Marina Carrasco-Llatas

16.1 Introduction to Orofacial Myofunctional Therapy: An Overview

The pathophysiological mechanisms of obstructive sleep apnea (OSA) are not fully known, and a multifactorial origin has been suggested [1]. In OSA, the interaction between anatomical and functional factors seems to determine whether the upper airway (UA) collapses as a result of an imbalance between the forces that tend to close and those that keep the UA open [2]. Since the studies of Remmers et al., it is believed that the forces that prevent pharyngeal obstruction are produced by the dilator muscles, the main dilator of the UA being the genioglossus muscle, and that these are involved in the pathogenesis of OSA [3–6]. Studies have found a ≈ 15% increase in the percentage of type IIA muscle fibers (fast-twitch fibers that use aerobic and anaerobic metabolism, but have a low fatigue threshold) in airway muscles such as the uvula in patients with OSA [7].

Guilleminault considered hypotony of the muscles of UA as the main pathophysiological reason for OSA, and this is the main therapeutic objective of the therapist. Orofacial myofunctional therapy (OMT) is one of the newest treatments for

---

Supplementary Information The online version contains supplementary material available at https://doi.org/10.1007/978-3-031-34992-8_16. The videos can be accessed individually by clicking the DOI link in the accompanying figure caption or by scanning this link with the SN More Media App.

C. O'Connor-Reina (✉)
Head of Otorhinolaryngology Department in Hospital Quironsalud Marbella, Marbella, Spain
e-mail: carlos.oconnor@quironsalud.es

M. Carrasco-Llatas
Department of Otorhinolaryngology, Hospital Universitario Dr. Peset, Valencia, Spain

Department of Otorhinolaryngology, IMED Hospital, Valencia, Spain

M. Delakorda, N. de Vries (eds.), *The Role of Epiglottis in Obstructive Sleep Apnea*, https://doi.org/10.1007/978-3-031-34992-8_16

sleep-disordered breathing (SDB) [8]. OMT is based on daily exercises with the aim of strengthening the oropharyngeal muscles and facilitating UA opening [9]. OSA originates from suboptimal function of the dilator muscles of the airway. OMT is a therapy designed, theoretically, to deal with the anatomical mechanism underlying this disease [10]. The patient is instructed to perform OMT exercises regularly for 20–40 min daily for at least 3 months under the supervision of a speech therapist. The exercises can be guided with the use of diagrams, apps, or videos. The idea of this therapy is to improve the tone of the UA muscles by reducing their volume and collapsibility. However, there is no evidence regarding who is the most suitable candidate for OMT.

16.1.1 Exercises

Suitable patients for this therapy should have no anatomical limitations and should be able to breathe through the nose. Therefore, short lingual frenulum, temporomandibular joint dysfunction, and the presence of anatomical nose obstruction can affect the results obtained from this therapy.

Classically, OMT exercises are based on isometric and isotonic contractions performed rhythmically, preferably before going to sleep (Fig. 16.1). The genioglossus is the main muscle activated. These exercises should be performed over the long term and adherence is important [11].

Different protocols for these exercises have been reported, and there is no consensus on which is most suitable. Most of these exercises are based on the randomized clinical trial (RCT) of Guimarães et al., in which the oropharyngeal exercises were based on those used to treat speech–language pathologies and included soft palate, tongue, and facial muscle exercises as well as stomatognathic function exercises [12].

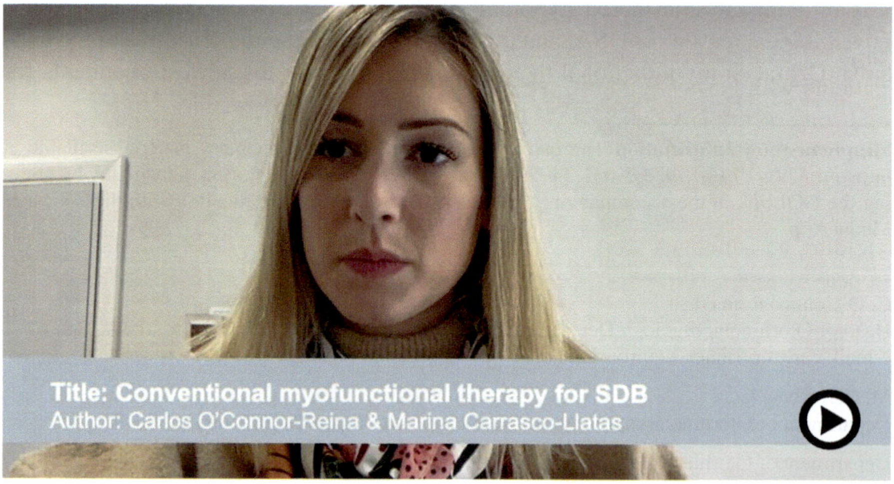

Fig. 16.1 (Video 16.1) An example of conventional orofacial myofunctional speech therapy for SDB (▶ https://doi.org/10.1007/000-bfg)

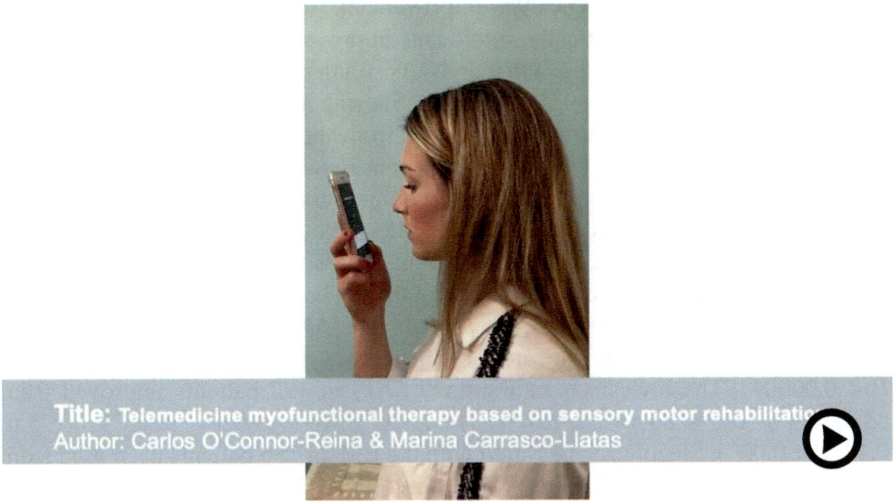

Fig. 16.2 (Video 16.2) Telemedicine orofacial myofunctional speech therapy based on sensory motor rehabilitation (▶ https://doi.org/10.1007/000-bfe)

Adherence to the OMT exercises is the main difficulty for patients. Some studies have reported adherence rates as low as 10% [11]. Newer concepts about the type of exercises have been reported recently, including the concept of sensory motor rehabilitation, which is based on the proprioceptive concept (Fig. 16.2) [13]. These authors consider this kind of exercise to be most suitable for patients with OSA with sensorial and motor deficits.

16.1.2 Scientific Evidence

In 2009, Guimarães et al. reported the first RCT to use OMT in the treatment of patients with OSA [12]. They used their exercise protocol to increase the strength and tone of the UA muscles and increase its patency. The patients were recently diagnosed with mild to moderate OSA and were aged 25–65 years. In the experimental group, 16 patients completed the study, giving an adherence rate of 84.25%; in the control group given sham therapy, only 15 patients completed the study, yielding an adherence rate of 75%. The parameters studied were sleep efficiency, apnea–hypopnea index (AHI) in the rapid eye movement (REM) and non-REM stages, and subjective values assessed using the Berlin and Epworth questionnaires. Guimarães et al. reported a significant reduction in the AHI from 22 ± 4.8 to 13.7 ± 8.5 events/h in the intervention group, but no significant change in the control group (22.4 ± 5.4 to 25.9 ± 8.5 events/h) [12].

The meta-analysis by Hsu et al. was based on nine studies with 394 adults and children diagnosed with mild to severe OSA. Eight of the nine studies measured the

AHI and reported an average 39% improvement from the baseline value after OMT. There was no statistically significant improvement in ESS from baseline ($P = 0.062$). Nevertheless, the Pittsburgh questionnaire score improved by −1.3 from 21 (95% CI = −2.4 to −0.2; P = 0.026). Snoring intensity also improved in the intervention group and differed significantly from the control group ($P = 0.044$). Hsu et al. concluded that OMT could be considered an alternative therapy for OSA. However, given the small number of studies included and the heterogeneity of the records, the conclusions may have been affected by bias [14].

Meghpara et al. published a meta-analysis of 15 studies with 237 patients who reported OSA outcomes before and after OMT. The mean AHI decreased from 28.0 ± 16.2 events/h to 18.6 ± 13.1 events/h. The AHI standard mean difference (SMD) was −1.34, which indicated a large effect (95% CI = −0.84 to −1.85; $P < 0.00001$). The lowest O_2 saturation (LSAT) in 197 patients improved from 83.18% ± 6.10% to 85.13% ± 7.01%. The LSAT SMD was 0.44 (95% CI = 0.75 to 0.12; $P < 0.007$). Sleepiness measured with the ESS in 156 patients decreased from 12.71 ± 5.73 to 8.78 ± 5.80 points. The ESS score SMD was −1.0 (95% CI = −0.50 to −1.50; $P < 0.0001$). The authors concluded that OMT in adults reduced the AHI by 34% and ESS score by 4 points and improved LSAT by 2%, and that OMT is a possible adjunct treatment for OSA [15].

Ieto et al. published the first RCT on the use of OMT to treat snoring in 39 patients randomly assigned to an intervention group that performed exercises or a control group. The intervention group performed exercises for 8 min three times/day, and the sham therapy involved breathing exercises. Both groups performed exercises for 3 months. The intensity and number of snores were analyzed. In the intervention group, snore index (snores >36 dB/h) decreased by ≈ 50% from 99.5 [49.6–221.3] to 48.2 [25.5–219.2] ($P = 0.017$) and the total snore index (total power of snore/h) decreased from 60.4 [21.8–220.6] to 31.0 [10.1–146.5] ($P = 0.033$) [16]. The results of some studies on OMT are summarized in Table 16.1 [12, 16, 18, 19].

Carrasco et al. reported that the available evidence demonstrates a positive effect of OMT in reducing OSA in adults as assessed using polysomnography (PSG) and clinical variables. The available evidence is solid for snoring reduction in adults. There is no evidence to support the use of OMT to treat UA resistance syndrome, including how long the effects last or which OMT protocol is better in children or adults. Despite these knowledge gaps, the available evidence indicates that OMT is safe. The available evidence for the use and safety of OMT suggests that OMT should be initially offered as a noninvasive therapy to patients with SDB [20].

Although there are other possible treatment options for some patients with OSA, such as oral appliances or surgery, Rueda et al. consider OMT to be noninvasive, inexpensive, and with no major risks. It may be a safe and acceptable option for many patients with OSA and would be economically accessible for lower-income people and countries [21].

Table 16.1 The results of some studies on OMT

	OSA	Intervention group			Control group		
	Mild OSA (AHI, 5–15 events/h); moderate OSA (AHI, 15–30 events/h); severe OSA (AHI > 30 events/h)	AHI basal	After treatment events/h	AHI change (%)	Basal AHI, event/h	After treatment events/h	AHI change (%)
Diaferia et al., 2013 [17]	26% mild	28.0 ± 22.7	13.9 ± 18.5	−50.4	27.8 ± 20.3	30.6 ± 21.8	10.1
	32% moderate						
	42% severe						
Guimarães et al., 2009 [12]	Moderate OSA	22.4 ± 4.8	13.7 ± 8.5	−38.8	22.4 ± 5.4	25.9 ± 8.5	15.6
Ieto et al., 2015 [16]	Mild to moderate OSA	22.4 ± 4.89	19.2 ± 6.44	−24.4%	25.7 ± 5.7	22.8 ± 7.33	−11.3
Kuo et al., 2017 [18]	Mild to moderate	16.5 ± 7.93	9.9 ± 3.56	−50.0	14.6 ± 5.2	15.18 ± 3.15	4.0
	$n = 14$ mild						
	$n = 11$ moderate						
Villa et al., 2015 [19]	Paediatric participants: AHI > 5 events/h for those with moderate to severe OSA	4.87 ± 2.96	1.84 ± 1.36	−62.2	4.56 ± 3.22	4.11 ± 2.73	−9.9

16.1.3 Clinical Impact Measurement

OMT is considered to be an optional therapy in adults and children with mild to moderate OSA (AHI < 15 events/h). It has been shown to be effective in reducing AHI, excessive sleepiness, and in improving quality of life, and adherence to other therapies such as continuous positive airway pressure (CPAP). Patients prescribed OMT should be examined weekly to assure adherence and proper performance of the exercises. There is no consensus on whether these exercises should be performed with a therapist or using other methods such as telemedicine. The impact of OMT by providing feedback to the patient has been evaluated using different methods [22–24].

Some authors have recommended the use of the Iowa Oral Performance Instrument (model 2.1; IOPI Medical LLC, Carnation, WA) (IOPI) or the tongue digital spoon (TDS) to measure objectively the muscle tone of the UA [22–24]. These instruments can provide objective feedback to patients about whether they are performing exercises properly and increasing the tone of the UA muscles. The IOPI is a portable tool that measures variables related to tongue and lip function by the amount of pressure exerted on a small air-filled bulb. Tongue strength is assessed by measuring the maximum pressure exerted when the patient presses a disposable standard-sized tongue bulb against the roof of the mouth. Lip strength is assessed by measuring the maximum pressure on the bulb located between the cheek and closed teeth, and the patient contracts the buccinator muscle without biting the bulb. The pressure obtained (kPa) is digitally displayed on an LCD panel on the instrument. A series of LED lights representing percentages in 10% increments of a manually set pressure baseline acts in combination with a built-in timer to measure endurance. As an instrument that measures tongue function, the IOPI has been used in several published experiments and has high inter- and intra-rater reliability [25, 26]. Reference values had been obtained from measurements in the population and are provided by the manufacturer [27, 28] (Fig. 16.3).

The digital spoon is used as a kitchen tool to estimate the weight (g) of food [24]. To develop the TDS, we used the Soehnle Cooking Star Digital Measuring Spoon, a hand scale with a spoon, with graduations from 0.1 g to 500 g. This TDS consists of a handle containing the tare and hold buttons. Pressing the hold button allows one to obtain the highest tared value, which is equivalent to the IOPI peak pressure (Fig. 16.4). To perform the measurements, the spoon is inverted and a 1 cm^2 circular

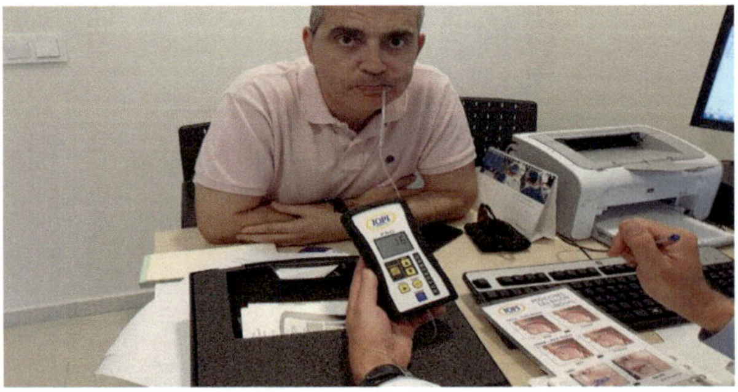

Fig. 16.3 Measurement of the lip strength with the IOPI

sticker is placed on the underside to provide a surface measurement (g/cm^2). The patient holds the spoon by the handle and, with the elbow resting on a flat surface, brings the spoon close to the tongue with an elbow angle of $\approx 30°$. The device is tared by pressing the hold key to mark 0.0 g. The patient then presses the vertex or tip of the tongue as strongly as possible on the marked circumference. When finished, using the index finger of the hand that holds the handle, the patient again presses the hold button. This test is performed fully by the patient to avoid any movements of the spoon that may interfere with the result. Our protocol recommends patients to use this spoon and act on their own control and the IOPI as an additional monthly control to confirm the changes in values as the patient performs the exercises over time. Also, it is a possible alternative method to stimulate patients (Fig. 16.5).

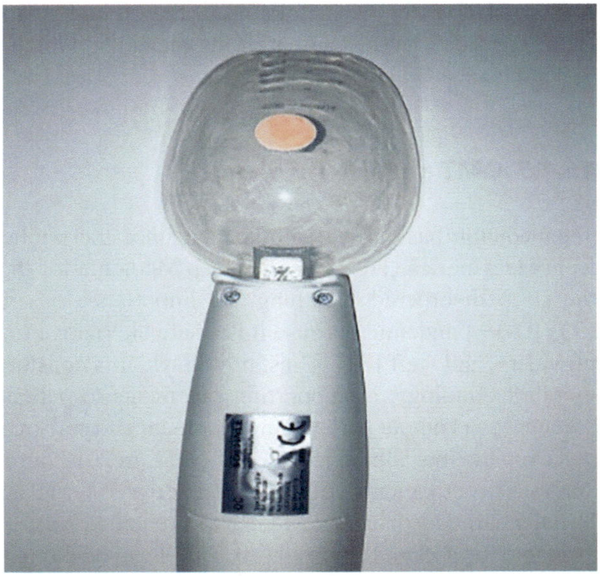

Fig. 16.4 Image of the TDS with a dot to show the patient where the tongue should be placed

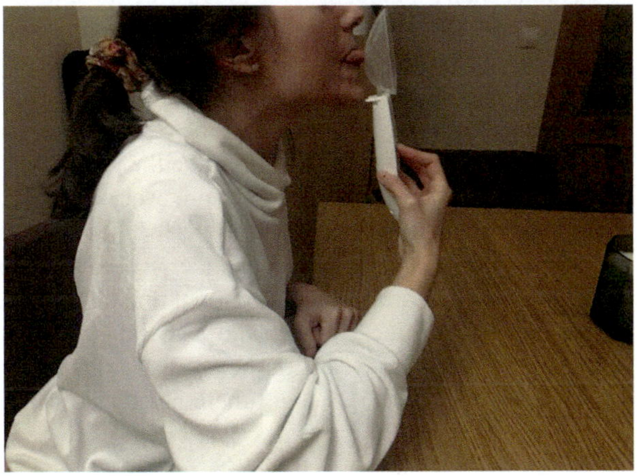

Fig. 16.5 Use of the TDS measuring the tongue strength

16.1.4 Side Effects, Adherence, and Compliance

Overall, OMT seems to be a safe treatment that has a low incidence of minor complications. Diaféria et al. reported that "there were very few side effects"; however, they did not provide details about them [17]. Randerath et al. performed an RCT of patients using passive OMT with electric stimulation of the tongue. Patients reported higher rates of erythema, skin irritation, and facial pain compared with patients in the placebo group [29]. In a study of patients following a mobile app OMT program, O'Connor et al. reported one case of tongue irritation, one case of temporomandibular joint disorder, and three cases of fatigue that led to rejection of the use of the app [30].

In children, OMT is a safe treatment according to the available evidence. Chuang et al. examined the use of passive OMT with an intraoral mandibular advancement device (MAD). At 1-year follow-up, they found an increase in the vertical facial growth and clockwise rotation of the mandible, which they attributed to the use of the oral device [31].

16.1.5 OMT and Telemedicine

Telemedicine has earned significance since the publication of the position paper from the American Academy of Sleep Medicine for the diagnosis and treatment of the sleep disordered breathing. Its importance has grown exponentially during COVID-19 pandemic because it is a safe alternative to provide wellness to patient, providers, and staff [32]. Thus, nowadays, it is considered a useful tool, especially mobile technology, in supporting treatments to patients with OSA because of its potential to promote patient empowerment and self-management.

Given the low adherence rates of OMT, in 2017 our research group developed an app to instruct patients with OSA in the use of OMT and to monitor their progress. Initially named Apnea Bye, it later was renamed AirwayGym®. The app is currently available for iOS and Android [10, 33]. It can be thought of as a portable fitness app except that its use is intended for OSA patients, rather than athletes, and that therapists, rather than trainers, provide the instructions. Its novelty is that it is the first app in the health-care market that allows the patient to interact directly with the smartphone without needing any other device. The app focuses on sleep apnea disease and improving proprioceptive deficits. When used with the app, the phone provides acoustic feedback on the efficacy of the exercises performed. It includes nine exercises based on OMT that aim to improve the tonicity of the muscles involved in the pathogenesis of OSA (Fig. 16.6). Before every exercise, an animated demonstration and a video show the patient how to perform the exercise. After each exercise, the patient receives visual, acoustic, and tactile feedback on the success of their performance as a point score. When the patient finishes the exercises, the results are saved on a networked online storage, and a therapist can evaluate the patient's performance of the exercises. Users of the app can follow the progress of their daily activity over time (Fig. 16.7). A chat function is available through which the patient can contact the therapist directly.

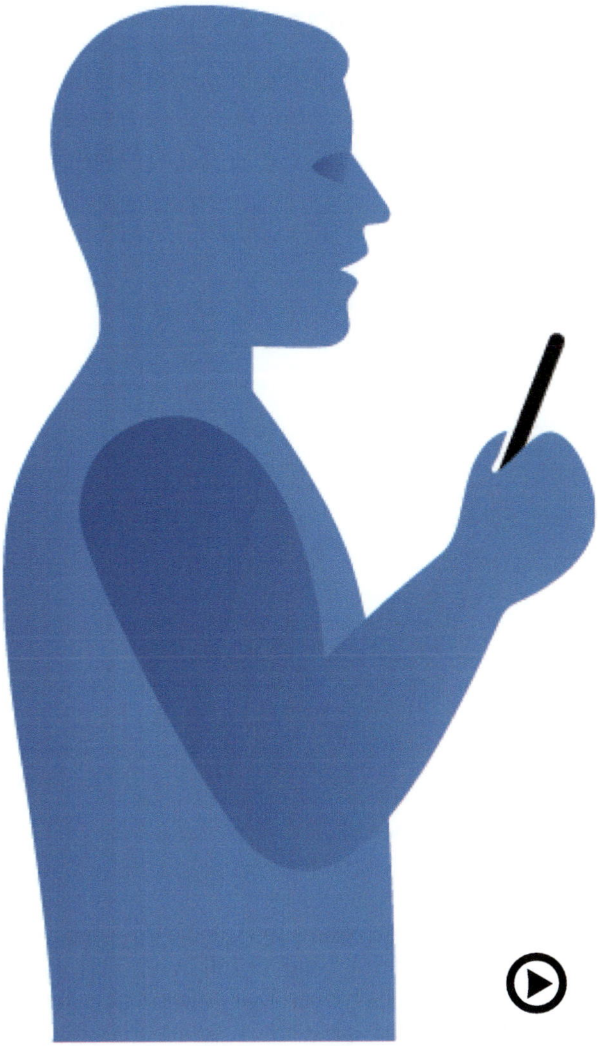

Fig. 16.6 (Video 16.3) An example of one of the exercises that the patient performs using the Airway Gym app (▶ https://doi.org/10.1007/000-bff)

The main objective of the exercises in the app is to increase the tone of the extrinsic muscles of the tongue (genioglossus, hyoglossus, styloglossus, and palatoglossus). The exercises are based on those described by Guimarães et al. and have been adapted to allow feedback using a smartphone [33]. The first results obtained with this app have been presented [33]. The app has been reported to be successful in an isolated clinical case [34] and in a preliminary series of 20 patients [30]. In the preliminary series, 15 of 20 (75%) patients adhered to the use of the OMT as indicated by their performance of the exercises 5 days a week. In patients who performed the exercises, the AHI decreased significantly from 25.78 ± 12.6 to 14.1 ± 7.7 events/h. The ESS scores also decreased from 18.2 ± 1.98 to 14.2 ± 7.7 and the minimum O_2 saturation decreased from 84.87% ± 7.02% to 89.27% ± 3.77%.

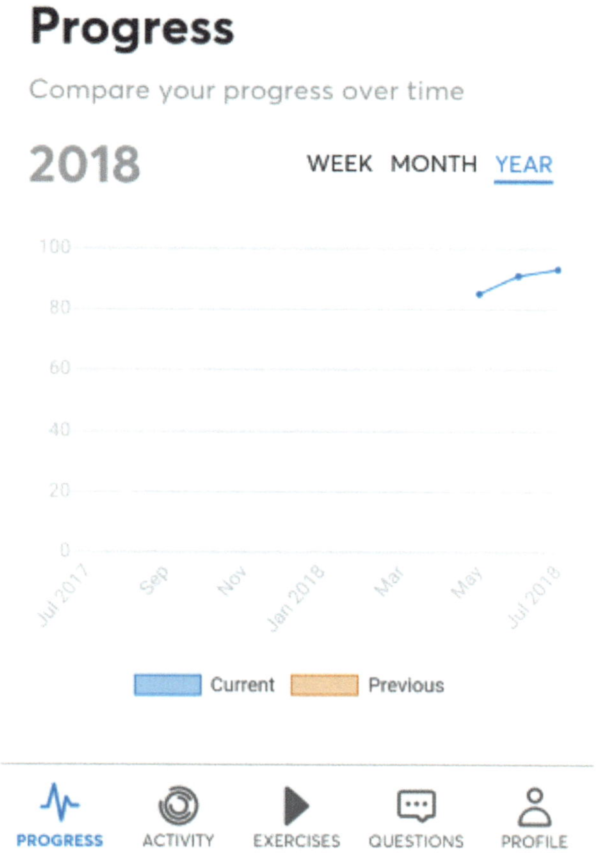

Fig. 16.7 Interface where patients can follow their own progress, also available for the doctor to confirm the patient compliance

A pilot RCT was conducted afterwards to evaluate the effects of these exercises in patients with severe OSA after a 3-month follow-up [35]. Forty patients with severe OSA (AHI > 30 events/h) were enrolled prospectively and randomized into an intervention group that used the app for 90 sessions or a control group. After the intervention, 28 patients remained adherent to OMT. No significant changes were observed in the control group. However, the intervention group showed significant improvements: AHI decreased by 53.4% from 44.7 to 20.88 events/h; the ESS score decreased from 10.33 to 5.37; and minimum O_2 saturation decreased by 46.5% from 36.31% to 19.4% (Fig. 16.8). The IOPI maximum tongue score increased from 39.83 to 59.06 kPa, and the IOPI maximum lip score increased from 27.89 to 44.11 kPa. The final AHI correlated significantly with the improvements in IOPI tongue and lip scores (Fig. 16.9). This was the first RCT performed with OMT in patients with severe OSA, and the results were similar to those obtained with other therapies [36].

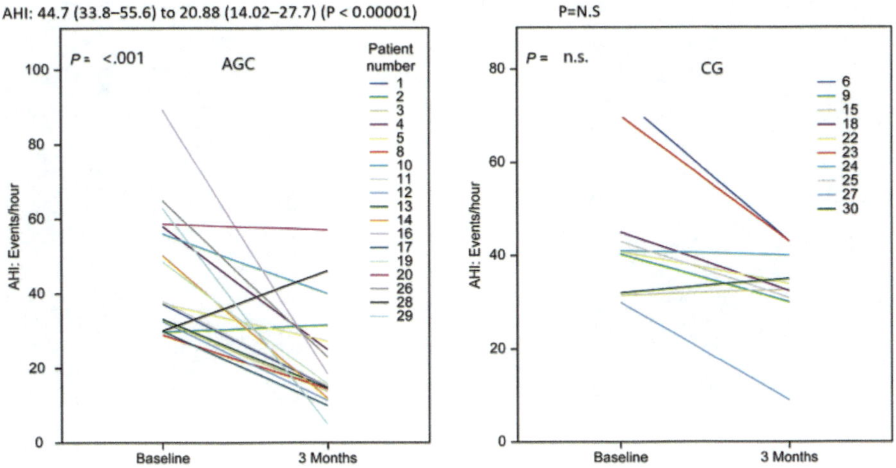

Fig. 16.8 Pre- and posttreatment AHI in the patients performing OMT (left side) or in the control group (right side). Only in the OMT there was a significant reduction in the AHI after therapy

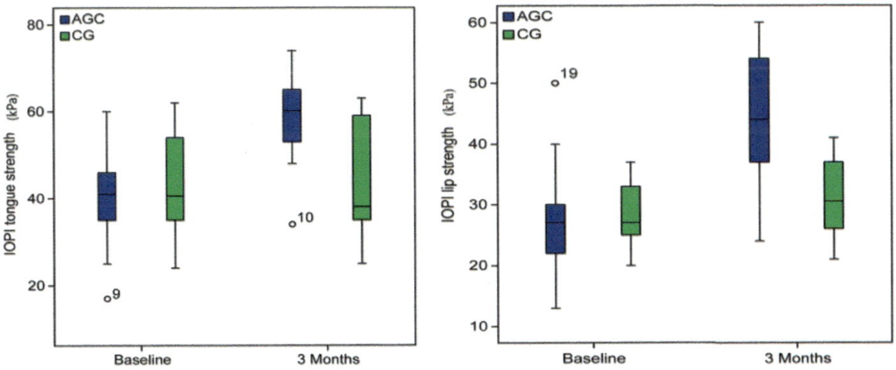

Fig. 16.9 Box plot showing the IOPI measurements of the tongue (right) and lips in the OMT and control groups

16.2 Diagnosis of Orofacial Myofunctional Disorders and Their Relationship with SDB

The diagnosis of an orofacial myofunctional disorder is based on an evaluation by a speech therapist. Orofacial myofunctional disorder is defined as one or a combination of the following: (1) abnormal thumb-, finger-, lip-, or tongue-sucking habits; (2) inappropriate mouth-open lips-open resting posture (lip incompetence); (3) forward interdental rest posture of the tongue; (4) forward rest position of the tongue against the maxillary incisors; (5) lateral posterior interdental tongue rest

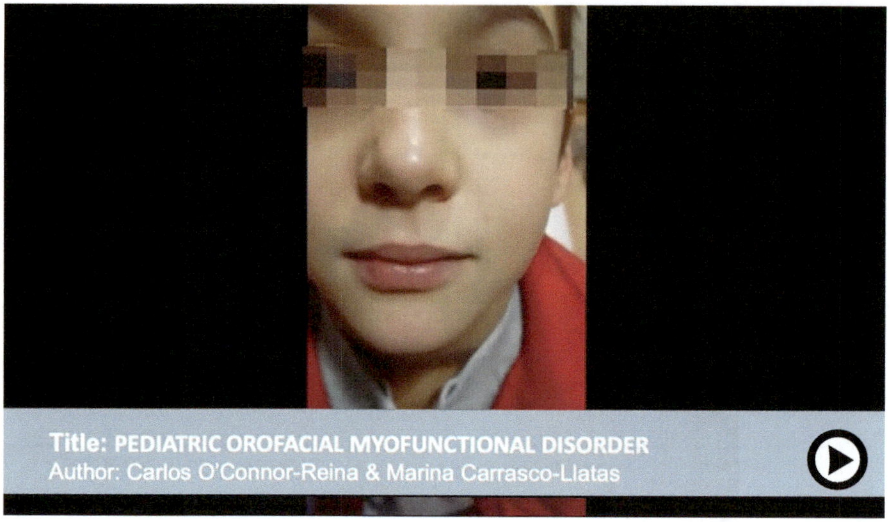

Fig. 16.10 (Video 16.4) Pediatric orofacial myofunctional disorder (▶ https://doi.org/10.1007/000-bfd)

posture; or (6) inappropriate thrusting of the tongue in speaking and/or swallowing (tongue thrusting) [37] (Fig. 16.10). Guilleminault and others consider that the presence of this disorder during childhood increases the risk of OSA in adulthood [38, 39].

The main test used to diagnose orofacial myofunctional disorder associated with OSA is the orofacial myofunctional evaluation expanded with scores (OMES), which includes several items and is administered by a speech therapist [40]. This test requires a well-trained speech therapist not available anywhere. Our group is conducting a case control study to evaluate the methods to select patients with OSA for OMT. Our evaluation uses the IOPI and TDS. Our hypothesis is that lower scores obtained with these instruments can complement the information obtained by the OMES questionnaire. We have started this study designed as a protocol to identify suitable patients for OMT [41].

In our practice, we use the results of drug-induced sleep endoscopy (DISE) to explain to the patient the reason for UA collapse and to improve adherence to OMT. Our group has published correlations between IOPI scores and tongue base and classification (T stage) during DISE [22]. Providing patients' information obtained by PSG, DISE, IOPI, TDS, and OMES gives them feedback on the state of their UA muscles and helps them to understand the disease. In our experience, the rate of adherence to OMT is 65%.

16.3 OMT Treatment and Epiglottic Collapse

Kuo et al. consider the epiglottis as a potential collapse site among multilevel obstructions in patients with moderate to severe OSA. They noted that the epiglottic length is highly sensitive for predicting epiglottis attachment to the posterior pharyngeal wall and found a cut-off value of 16.6 mm. Patients with epiglottic collapse have significantly lower body mass index (BMI) that does not correspond with the severity of OSA. Patients with epiglottic collapse are expected to respond well to oral devices or positional therapy [42].

Floppy epiglottis causing a trapdoor collapse is one of the most challenging conditions for sleep surgeons [43]. Its diagnosis is based on the results of DISE, which allow the surgeon to identify the site of obstruction causing OSA [44]. Until now, the only effective treatment has been surgery to remove the epiglottis totally or partially. However, this surgery involves serious risks such as permanent bronchoaspiration, inspiratory dyspnea, or fixed swallowing problems. Using OMT, we have confirmed that some patients with epiglottic collapse have improved.

The first patient reported was a 50-year-old man who came to our ear, nose, and throat (ENT) department, as recommended by his pneumologist, after diagnosed with OSA because he could not tolerate CPAP or MAD. He complained of progressive somnolence and headaches. He had had two heart infarctions and bypass surgery 3 years previously. He was taking anticoagulant medication and had high blood pressure, which was controlled with calcium channel blockers. The ENT examination showed no anatomical findings to explain his OSA. The patient had Friedman stage 1 and tonsil size grade 1. An examination showed no obstruction and a normal size of the tongue. In a sleep study performed using PSG, his AHI was 31.2 events/h. His BMI was 22.1 kg/m^2, ESS score was 22, minimal O_2 saturation was 91.3%, tongue IOPI score was 34 kPa, and lips score was 15 kPa. Given this history, we offered him to perform DISE, which revealed a floppy, "trap door" type of epiglottis closure. Three expert sleep surgeons evaluated the video and considered that the only viable option was a partial epiglottectomy or epiglottoplasty under general anesthesia. For personal reasons, the patient declined surgery and did not tolerate the use of MAD. After obtaining his consent for OMT, he started using Airway Gym app for 90 sessions and arranged periodic follow-up. The patient noticed that his headaches and somnolence decreased gradually. His IOPI score improved monthly and reached a tongue score of 51 kPa and lips score of 25 kPa. DISE was repeated after 3 months and found that the epiglottis collapse had improved (Fig. 16.11). A new sleep study found that his AHI had decreased to 17.2 events/h, minimal O_2 saturation improved to 95.1%, and ESS score decreased to 15. There was no change in his BMI. The patient is still performing the exercises and a MAD was recommended to improve the residual OSA [33].

The second patient was a 36-year-old man who came to our ENT department with the same problem. The patient exhibited severe OSA with an AHI of 44

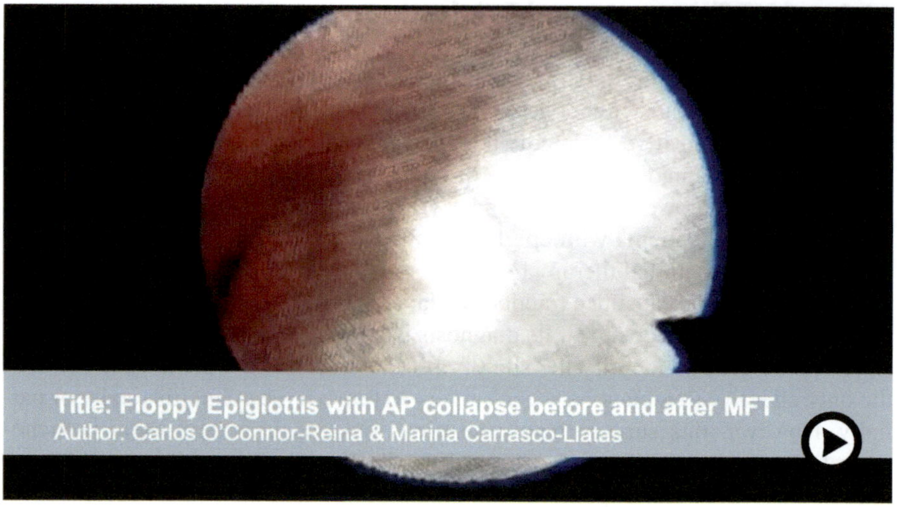

Fig. 16.11 (Video 16.5) Floppy epiglottis with anteroposterior collapse before and after 90 sessions of OMT (▶ https://doi.org/10.1007/000-bfh)

events/h, minimum O_2 saturation of 81%, Friedman stage 2, tongue IOPI score of 38 kPa, and lips score of 21 kPa. He did not tolerate CPAP or MAD, and DISE was performed. In this DISE, a lateral type of epiglottis collapse was observed. Surgery was offered to the patient, but he rejected it. Therefore, OMT for 90 sessions was suggested and the patient improved progressively. His IOPI tongue score increased to 48 kPa and lips score to 30 kPa. His AHI decreased to 29 events/h and his minimum O_2 saturation improved to 90%. DISE was repeated and it was observed that the collapsibility during an Esmarch maneuver disappeared. Likewise, a recommendation was made to the patient to use his MAD again (Fig. 16.12). A new sleep study with MAD showed that his AHI was 12 events/h and his minimum O_2 saturation was 92%. The patient continues to decline surgery (Unpublished data).

These are the two first cases reported for which the anatomical changes (type of epiglottis collapse) that patients experience after OMT were documented with DISE. The mechanism that explains how these exercises modify the epiglottis collapse is unknown. However, in patients who are noncompliant with other treatments, OMT could be a helpful therapy with few side effects, as has been demonstrated in these patients [34] Nevertheless, the real-life effect needs to be confirmed in larger series.

In conclusion, OMT is a comprehensive approach that begins by creating awareness of the reciprocal impact of OSA on the orofacial musculature and oronasal functions. OMT is a reasonable option for increasing adherence to conventional therapies and, in selected patients, may offer a valid option for treating OSA [45].

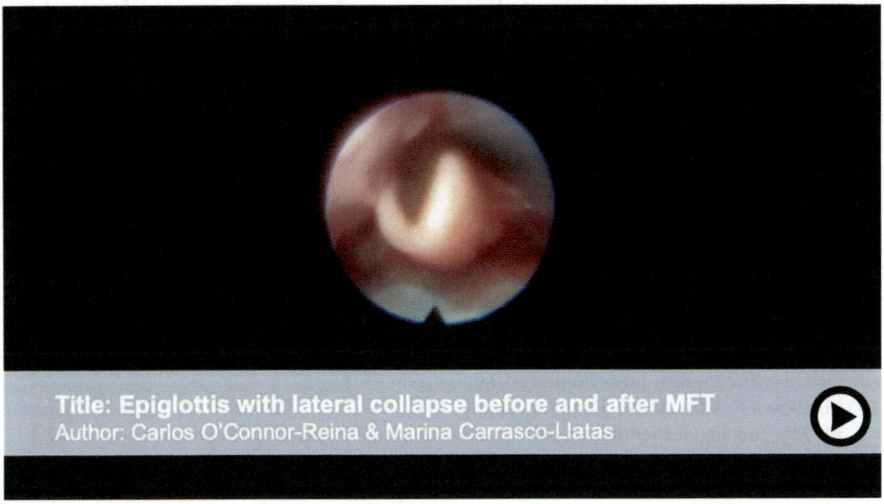

Fig. 16.12 (Video 16.6) DISE video showing the epiglottis with lateral collapse before and after OMT (▶ https://doi.org/10.1007/000-bfj)

References

1. Eckert DJ, White DP, Jordan AS, Malhotra A, Wellman A. Defining phenotypic causes of obstructive sleep apnea. Identification of novel therapeutic targets. Am J Respir Crit Care Med. 2013;188(8):996–1004. https://doi.org/10.1164/rccm.201303-0448OC.
2. White DP. Pathogenesis of obstructive and central sleep apnea. Am J Respir Crit Care Med. 2005;172(11):1363–70. https://doi.org/10.1164/rccm.200412-1631SO. Epub 2005 Aug 11.
3. Remmers JE, deGroot WJ, Sauerland EK, Anch AM. Pathogenesis of upper airway occlusion during sleep. J Appl Physiol Respir Environ Exerc Physiol. 1978;44(6):931–8. https://doi.org/10.1152/jappl.1978.44.6.931.
4. Remmers JE, Anch AM, deGroot WJ, Baker JP Jr, Sauerland EK. Oropharyngeal muscle tone in obstructive sleep apnea before and after strychnine. Sleep. 1980;3(3–4):447–53. https://doi.org/10.1093/sleep/3.3-4.447.
5. Isoni S, Feroah TR, Hajduk EA, Morrison DL, Launois SH, Issa FG, Whitelaw WA, Remmers JE. Anatomy of the pharyngeal airway in sleep apneics: separating anatomic factors from neuromuscular factors. Sleep. 1993;16(8 Suppl):S80–4. https://doi.org/10.1093/sleep/16.suppl_8.s80.
6. Malhotra A, Fogel RB, Edwards JK, Shea SA, White DP. Local mechanisms drive genioglossus activation in obstructive sleep apnea. Am J Respir Crit Care Med. 2000;161(5):1746–9. https://doi.org/10.1164/ajrccm.161.5.9907109.
7. Sériès F, Côté C, Simoneau JA, Gélinas Y, St Pierre S, Leclerc J, Ferland R, Marc I. Physiologic, metabolic, and muscle fiber type characteristics of musculus uvulae in sleep apnea hypopnea syndrome and in snorers. J Clin Invest. 1995;95(1):20–5. https://doi.org/10.1172/JCI117640.
8. Guilleminault C, Huang YS, Quo S. Apraxia in children and adults with obstructive sleep apnea syndrome. Sleep. 2019;42(12):zsz168. https://doi.org/10.1093/sleep/zsz168.
9. Garliner D. Myofunctional therapy. Gen Dent. 1976;24(1):30–40.

10. Amat P, O'Connor-Reina C, Plaza G. Rééducation myofonctionnelle _ orofaciale et syndrome d'apnées obstructives du sommeil: l'apport de la santé connectée. Revue d'Orthopédie Dento Faciale. 2021;55:457–76.
11. Mario Diaz S, Ana Salazar C, Felipe Bravo G, Ocampo-Garcés A. Tratamiento del síndrome de apneas e hipopneas obstructivas del sueño con terapia miofuncional orofaríngea: Experiencia en hospital público de Chile. Rev Otorrinolaringol Cir Cabeza Cuello. 2019;79:395–403.
12. Guimarães KC, Drager LF, Genta PR, Marcondes BF, Lorenzi-Filho G. Effects of oropharyngeal exercises on patients with moderate obstructive sleep apnea syndrome. Am J Respir Crit Care Med. 2009;179(10):962–6. https://doi.org/10.1164/rccm.200806-981OC.
13. Rodríguez-Alcalá L, Martínez JM, Baptista P, Ríos Fernández R, Javier Gómez F, Parejo Santaella J, Plaza G. Sensorimotor tongue evaluation and rehabilitation in patients with sleep-disordered breathing: a novel approach. J Oral Rehabil. 2021;48(12):1363–72. https://doi.org/10.1111/joor.13247.
14. Hsu B, Emperumal CP, Grbach VX, Padilla M, Enciso R. Effects of respiratory muscle therapy on obstructive sleep apnea: a systematic review and meta-analysis. J Clin Sleep Med. 2020;16(5):785–801. https://doi.org/10.5664/jcsm.8318.
15. Meghpara S, Chohan M, Bandyopadhyay A, Kozlowski C, Casinas J, Kushida C, Camacho M. Myofunctional therapy for OSA: a meta-analysis. Expert Rev Respir Med. 2021;22:1–7. https://doi.org/10.1080/17476348.2021.2001332.
16. Ieto V, Kayamori F, Montes MI, Hirata RP, Gregório MG, Alencar AM, Drager LF, Genta PR, Lorenzi-Filho G. Effects of oropharyngeal exercises on snoring: a randomized trial. Chest. 2015;148(3):683–91. https://doi.org/10.1378/chest.14-2953.
17. Diaféria G, Santos-Silva R, Truksinas E, Haddad FLM, Santos R, Bommarito S, Gregório LC, Tufik S, Bittencourt L. Myofunctional therapy improves adherence to continuous positive airway pressure treatment. Sleep Breath. 2017;21(2):387–95. https://doi.org/10.1007/s11325-016-1429-6.
18. Kuo YC, Song TT, Bernard JR, Liao YH. Short-term expiratory muscle strength training attenuates sleep apnea and improves sleep quality in patients with obstructive sleep apnea. Respir Physiol Neurobiol. 2017;243:86–91. https://doi.org/10.1016/j.resp.2017.05.007.
19. Villa MP, Evangelisti M, Martella S, Barreto M, Del Pozzo M. Can myofunctional therapy increase tongue tone and reduce symptoms in children with sleep-disordered breathing? Sleep Breath. 2017;21(4):1025–32. https://doi.org/10.1007/s11325-017-1489-2.
20. Carrasco-Llatas M, O'Connor-Reina C, Calvo-Henríquez C. The role of Myofunctional therapy in treating sleep-disordered breathing: a state-of-the-art review. Int J Environ Res Public Health. 2021;18(14):7291. https://doi.org/10.3390/ijerph18147291.
21. Rueda JR, Mugueta-Aguinaga I, Vilaró J, Rueda-Etxebarria M. Myofunctional therapy (oropharyngeal exercises) for obstructive sleep apnoea. Cochrane Database Syst Rev. 2020;11(11):CD013449. https://doi.org/10.1002/14651858.CD013449.pub2.
22. O'Connor-Reina C, Plaza G, Garcia-Iriarte MT, Ignacio-Garcia JM, Baptista P, Casado-Morente JC, De Vicente E. Tongue peak pressure: a tool to aid in the identification of obstruction sites in patients with obstructive sleep apnea/hypopnea syndrome. Sleep Breath. 2020;24(1):281–6. https://doi.org/10.1007/s11325-019-01952-x.
23. Suzuki M, Okamoto T, Akagi Y, Matsui K, Sekiguchi H, Satoya N, Inoue Y, Tatsuta A, Hagiwara N. Efficacy of oral myofunctional therapy in middle-aged to elderly patients with obstructive sleep apnoea treated with continuous positive airway pressure. J Oral Rehabil. 2021;48(2):176–82. https://doi.org/10.1111/joor.13119.
24. Rodríguez-Alcalá L, Martín-Lagos Martínez JO, Connor-Reina C, Plaza G. Assessment of muscular tone of the tongue using a digital measure spoon in a healthy population: a pilot study. PLoS One. 2021;16(2):e0245901. https://doi.org/10.1371/journal.pone.0245901.
25. Youmans SR, Stierwalt JA. Measures of tongue function related to normal swallowing. Dysphagia. 2006;21(2):102–11. https://doi.org/10.1007/s00455-006-9013-z.
26. Clark HM, Solomon NP. Age and sex differences in orofacial strength. Dysphagia. 2012 Mar;27(1):2–9. https://doi.org/10.1007/s00455-011-9328-2.

27. Clark HM, O'Brien K, Calleja A, Corrie SN. Effects of directional exercise on lingual strength. J Speech Lang Hear Res. 2009;52(4):1034–47. https://doi.org/10.1044/1092-4388(2009/08-0062).
28. IOPI Medical. Qualitative guidelines for interpreting tongue elevation strength (P_{max}). 2021; https://iopimedical.com/normal-values/. Accessed 10 Nov 2021.
29. Randerath WJ, Galetke W, Domanski U, Weitkunat R, Ruhle KH. Tongue-muscle training by intraoral electrical neurostimulation in patients with obstructive sleep apnea. Sleep. 2004;27(2):254–9. https://doi.org/10.1093/sleep/27.2.254.
30. O'Connor Reina C, Plaza G, Ignacio-Garcia JM, Baptista P, Garcia Iriarte MT, Casado JC, et al. New mHealth application software based on myofunctional therapy applied to sleep-disordered breathing in non-compliant subjects. Sleep Sci Pract. 2020;4, 3:1. https://doi.org/10.1186/s41606-019-0040-8.
31. Chuang LC, Hwang YJ, Lian YC, Hervy-Auboiron M, Pirelli P, Huang YS, Guilleminault C. Changes in craniofacial and airway morphology as well as quality of life after passive myofunctional therapy in children with obstructive sleep apnea: a comparative cohort study. Sleep Breath. 2019;23(4):1359–69. https://doi.org/10.1007/s11325-019-01929-w.
32. Shamim-Uzzaman QA, Bae CJ, Ehsan Z, Setty AR, Devine M, Dhankikar S, Donskoy I, Fields B, Hearn H, Hwang D, Jain V, Kelley D, Kirsch DB, Martin W, Troester M, Trotti LM, Won CH, Epstein LJ. The use of telemedicine for the diagnosis and treatment of sleep disorders: an American Academy of sleep medicine update. J Clin Sleep Med. 2021;17(5):1103–7. https://doi.org/10.5664/jcsm.9194.
33. O'Connor Reina C, García Iriarte MT, Casado-Morente JC, Plaza Mayor G, Baptista PM, Vicente GE. New app "apnea bye" increases adherence in myofunctional therapy to treat sleep disordered breathing. Otolaryngol Neck Surg. 2018;159(1_suppl):P326–7.
34. O'Connor Reina C, Plaza Mayor G, Ignacio-Garcia JM, Baptista Jardin P, Garcia-Iriarte MT, Casado-Morente JC. Floppy closing door epiglottis treated successfully with an Mhealth application based on Myofunctional therapy: a case report. Case Rep Otolaryngol. 2019;2019:4157898. https://doi.org/10.1155/2019/4157898.
35. O'Connor-Reina C, Ignacio Garcia JM, Rodriguez Ruiz E, Morillo Dominguez MDC, Ignacio Barrios V, Baptista Jardin P, Casado Morente JC, Garcia Iriarte MT, Plaza G. Myofunctional therapy app for severe apnea-hypopnea sleep obstructive syndrome: pilot randomized controlled trial. JMIR Mhealth Uhealth. 2020;8(11):e23123. https://doi.org/10.2196/23123.
36. Strollo PJ Jr, Gillespie MB, Soose RJ, Maurer JT, de Vries N, Cornelius J, Hanson RD, Padhya TA, Steward DL, Woodson BT, Verbraecken J, Vanderveken OM, Goetting MG, Feldman N, Chabolle F, Badr MS, Randerath W, Strohl KP, Stimulation Therapy for Apnea Reduction (STAR) Trial Group. Upper airway stimulation for obstructive sleep apnea: durability of the treatment effect at 18 months. Sleep. 2015;38(10):1593–8. https://doi.org/10.5665/sleep.5054.
37. Mason RM, Franklin H. Orofacial myofunctional disorders and otolaryngologists. Otolaryngol (Sunnyvale). 2010;4:e110. https://doi.org/10.4172/2161-119X.1000e110.
38. Guilleminault C, Huseni S, Lo L. A frequent phenotype for paediatric sleep apnoea: short lingual frenulum. ERJ Open Res. 2016;2(3):00043–2016. https://doi.org/10.1183/23120541.00043-2016.
39. Yuen HM, Au CT, Chu WCW, Li AM, Chan KC. Reduced tongue mobility: an unrecognised risk factor of childhood obstructive sleep Apnoea. Sleep. 2021;45:zsab217. https://doi.org/10.1093/sleep/zsab217.
40. de Felício CM, Medeiros AP, de Oliveira MM. Validity of the 'protocol of oro-facial myofunctional evaluation with scores' for young and adult subjects. J Oral Rehabil. 2012;39(10):744–53. https://doi.org/10.1111/j.1365-2842.2012.02336.x.
41. Borrmann PF, O'Connor-Reina C, Ignacio JM, Rodriguez Ruiz E, Rodriguez Alcala L, Dzembrovsky F, Baptista P, Garcia Iriarte MT, Casado Alba C, Plaza G. Muscular assessment in patients with severe obstructive sleep apnea syndrome: protocol for a case-control study. JMIR Res Protoc. 2021;10(8):e30500. https://doi.org/10.2196/30500.

42. Kuo IC, Hsin LJ, Lee LA, Fang TJ, Tsai MS, Lee YC, Shen SC, Li HY. Prediction of Epiglottic collapse in obstructive sleep apnea patients: epiglottic length. Nat Sci Sleep. 2021;13:1985–92. https://doi.org/10.2147/NSS.S336019.
43. Kim HY, Sung CM, Jang HB, Kim HC, Lim SC, Yang HC. Patients with epiglottic collapse showed less severe obstructive sleep apnea and good response to treatment other than continuous positive airway pressure: a case-control study of 224 patients. J Clin Sleep Med. 2021;17(3):413–9. https://doi.org/10.5664/jcsm.8904.
44. Kanemaru S, Kojima H, Fukushima H, Tamaki H, Tamura Y, Yamashita M, Umeda H, Ito J. A case of floppy epiglottis in adult: a simple surgical remedy. Auris Nasus Larynx. 2007;34(3):409–11. https://doi.org/10.1016/j.anl.2007.01.009.
45. Moeller M, Weber S, Coceani-Paskay L, Amat P, Bianchini E, Botzer E, et al. Déclaration de consensus sur l'évaluation et la rééducation myofonctionnelles orofaciales chez les patients souffrants de SAOS: proposition d'un processus international par la méthode Delphi. Rev Orthop Dento Faciale. 2021;55(4):513–21. https://doi.org/10.1051/odf/2021035.

Oral Appliance Therapy 17

Eli Van de Perck, Peter A. Cistulli, and Olivier M. Vanderveken

17.1 Introduction

Oral appliances are being increasingly prescribed for treating obstructive sleep apnea (OSA). They are worn at night and can be broadly classified into two groups (Fig. 17.1).

- Tongue retaining devices (TRD) use suction pressure to hold the tongue in a forward position.
- Mandibular advancement devices (MAD) mechanically protrude the lower jaw. Many designs are commercially available, but custom-made, titratable devices are generally preferred.

As most clinical evidence pertains to the latter type [1], this chapter will focus on MAD.

E. Van de Perck (✉)
Department of Otolaryngology—Head and Neck Surgery, Antwerp University Hospital, Edegem, Belgium
e-mail: eli.vandeperck@uza.be

P. A. Cistulli
Centre for Sleep Health and Research, Royal North Shore Hospital, Sydney, NSW, Australia

Charles Perkins Centre, The University of Sydney, Sydney, NSW, Australia

O. M. Vanderveken
Department of Otolaryngology—Head and Neck Surgery, Antwerp University Hospital, Edegem, Belgium

Faculty of Medicine and Health Sciences, University of Antwerp, Wilrijk, Belgium

M. Delakorda, N. de Vries (eds.), *The Role of Epiglottis in Obstructive Sleep Apnea*, https://doi.org/10.1007/978-3-031-34992-8_17

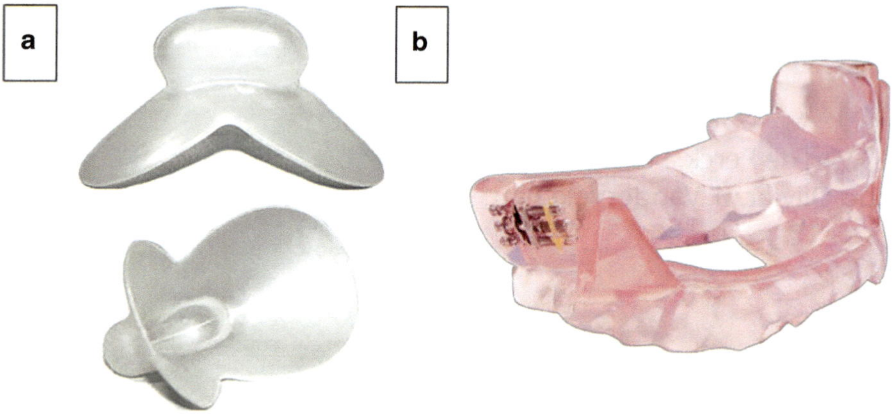

Fig. 17.1 Examples of oral appliances for obstructive sleep apnea. (**a**) tongue retaining device (Good Morning Snore Solution [28], MPowrx Health and Welness Products, Canada). (**b**) mandibular advancement device (SomnoDent Flex [29], SomnoMed AG, Australia)

Treatment with MAD reduces the severity of OSA by an average of 50% to 70% and completely eliminates OSA in approximately half of treated patients [2]. Although its efficacy is inferior to that of continuous positive airway pressure therapy (CPAP), MAD are generally better tolerated and accepted by patients. This causes both treatments to be equally effective [3, 4] and to yield similar health benefits in terms of sleepiness, blood pressure, and quality of life [5, 6]. A drawback of MAD, however, are the variable results in outcome across nonselected patients. Therefore, accurate predictive models are a clinical priority.

Both anatomical and nonanatomical factors can affect MAD outcome. A full description of these factors is beyond the scope of this chapter (see references [7, 8] for a comprehensive review). The sites and mechanisms of upper airway collapse are important anatomical traits known to affect the outcome of different treatment modalities [9, 10]. Previous sleep-endoscopic studies have demonstrated that subjects with tongue-related collapse are more likely to experience a beneficial outcome with MAD [11, 12]. This chapter will further discuss the relationship between MAD therapy and epiglottis collapse.

17.2 Mechanism of Action

MAD essentially reduce upper airway collapsibility by advancing the mandible. Nevertheless, the specific biomechanical changes that underlie this therapeutic effect are far less evident. There is some evidence from imaging and endoscopic studies that MAD primarily improve the patency of the retropalatal airway [13–15], which is the most common site of upper airway obstruction and flow limitation in patients with OSA. This effect is most pronounced in the laterolateral dimension. The exact mechanism has not been fully clarified, but seems to be related to direct soft tissue connections between the mandible, tongue base, pharyngeal wall, and soft palate, which may be stretched by mandibular advancement, thus stabilizing the velopharynx [16]. Additionally, mandibular advancement causes anterior repositioning or elongation of the tongue base depending on the severity of OSA and local mechanics [15, 16]. Hence, MAD outcome is not only determined by the degree of mandibular protrusion [17], but also by individual anatomic and physiologic differences (e.g., mandibular profile, hyoid position, neck circumference, length of the soft palate, and pharyngeal airway space) [8].

Theoretically, MAD can affect epiglottis collapse in two ways: either directly or indirectly. The hyoid bone gives insertion to numerous muscles and ligaments in the pharyngeal region and is both connected to the mandible and epiglottis. Cephalometric studies have shown that mandibular advancement leads to an anterosuperior displacement of the hyoid bone, although to varying degrees in different individuals [18]. Comparable with the effect on the velopharynx, MAD may stretch the soft tissue connections between the epiglottis and mandible (Fig. 17.2), directly

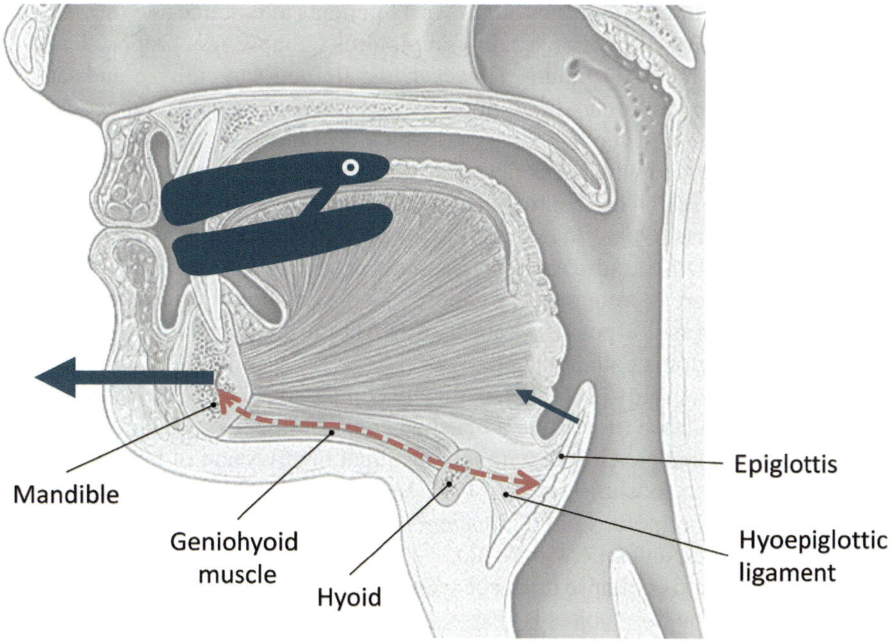

Fig. 17.2 The hyoid bone is connected to the mandible through several muscles (including the geniohyoid and mylohyoid muscles). As a result, MAD may pull the hyoid bone upward and forward. This mechanical force may extend to the epiglottis through the hyoepiglottic ligament

changing the position and/or inclination of the epiglottis. Furthermore, being the most inferior portion of the collapsible segment in the upper airway, the epiglottis is susceptible to the build-up of negative pressure generated by upstream collapse sites. Thus, MAD may indirectly neutralize epiglottis collapse by restoring pharyngeal patency and reducing intraluminal pressure levels. This theory may explain why surgical interventions of the soft palate and tongue base are equally effective in patients with and without epiglottis collapse [19].

17.3 Role of MAD in Cases with Epiglottis Collapse

Because epiglottis collapse is a dynamic phenomenon that occurs almost exclusively during sleep, most of the evidence is derived from sleep-endoscopic studies. At present, drug-induced sleep endoscopy (DISE) evaluation (see Chap. 8) usually includes a chin-lift or jaw-thrust maneuver to visualize upper airway changes associated with mandibular advancement. Most of the studies have demonstrated positive effects of such maneuvers, with a resolution of epiglottis collapse in 67–93% of cases [20–23].

Only few studies have assessed the relationship between epiglottis collapse and MAD outcome. *Kent* et al. performed DISE in 35 patients with incomplete response to MAD and identified epiglottis collapse in 11 patients at baseline and in 7 patients with MAD [24]. Based on these findings, epiglottis collapse was proposed as possible contributor to MAD failure. However, the limited sample size and lack of control group are important limitations of this study. Likewise, *Vroegop* et al. showed that collapse at the hypopharynx, which encompassed collapse of the epiglottis, was associated with a less favorable outcome [25].

More recent research has contradicted the findings above. In a prospective cohort study of 72 patients, *Op de Beeck* et al. reported no association between epiglottis collapse during DISE and treatment response or deterioration with MAD [11]. These findings were corroborated by endoscopic observations during natural sleep, which even suggested a positive impact of MAD on pharyngeal collapsibility in patients with epiglottis collapse [12].

In a case-control study [26], we specifically compared MAD outcome in patients with epiglottis collapse ($n = 20$) and matched controls ($n = 40$). Epiglottis collapse was defined as complete closure without any direct involvement of the tongue base or other structures. As shown in Fig. 17.3, MAD therapy was equally effective in both groups. Furthermore, 4 out of 5 patients with isolated epiglottis collapse experienced a beneficial outcome with MAD.

Overall, epiglottis collapse does not seem to affect MAD therapy. However, the current evidence on this subject is sparse, precluding any firm conclusions.

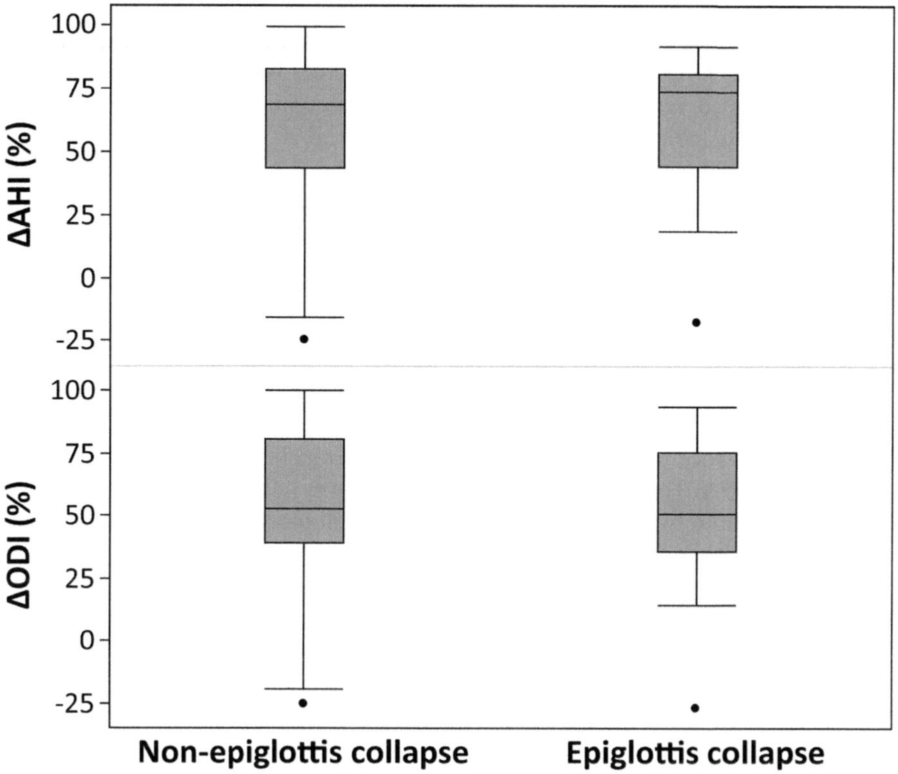

Fig. 17.3 Treatment outcome with MAD. Δ-values were calculated as the percentage difference between baseline and follow-up. *AHI* apnea-hypopnea index, *ODI* oxygen desaturation index

17.4 Future Directions

There is a paucity of high-quality evidence on the exact mechanisms by which MAD resolve upper airway collapse in patients with OSA. Most of the previous observations were made during wakefulness and may not accurately reflect the dynamic changes that occur during sleep [13–16, 18]. This is especially the case for epiglottis collapse, which is a sleep-specific finding. Thus, future research is needed to assess the mechanical effects of mandibular advancement during natural and drug-induced sleep. This can be achieved, for instance, by using ultrafast, dynamic imaging modalities, and remotely controlled systems for mandibular protrusion. Such data may not only provide more insight into the mechanism of action, but may also improve the current patient selection models for MAD.

Flow shape analysis is an emerging method to noninvasively estimate the sites of upper airway collapse. It is based on the premise that different patterns of upper airway collapse produce recognizable patterns of flow limitation. Epiglottis collapse, for instance, is characterized by an abrupt discontinuity in inspiratory flow. Recent research indicated that certain flow features of velopharyngeal collapse increase the likelihood of nonresponse to MAD therapy [27]. The same study found no associations between epiglottis-specific flow features and MAD outcome. Although these findings need further validation and development, they may provide a noninvasive means to assess upper airway collapse during sleep and may prove useful in upfront response prediction of MAD therapy.

17.5 Conclusion

Mandibular advancement devices are the leading therapeutic alternative to CPAP in patients with OSA. They may stabilize the collapsing epiglottis either by repositioning the structure or by reducing negative intraluminal pressure. According to some case studies, CPAP can aggravate epiglottis collapse (see Chap. 15). By contrast, MAD therapy is neither positively nor negatively affected by epiglottis collapse. However, the evidence on this subject is limited and requires further research.

References

1. Ramar K, Dort LC, Katz SG, et al. Clinical practice guideline for the treatment of obstructive sleep apnea and snoring with Oral appliance therapy: an update for 2015. J Clin Sleep Med. 2015;11(7):773–827.
2. Sutherland K, Vanderveken OM, Tsuda H, et al. Oral appliance treatment for obstructive sleep apnea: an update. J Clin Sleep Med. 2014;10(2):215–27.
3. Vanderveken OM, Dieltjens M, Wouters K, De Backer WA, Van de Heyning PH, Braem MJ. Objective measurement of compliance during oral appliance therapy for sleep-disordered breathing. Thorax. 2013;68(1):91–6.
4. Hamoda MM, Kohzuka Y, Almeida FR. Oral appliances for the management of OSA: an updated review of the literature. Chest. 2018;153(2):544–53.
5. Bratton DJ, Gaisl T, Schlatzer C, Kohler M. Comparison of the effects of continuous positive airway pressure and mandibular advancement devices on sleepiness in patients with obstructive sleep apnoea: a network meta-analysis. Lancet Respir Med. 2015;3(11):869–78.
6. Bratton DJ, Gaisl T, Wons AM, Kohler M. CPAP vs mandibular advancement devices and blood pressure in patients with obstructive sleep apnea: a systematic review and meta-analysis. JAMA. 2015;314(21):2280–93.
7. Cistulli PA, Sutherland K. Phenotyping obstructive sleep apnoea-bringing precision to oral appliance therapy. J Oral Rehabil. 2019;46(12):1185–91.
8. Chen H, Eckert DJ, van der Stelt PF, et al. Phenotypes of responders to mandibular advancement device therapy in obstructive sleep apnea patients: a systematic review and meta-analysis. Sleep Med Rev. 2020;49:101229.
9. Vanderveken OM, Maurer JT, Hohenhorst W, et al. Evaluation of drug-induced sleep endoscopy as a patient selection tool for implanted upper airway stimulation for obstructive sleep apnea. J Clin Sleep Med. 2013;9(5):433–8.

10. Koutsourelakis I, Safiruddin F, Ravesloot M, Zakynthinos S, de Vries N. Surgery for obstructive sleep apnea: sleep endoscopy determinants of outcome. Laryngoscope. 2012;122(11):2587–91.
11. Op de Beeck S, Dieltjens M, Verbruggen AE, et al. Phenotypic labelling using drug-induced sleep endoscopy improves patient selection for mandibular advancement device outcome: a prospective study. J Clin Sleep Med. 2019;15(8):1089–99.
12. Marques M, Genta PR, Azarbarzin A, et al. Structure and severity of pharyngeal obstruction determine oral appliance efficacy in sleep apnoea. J Physiol. 2019;597(22):5399–410.
13. Ryan CF, Love LL, Peat D, Fleetham JA, Lowe AA. Mandibular advancement oral appliance therapy for obstructive sleep apnoea: effect on awake calibre of the velopharynx. Thorax. 1999;54(11):972–7.
14. Chan AS, Lee RW, Srinivasan VK, Darendeliler MA, Grunstein RR, Cistulli PA. Nasopharyngoscopic evaluation of oral appliance therapy for obstructive sleep apnoea. Eur Respir J. 2010;35(4):836–42.
15. Chan AS, Sutherland K, Schwab RJ, et al. The effect of mandibular advancement on upper airway structure in obstructive sleep apnoea. Thorax. 2010;65(8):726–32.
16. Brown EC, Cheng S, McKenzie DK, Butler JE, Gandevia SC, Bilston LE. Tongue and lateral upper airway movement with mandibular advancement. Sleep. 2013;36(3):397–404.
17. Bamagoos AA, Cistulli PA, Sutherland K, et al. Dose-dependent effects of mandibular advancement on upper airway collapsibility and muscle function in obstructive sleep apnea. Sleep. 2019;42(6):zsz049.
18. Battagel JM, Johal A, L'Estrange PR, Croft CB, Kotecha B. Changes in airway and hyoid position in response to mandibular protrusion in subjects with obstructive sleep apnoea (OSA). Eur J Orthod. 1999;21(4):363–76.
19. Kwon OE, Jung SY, Al-Dilaijan K, Min JY, Lee KH, Kim SW. Is epiglottis surgery necessary for obstructive sleep apnea patients with epiglottis obstruction? Laryngoscope. 2019;129(11):2658–62.
20. Vonk PE, Ravesloot MJL, Kasius KM, van Maanen JP, de Vries N. Floppy epiglottis during drug-induced sleep endoscopy: an almost complete resolution by adopting the lateral posture. Sleep Breath. 2020;24(1):103–9.
21. Eichler C, Sommer JU, Stuck BA, Hormann K, Maurer JT. Does drug-induced sleep endoscopy change the treatment concept of patients with snoring and obstructive sleep apnea? Sleep Breath. 2013;17(1):63–8.
22. Park D, Kim JS, Heo SJ. The effect of the modified jaw-thrust maneuver on the depth of sedation during drug-induced sleep endoscopy. J Clin Sleep Med. 2019;15(10):1503–8.
23. Kim HY, Sung CM, Jang HB, Kim HC, Lim SC, Yang HC. Patients with epiglottic collapse showed less severe obstructive sleep apnea and good response to treatment other than continuous positive airway pressure: a case-control study of 224 patients. J Clin Sleep Med. 2021;17(3):413–9.
24. Kent DT, Rogers R, Soose RJ. Drug-induced sedation endoscopy in the evaluation of OSA patients with incomplete Oral appliance therapy response. Otolaryngol Head Neck Surg. 2015;153(2):302–7.
25. Vroegop AV, Vanderveken OM, Dieltjens M, et al. Sleep endoscopy with simulation bite for prediction of oral appliance treatment outcome. J Sleep Res. 2013;22(3):348–55.
26. Van de Perck E, Dieltjens M, et al. Mandibular advancement device therapy in patients with epiglottic collapse. Sleep Breath. 2022;26(4). https://doi.org/10.1007/s11325-021-02532-8
27. Vena D, Azarbarzin A, Marques M, et al. Predicting sleep apnea responses to oral appliance therapy using polysomnographic airflow. Sleep. 2020;43:zsaa004.
28. Dort L, Brant R. A randomized, controlled, crossover study of a noncustomized tongue retaining device for sleep disordered breathing. Sleep Breath. 2008;12(4):369–73.
29. Zeng B, Ng AT, Darendeliler MA, Petocz P, Cistulli PA. Use of flow-volume curves to predict oral appliance treatment outcome in obstructive sleep apnea. Am J Respir Crit Care Med. 2007;175(7):726–30.

Treatment of Epiglottic Collapse with Positional Therapy

18

Mickey Leentjens, Patty E. Vonk, and Nico de Vries

18.1 Introduction

It has been found that the majority of patients with obstructive sleep apnea (OSA) have a higher frequency and duration of apneic events in the supine position [1–3]. In literature, many definitions of position-dependent OSA (POSA) have been applied. The most common approach is to categorize patients in two groups: positional (PP) and non-positional (NPP) OSA patients [1, 2, 4, 5]. In PP, apneic events appear almost exclusively in supine position and the severity of disease is to a large extent dependent on the time spent sleeping in this posture [1, 2, 6–9]. Patients are classified as being NPP or PP using modified versions of Cartwright's criteria [1]. In this definition, there should be a difference of 50% or more in apnea-hypopnea index (AHI) between supine and non-supine positions with a total sleeping time in worst sleeping position of >10% and < 90%. In PP, a further distinction can be made between supine isolated OSA (non-supine AHI <5 events/hour) and supine predominant OSA (non-supine AHI ≥5 events/hour) [10, 11].

Overall, 56% to 75% of patients with OSA are classified as being positional [2, 3, 7, 9, 12]. POSA is in particular prevalent in mild to moderate OSA, as the

M. Leentjens (✉)
Department of Otorhinolaryngology, OLVG, location West, Amsterdam, The Netherlands
e-mail: M.Leentjens@olvg.nl

P. E. Vonk
Department of Otorhinolaryngology, Academic Medical Center, Amsterdam, The Netherlands

N. de Vries
Jan Tooropstraat, Onze Lieve Vrouwe Gasthuis, Amsterdam, The Netherlands
e-mail: n.vries@olvg.nl

M. Delakorda, N. de Vries (eds.), *The Role of Epiglottis in Obstructive Sleep Apnea*, https://doi.org/10.1007/978-3-031-34992-8_18

majority of PP (70–80%) is afflicted with this form [2, 7, 8, 13]. In addition, the prevalence of POSA decreases as the severity of OSA increases. There are also several studies that have shown clinical differences in patient characteristics between PP and NPP. For example, PP are younger and have a lower body mass index (BMI) compared with NPP [2, 7, 8, 14]. In addition, the prevalence of POSA is higher in Asian populations [15–17].

18.2 Epiglottic Collapse in PP

In PP, the severity of OSA is to a large extent dependent on the total sleeping time (TST) spent in the supine position. The effect of gravitational forces on the upper airway (UA) when adopting the supine position is thought to be responsible for the increase in UA collapse observed in this position [18]. One of the structures which can be responsible for UA narrowing and obstruction is the epiglottis.

As discussed in Part 2 of this book, many different definitions of epiglottic collapse (EC) are used. An EC can occur in two configurations: anteroposterior (A-P) or, less common, lateral. An A-P collapse can result in posterior displacement of the entire epiglottis against the posterior pharyngeal wall due to various causes. First, an EC can occur isolated in A-P configuration, which is also called a floppy epiglottis (FE) or trapdoor phenomenon. This collapse pattern often appears to be related to decreased structural rigidity of the epiglottis. Second, an EC can be secondary to an A-P collapse of the tongue base. Less common is a secondary collapse of the epiglottis due to a vallecular cyst. Third, a lateral collapse can be caused by anatomical variation or due to underdevelopment of the epiglottis itself.

It has been suggested that a collapse at this level, in particular FE, is influenced by sleeping position and seems to occur more often in the supine position compared to non-supine position [19, 20]. The increased usage of DISE and performing this procedure in different body positions have given more insight into the involvement of the epiglottis in OSA, with in particular an isolated EC (e.g., FE). In a study by Vonk et al., the authors observed that a FE seems to be a position-dependent phenomenon. This study showed that this phenomenon appears almost exclusively in the supine position and to a lesser extent during lateral head (and trunk) rotation [21].

Previously, several studies had already shown that base of tongue and epiglottic collapse are more common in PP [7, 22]. Victores et al. found an overall improvement in UA collapse in PP while moving to lateral sleep position, this in contrast to NPP. Moreover, the biggest improvement of UA obstruction in PP involved the tongue base and epiglottis [19]. In addition, Safiruddin et al. examined the influence of different head positions during DISE in patients with OSA and PP. They observed a positive effect of lateral head rotation on UA patency in EC, predominantly in PP [23].

18.3 Treatment Options for EC

Over the past few years, interest in EC has been increasing. However, treatment of patients with a FE remains challenging. A variety of treatment methods have been attempted to resolve this, but both conservative and surgical treatment are hampered by differences in success rates and possible complications accompanied with surgical interventions. As discussed in the previous chapters of this part of the book, conservative treatment includes continuous positive airway pressure (CPAP), mandibular advancement device (MAD) treatment, and to a lesser extent myofunctional therapy.

Besides conventional treatments, several surgical techniques have been applied to resolve an EC and will be described in Part 4. Various small-scale studies have been published about techniques, success rates, and complications of epiglottis surgery [24–26]. Many sleep surgeons are hesitant to embark on epiglottis surgery, because of the risk of irreversible dysphagia after partial or total epiglottectomy. The risk of sequelae must be weighed individually, depending on, for example, the severity of the disease.

18.4 Positional Therapy

Positional therapy (PT) aims at preventing patients from sleeping in supine position. Various techniques have been described. The majority of studies on PT use the old fashioned, so-called tennis-ball technique (TBT) [12]. This technique uses a passive object, a bulky mass, which is strapped to the patients' back avoiding them from sleeping in the supine position. The advantage of TBT is that it is a simple and inexpensive treatment. More importantly, it has proven its effectiveness in reducing the percentage of TST in supine position and therefore the total AHI in PP. However, the long-term compliance of TBT is poor. The poor compliance can be mainly explained by backache, discomfort and no improvement, or even deterioration, of sleep quality and daytime alertness [27]. Another drawback is the inability to do anything else in bed with such device installed, e.g., read, which means it must be installed just before actually falling asleep. Compliance rates of TBT reported in literature range from 40 to 70% short-term to only 10% long-term [12, 28, 29]. This old school positional therapy is therefore obsolete and should be discouraged.

Hereafter, a new generation of small, lightweight, battery-powered vibro-tactile devices was developed. These devices are either worn around the chest or secured to the skin of the neck [30, 31]. When the supine position is identified, these devices provide a vibrating stimulus aiming to turn the patient to a non-supine sleeping position. Several studies have shown that PT with new-generation devices is effective in reducing the percentage of supine sleep in PP as well [32–35]. Data for studies reporting on the effect of new-generation devices for PT were combined in a recent meta-analysis [35]. The pooled mean reduction in AHI was 11.3 events/hour (54%) and the pooled mean reduction in percentage of TST in supine position was 33.6%; a mean difference of 84% [35]. Short-term compliance is high, varying from 76% to 96%, when defined as at least 4 h of use per night during 7 days a week [4, 31, 34]. Long-term compliance is varying among studies between 64.4% and 75.5% [33, 36]. In another study, the proportion of patients using their device more than 4 h during 5 days a week after 12 months of follow-up was 100% [37].

18.4.1 The Amsterdam Positional Obstructive Sleep Apnea Classification

To determine which patients are suitable candidates for PT, the Amsterdam Positional Obstructive Sleep Apnea Classification (APOC) was introduced [8]. This classification system gives a description of patients who probably will or will not achieve clinical improvement of their OSA with PT. The APOC discriminates between three categories: the true PP, the NPP, and the multifactorial patient (Fig. 18.1). The true PP can be cured by PT alone and is categorized as APOC I. Patients categorized as APOC II or III could benefit from PT, but will not be cured. These patients may benefit from a combination of PT with, for example, less invasive UA surgery, or a MAD. Obviously, the NPP will not benefit from PT since the severity of OSA is not influenced by sleeping position.

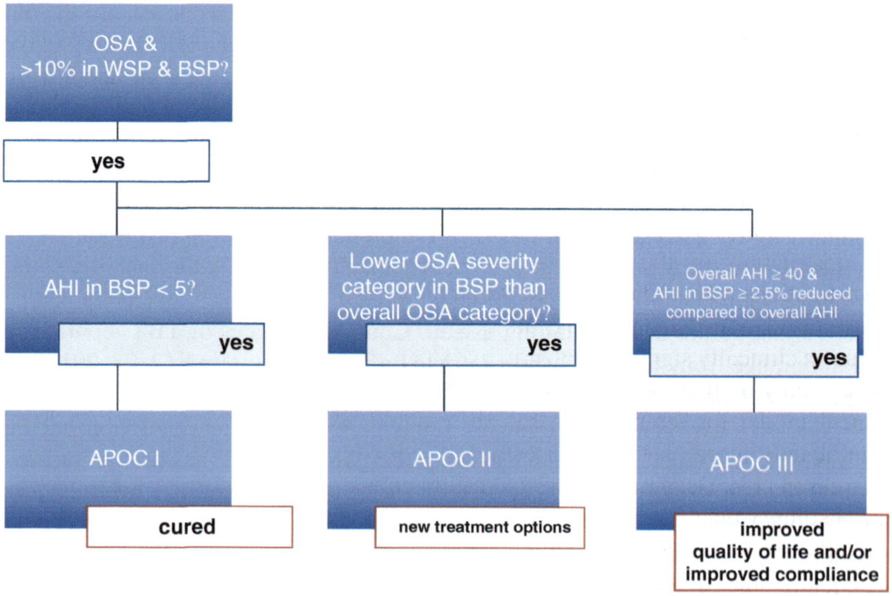

Fig. 18.1 Flow chart for the Amsterdam Positional Obstructive Apnea Classification (APOC). The red boxes show the best possible outcome for these patients with successful positional therapy (PT)

18.5 EC and PT

As described earlier in this chapter, it has been suggested that obstruction by an isolated EC is enhanced by sleeping position and occurs more often in the supine position compared to non-supine position [19, 20]. Vonk et al. described that a FE appears almost exclusively in the supine position [21]. Therefore, avoiding the supine position might be a rational and promising option that could be used as a standalone treatment in patients with a FE.

As mentioned above, the multifactorial patient could benefit from PT, as the severity of disease is influenced, in part, by sleeping position. In APOC II, the patients have a best sleeping position (BSP) AHI in a lower OSA severity category than the overall AHI. Theoretically, the patients can decrease overall AHI and OSA severity category when treated with PT. Consequently, patients could potentially be treated with less aggressive treatment. Studies report that 42–75% of NPP improve to less severe PP after UA surgery [32, 38–44]. The effect of UA surgery is thought to be greater in the lateral position. This might result in residual OSA in the supine position post-surgery. In patients with partial effective surgery, additional treatment with PT could be offered as adjuvant therapy. Catalfumo et al. evaluated 104 patients who underwent uvulopalatopharyngoplasty (UPPP) with postoperative persistent OSA. Using awake fiberoptic endoscopy, they observed 11.5% of these patients to have an abnormal position of the epiglottis as it was pushed against the posterior pharyngeal wall further down into the laryngeal inlet during inspiration [24]. Patients with a postoperative persistent EC could benefit from PT, as the epiglottis has previously been identified as a primary site to improve in the lateral position [19]. Several studies observed beneficial effect of adjuvant PT in patients with post-operative persistent POSA [32, 40].

In APOC III, patients have an overall AHI of at least 40 events/hour and at least a 25% lower BSP AHI. CPAP is undoubtedly regarded as the gold standard treatment in these patients. The patient would remain in the same OSA severity category when avoiding the supine position, but as the AHI decreases, so does the CPAP pressure needed, which potentially leads to better compliance. In case the patient does not tolerate CPAP or MAD, PT can be considered as salvage therapy since this could lower the AHI.

18.6 Further Considerations

There are a few considerations that need to be kept in mind when choosing PT as a treatment option. As described above, the distinction between PP and NPP is crucial. The NPP patient will not benefit from PT, since UA narrowing will be present in both supine and non-supine sleeping position. Also, patients are not good candidates for PT when they are unable to sleep in the lateral position due to physical discomfort (e.g., neck or shoulder problems) or any other disabilities that interfere when sleeping in lateral position. It is important to take into account that the effectiveness of a treatment depends not only on the effect on UA obstruction, but also on compliance. Last, PT may not be the treatment of choice when the patient's main complaint is snoring in all body positions.

18.7 Conclusion

In this chapter, we described the role of the epiglottis in PP. For PP, avoiding the supine position is key. A primary EC (e.g., FE), not secondary to collapse of the base of tongue, is a phenomenon that appears almost exclusively in supine position and disappears when the patient is positioned in lateral position [21]. Therefore, these patients are suitable candidates for PT. Also, tongue base and epiglottic collapse have been shown to improve in the lateral position [7, 22]. The multifactorial patient could also benefit from PT, by going down in OSA class (APOC II) or a decrease in AHI (APOC III). Postoperative residual POSA, which may possibly be due to an EC, can be a good indication for additional PT as well.

References

1. Cartwright RD. Effect of sleep position on sleep apnea severity. Sleep. 1984;7(2):110–4.
2. Oksenberg A, Silverberg DS, Arons E, Radwan H. Positional vs nonpositional obstructive sleep apnea patients: anthropomorphic, nocturnal polysomnographic, and multiple sleep latency test data. Chest. 1997;112(3):629–39.
3. Ravesloot MJ, Frank MH, van Maanen JP, Verhagen EA, de Lange J, de Vries N. Positional OSA part 2: retrospective cohort analysis with a new classification system (APOC). Sleep Breath. 2016;20(2):881–8.
4. Eijsvogel MM, Ubbink R, Dekker J, Oppersma E, de Jongh FH, van der Palen J, et al. Sleep position trainer versus tennis ball technique in positional obstructive sleep apnea syndrome. J Clin Sleep Med. 2015;11(2):139–47.
5. Marklund M, Persson M, Franklin KA. Treatment success with a mandibular advancement device is related to supine-dependent sleep apnea. Chest. 1998;114(6):1630–5.
6. Oksenberg A, Gadoth N. Are we missing a simple treatment for most adult sleep apnea patients? The avoidance of the supine sleep position. J Sleep Res. 2014;23(2):204–10.
7. Richard W, Kox D, den Herder C, Laman M, van Tinteren H, de Vries N. The role of sleep position in obstructive sleep apnea syndrome. Eur Arch Otorhinolaryngol. 2006;263(10):946–50.
8. Frank MH, Ravesloot MJ, van Maanen JP, Verhagen E, de Lange J, de Vries N. Positional OSA part 1: towards a clinical classification system for position-dependent obstructive sleep apnoea. Sleep Breath. 2015;19(2):473–80.
9. Heinzer R, Petitpierre NJ, Marti-Soler H, Haba-Rubio J. Prevalence and characteristics of positional sleep apnea in the HypnoLaus population-based cohort. Sleep Med. 2018;48:157–62.
10. Kim KT, Cho YW, Kim DE, Hwang SH, Song ML, Motamedi GK. Two subtypes of positional obstructive sleep apnea: supine-predominant and supine-isolated. Clin Neurophysiol. 2016;127(1):565–70.
11. Lee SA, Paek JH, Chung YS, Kim WS. Clinical features in patients with positional obstructive sleep apnea according to its subtypes. Sleep Breath. 2017;21(1):109–17.
12. Ravesloot MJ, van Maanen JP, Dun L, de Vries N. The undervalued potential of positional therapy in position-dependent snoring and obstructive sleep apnea-a review of the literature. Sleep Breath. 2013;17(1):39–49.
13. Mador MJ, Kufel TJ, Magalang UJ, Rajesh SK, Watwe V, Grant BJ. Prevalence of positional sleep apnea in patients undergoing polysomnography. Chest. 2005;128(4):2130–7.

14. Itasaka Y, Miyazaki S, Ishikawa K, Togawa K. The influence of sleep position and obesity on sleep apnea. Psychiatry Clin Neurosci. 2000;54(3):340–1.
15. Mo JH, Lee CH, Rhee CS, Yoon IY, Kim JW. Positional dependency in Asian patients with obstructive sleep apnea and its implication for hypertension. Arch Otolaryngol Head Neck Surg. 2011;137(8):786–90.
16. Teerapraipruk B, Chirakalwasan N, Simon R, Hirunwiwatkul P, Jaimchariyatam N, Desudchit T, et al. Clinical and polysomnographic data of positional sleep apnea and its predictors. Sleep Breath. 2012;16(4):1167–72.
17. Tanaka F, Nakano H, Sudo N, Kubo C. Relationship between the body position-specific apnea-hypopnea index and subjective sleepiness. Respiration. 2009;78(2):185–90.
18. Oksenberg A, Silverberg DS. The effect of body posture on sleep-related breathing disorders: facts and therapeutic implications. Sleep Med Rev. 1998;2(3):139–62.
19. Victores AJ, Hamblin J, Gilbert J, Switzer C, Takashima M. Usefulness of sleep endoscopy in predicting positional obstructive sleep apnea. Otolaryngol Head Neck Surg. 2014;150(3):487–93.
20. Marques M, Genta PR, Sands SA, Azarbazin A, de Melo C, Taranto-Montemurro L, et al. Effect of sleeping position on upper airway patency in obstructive sleep apnea is determined by the pharyngeal structure causing collapse. Sleep. 2017;40(3):zsx005.
21. Vonk PE, Ravesloot MJL, Kasius KM, van Maanen JP, de Vries N. Floppy epiglottis during drug-induced sleep endoscopy: an almost complete resolution by adopting the lateral posture. Sleep Breath. 2020;24(1):103–9.
22. Ravesloot MJ, de Vries N. One hundred consecutive patients undergoing drug-induced sleep endoscopy: results and evaluation. Laryngoscope. 2011;121(12):2710–6.
23. Safiruddin F, Koutsourelakis I, de Vries N. Analysis of the influence of head rotation during drug-induced sleep endoscopy in obstructive sleep apnea. Laryngoscope. 2014;124(9):2195–9.
24. Catalfumo FJ, Golz A, Westerman ST, Gilbert LM, Joachims HZ, Goldenberg D. The epiglottis and obstructive sleep apnoea syndrome. J Laryngol Otol. 1998;112(10):940–3.
25. Golz A, Goldenberg D, Westerman ST, Catalfumo FJ, Netzer A, Westerman LM, et al. Laser partial epiglottidectomy as a treatment for obstructive sleep apnea and laryngomalacia. Ann Otol Rhinol Laryngol. 2000;109(12 Pt 1):1140–5.
26. Bourolias C, Hajiioannou J, Sobol E, Velegrakis G, Helidonis E. Epiglottis reshaping using CO2 laser: a minimally invasive technique and its potent applications. Head Face Med. 2008;4:15.
27. Ravesloot MJL, Benoist L, van Maanen P, de Vries N. Novel positional devices for the treatment of positional obstructive sleep apnea, and how this relates to sleep surgery. Adv Otorhinolaryngol. 2017;80:28–36.
28. Oksenberg A, Silverberg D, Offenbach D, Arons E. Positional therapy for obstructive sleep apnea patients: a 6-month follow-up study. Laryngoscope. 2006;116(11):1995–2000.
29. Bignold JJ, Deans-Costi G, Goldsworthy MR, Robertson CA, McEvoy D, Catcheside PG, et al. Poor long-term patient compliance with the tennis ball technique for treating positional obstructive sleep apnea. J Clin Sleep Med. 2009;5(5):428–30.
30. van Maanen JP, Richard W, Van Kesteren ER, Ravesloot MJ, Laman DM, Hilgevoord AA, et al. Evaluation of a new simple treatment for positional sleep apnoea patients. J Sleep Res. 2012;21(3):322–9.
31. Levendowski DJ, Seagraves S, Popovic D, Westbrook PR. Assessment of a neck-based treatment and monitoring device for positional obstructive sleep apnea. J Clin Sleep Med. 2014;10(8):863–71.
32. Benoist LBL, Verhagen M, Torensma B, van Maanen JP, de Vries N. Positional therapy in patients with residual positional obstructive sleep apnea after upper airway surgery. Sleep Breath. 2017;21(2):279–88.
33. van Maanen JP, de Vries N. Long-term effectiveness and compliance of positional therapy with the sleep position trainer in the treatment of positional obstructive sleep apnea syndrome. Sleep. 2014;37(7):1209–15.
34. van Maanen JP, Meester KA, Dun LN, Koutsourelakis I, Witte BI, Laman DM, et al. The sleep position trainer: a new treatment for positional obstructive sleep apnoea. Sleep Breath. 2013;17(2):771–9.

35. Ravesloot MJL, White D, Heinzer R, Oksenberg A, Pepin JL. Efficacy of the new generation of devices for positional therapy for patients with positional obstructive sleep apnea: a systematic review of the literature and meta-analysis. J Clin Sleep Med. 2017;13(6):813–24.
36. Laub RR, Tonnesen P, Jennum PJ. A sleep position trainer for positional sleep apnea: a randomized, controlled trial. J Sleep Res. 2017;26(5):641–50.
37. de Ruiter MHT, Benoist LBL, de Vries N, de Lange J. Durability of treatment effects of the sleep position trainer versus oral appliance therapy in positional OSA: 12-month follow-up of a randomized controlled trial. Sleep Breath. 2018;22(2):441–50.
38. Lee CH, Kim SW, Han K, Shin JM, Hong SL, Lee JE, et al. Effect of uvulopalatopharyngoplasty on positional dependency in obstructive sleep apnea. Arch Otolaryngol Head Neck Surg. 2011;137(7):675–9.
39. Kastoer C, Benoist LBL, Dieltjens M, Torensma B, de Vries LH, Vonk PE, et al. Comparison of upper airway collapse patterns and its clinical significance: drug-induced sleep endoscopy in patients without obstructive sleep apnea, positional and non-positional obstructive sleep apnea. Sleep Breat. 2018;22(4):939–48.
40. van Maanen JP, Witte BI, de Vries N. Theoretical approach towards increasing effectiveness of palatal surgery in obstructive sleep apnea: role for concomitant positional therapy? Sleep Breath. 2014;18(2):341–9.
41. Lee YC, Eun YG, Shin SY, Kim SW. Change in position dependency in non-responders after multilevel surgery for obstructive sleep apnea: analysis of polysomnographic parameters. Eur Arch Otorhinolaryngol. 2014;271(5):1081–5.
42. Li HY, Cheng WN, Chuang LP, Fang TJ, Hsin LJ, Kang CJ, et al. Positional dependency and surgical success of relocation pharyngoplasty among patients with severe obstructive sleep apnea. Otolaryngol Head Neck Surg. 2013;149(3):506–12.
43. van Maanen JP, Ravesloot MJ, Witte BI, Grijseels M, de Vries N. Exploration of the relationship between sleep position and isolated tongue base or multilevel surgery in obstructive sleep apnea. Eur Arch Otorhinolaryngol. 2012;269(9):2129–36.
44. Katsantonis GP, Miyazaki S, Walsh JK. Effects of uvulopalatopharyngoplasty on sleep architecture and patterns of obstructed breathing. Laryngoscope. 1990;100(10 Pt 1):1068–72.

Part V

Surgical Treatment of Epiglottis Collapse

Epiglottectomy

19

Bhik T. Kotecha

19.1 Introduction

Hypopharynx is a challenging anatomical upper airway segment from a surgical perspective. It is crucial that the evaluation of the obstructive upper airway is conducted very carefully in order to identify exactly where the problem is. Drug-induced sleep endoscopy (DISE) has been pivotal in the evaluation process of the upper airway obstruction [1, 2]. This technique allows a three-dimensional visualisation of the dynamic upper airway during sedation and enables identification of the epiglottic obstruction be this as the only obstructive element or indeed as part of multi-level obstruction and this is particularly important in patients who have failed CPAP therapy [3].

Epiglottic collapse is now more actively sought for and the finding is more common than previously thought with the prevalence range of 12.5% to just above 70% [4, 5]. Epiglottic surgery is surrounded by fear of potential complications that could result, namely that of excessive bleeding into the airway and of course the risk of swallowing difficulty and/or aspiration. With regard to swallowing, there are reports to confirm that process of swallowing is not significantly affected [6, 7]. Advance in technology has aided in performing the procedure in a safer manner and these include surgical tools such as coblation, laser and the trans-oral robotic approach [7].

Supplementary Information The online version contains supplementary material available at https://doi.org/10.1007/978-3-031-34992-8_19. The videos can be accessed individually by clicking the DOI link in the accompanying figure caption or by scanning this link with the SN More Media App.

B. T. Kotecha (✉)
Nuffield Health Brentwood, Essex, UK

M. Delakorda, N. de Vries (eds.), *The Role of Epiglottis in Obstructive Sleep Apnea*, https://doi.org/10.1007/978-3-031-34992-8_19

19.2 Indications/Rationale

As with any other surgical intervention, careful patient selection is of utmost importance. Clinical evaluation of the upper airway particularly in patients who have failed CPAP therapy may reveal the problem to be at the level of the epiglottis and this could be identified by awake endoscopy, DISE or indeed by MRI studies. Awake endoscopy for example may demonstrate a very retractile epiglottis almost impinging on the posterior pharyngeal wall and likewise DISE could reveal a trapdoor phenomenon whereby the laryngeal lumen is almost completely occluded. The trapdoor phenomenon seen during DISE is due to the high negative intra-luminal pressure sucking the floppy epiglottis inwards towards the laryngeal inlet (Fig. 19.1). In this case, the glosso-epiglottic fold is quite long and the vallecula appears somewhat deeper and very easily visible. In addition, the anatomy and shape of epiglottis such as omega shaped, normally curved, flat will determine the type of specific obstruction and hence the surgical procedure deemed necessary [8]. However, at times one may see that the base of tongue is rather bulky and that may be pushing the epiglottis posteriorly and inferiorly to occlude the larynx. In these cases, the glosso-epiglottic fold is fairly short and the vallecula rather narrow. Imaging techniques such as MRI scans are useful for soft tissue analysis and could potentially pick up compromised retro-glossal component due to prominence of tongue base and/or epiglottis. Laryngomalacia is not uncommonly seen in the paediatric population and is occasionally encountered in adults with sleep disordered breathing where there is redundant soft tissue around the ary-epiglottic folds and some in-curling of the epiglottis which compromises the airway during inspiration.

It is prudent that the patient is fully informed and consented prior to undergoing surgery and during this process, it is important to discuss risks such as bleeding, infections and swallowing difficulties in the earlier phase and possibility of laryngeal penetration or aspiration. In some cases, if the airway gets significantly compromised from bleeding and/or swelling, then it may be necessary to perform a

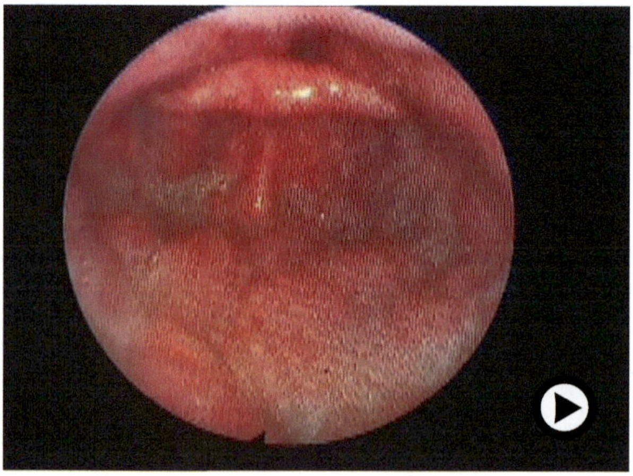

Fig. 19.1 (Video 19.1) DISE demonstrating epiglottic trap door phenomenon (► https://doi.org/10.1007/000-bfm)

temporary tracheotomy and the patient ought to be made aware of this. This may particularly be the case if surgery to the epiglottis is combined with procedure on the tongue at the same time.

19.3 Contraindications

Patient selection is crucial for all surgical procedures and the case in epiglottectomy is no exception. In patients with co-existing neurological conditions, the risks of aspiration may be greater, so this would need to be taken into consideration. General co-morbidities of the individual patient should also be considered and factors such as obesity would make the outcome from surgery less favourable.

19.4 Surgical Technique

Pre-operative assessment should also include a full and thorough evaluation by the anaesthetist and the discussion between the surgeon and the anaesthetist should include the type of endotracheal intubation tube to be used. From a safety perspective, a metallic laser tube is recommended for laser surgery and furthermore, the insertion of the tube may have to be via the naso-tracheal approach if combined surgery of the tongue and epiglottis is being considered. If laser tubes are unavailable, then it may be possible to use a rubber endotracheal tube with a protective foil, but in terms of safety this is not as good as the metallic laser tube.

For surgery on epiglottis solely, an oro-tracheal intubation may suffice and the standard endo-laryngeal surgery using suspension microlaryngoscopy is the preferred option. The patient is placed in the supine position with the head in the "sniffing the morning air" position with the head extended and the neck flexed. This could be attained with an appropriate positioning of a pillow half under the shoulders with or without the use of a head-ring depending on the size and flexibility of the neck. While draping the patient, if laser is to be used then the standard laser safety precautionary measures should be taken including applying wet gauze swabs around the face.

A variety of rigid laryngoscopes are available and include Dedo, Lindholm, Holinger and Sataloff. The choice of scope would be determined by the anatomy and of course the personal preference. Surgical exposure is of utmost importance and hence the use of the appropriate laryngoscope to accommodate the anatomy is equally important. Illumination of the surgical field is initially attained with a good light source and cable followed by the light from the microscope or rigid endoscope if that is preferred. While inserting the laryngoscope, great care should be taken to protect the dentition with a plastic guard and unnecessary aggressive levering of the laryngoscope on the teeth should be avoided in order to prevent dental trauma. The beak of the laryngoscope is placed in the vallecula to expose the epiglottis adequately. A micro-laryngoscopy Lewy suspension system is utilised to allow bimanual surgery and a Mayo stand may be used to support the surgeon's arms. While

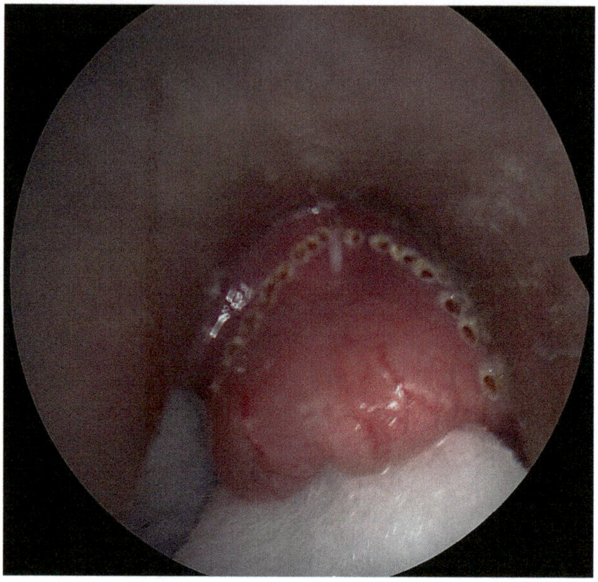

Fig. 19.2 Epiglottis exposed and the undersurface covered by wet swab. The excision margin of inverted "V" is marked out with the microscope mounted laser

some surgeons may choose to use a rigid endoscope to be inserted via the rigid laryngoscope, the author prefers the use of a microscope with a 400 mm lens and a micromanipulator for attachment of the CO_2 laser to it and this technique will be described first.

Once the epiglottis has been exposed, the choice of excision is dependent on how the epiglottis is obstructing the upper airway. In most cases of the trapdoor phenomenon, a laser wedge resection in the shape of an inverted "V" would appropriately resolve the problem. This is the author's preferred practice and is demonstrated by Fig. 19.2. Inadvertent lasering of the posterior pharyngeal surface is avoided by inserting a wet swab or surgical patties underneath the epiglottis. The CO_2 laser is set on 5–10 W power in the continuous mode and using the micromanipulator to control the fine laser beam and pushing the foot pedal to deliver the laser energy, the outline is first marked as shown in Fig. 19.2. Smoke aspirator is connected alongside the shaft of the laryngoscope which aids in sucking the smoke and thus providing a constantly satisfactory view. Further careful lasering is continued to resect the wedge alongside one of the edges of the triangle (Fig. 19.3) and then the other edge likewise. Hardly any bleeding is encountered, but should this become an issue then de-focussing the laser beam and addressing the bleeding point with this should rectify the problem. Alternatively, adrenaline-soaked surgical patties would also be helpful. Figure 19.4 demonstrates the clear view of the larynx after resection. Figure 19.5 demonstrates the six-week post-operative view with a flexible nasendoscope illustrating the patent laryngeal inlet. However, the surgical technique may need modification if in-curling of the epiglottis is noted during DISE [9]. In these cases, the lateral borders of the omega-shaped epiglottis are trimmed from the pharyngo-epiglottic fold with preservation of mucosa using the transoral robotic

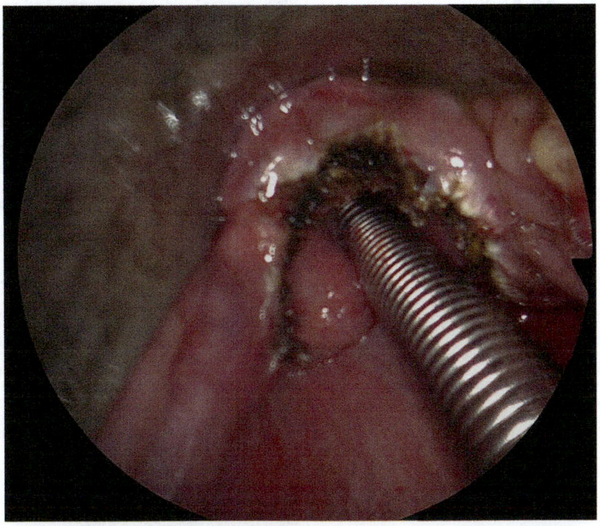

Fig. 19.3 Some of the epiglottis resected, but vocal cords still not seen clearly

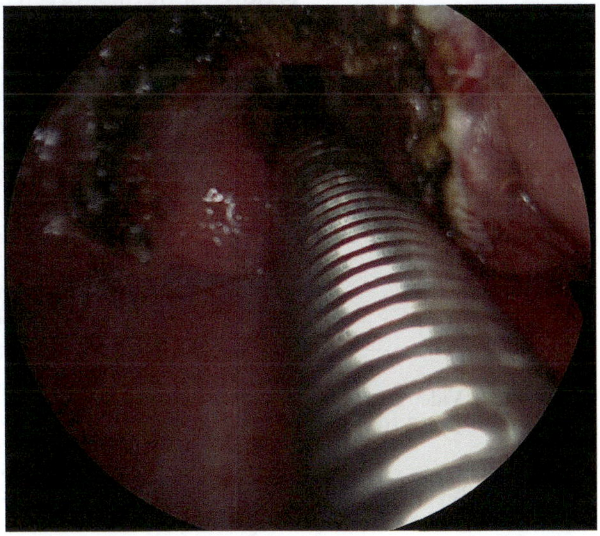

Fig. 19.4 Clear view of the larynx following laser wedge resection

approach. Robotic approach is also usefully applied in cases where both the tongue and the epiglottis need addressing [7].

Alternative techniques using different surgical tools if laser is unavailable and endoscopes rather than the operating microscope have been described. Endoscopic diathermy epiglottectomy has been reported in four cases of sleep disordered breathing [10]. They used a microdissection monopolar scissors to excise most of the epiglottis leaving behind approximately 3 mm of the suprahyoid epiglottis. They reported that the view was satisfactory without the microscope and in any case, if the microscope was to be used then it was more difficult to manoeuvre the scissors.

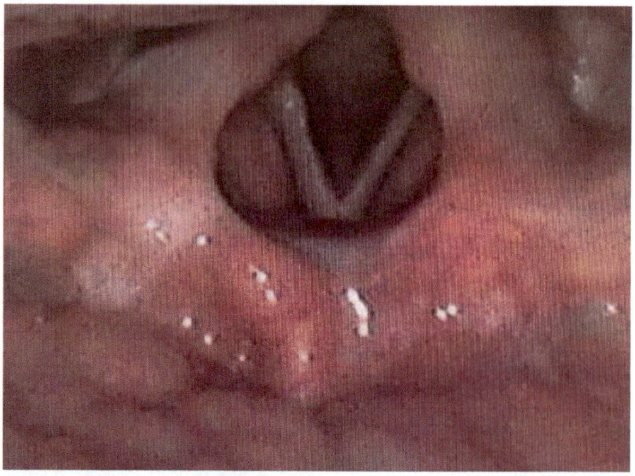

Fig. 19.5 Six-week post-operative view of the larynx demonstrating the epiglottic remnant and a very clear view of the larynx

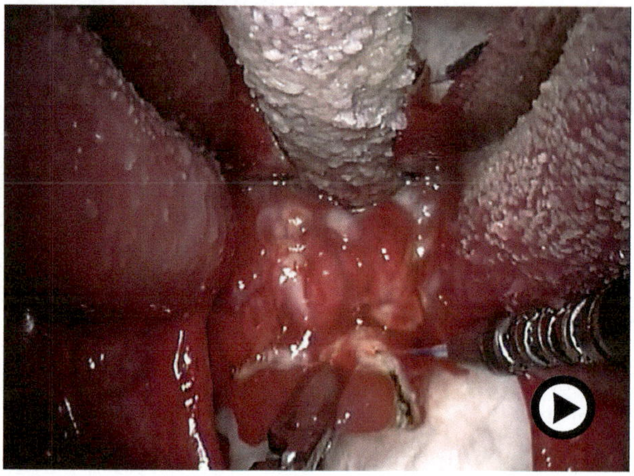

Fig. 19.6 (Video 19.2) TORS epiglottic resection with thulium laser (▶ https://doi.org/10.1007/000-bfk)

Similarly, endoscopic coblator-assisted epiglottic surgery has been reported [11]. This describes the use of a 30^0 rigid laryngeal 5 mm endoscope, inserted via a broad lumen laryngoscope suspended with Lewy laryngoscope holder and fixed to a Mayo table. A PROcise™ Plasma wand connected to the Coblator II surgical system is utilised, but an epiglottoplasty rather than epiglottectomy is performed. However, there is no reason why the excision of the epiglottis cannot be carried out with this technique.

If base of tongue surgery is also required in addition to the epiglottic resection, then the author modifies the approach and utilises the trans-oral robotic surgery [7]. In this case, the microscope is no longer required and da Vinci robotic system is used. The laser used here is the thulium laser available in the fibre mode and hence very easy to use through one of the robotic ports via an introducer. The excision of the epiglottis is carried out with thulium laser set at 15 W (Fig. 19.6). The setup is somewhat different; as there is no microscope, a Boyle-Davis gag is used to keep the mouth open and wet swabs are used as a protective measure on the pharyngeal wall and also underneath the epiglottis to prevent inadvertent lasering. During the procedure with any of the above, it is prudent to give the patient intravenous prophylactic antibiotics (500/125 mg of amoxicillin-clavulonic acid if not allergic to penicillin) and 8 mg of intravenous dexamethasone to prevent swelling.

19.5 Post-Operative Care and Complications

Post-operatively, one would look out for bleeding or breathing difficulty with close monitoring. The patient would be kept in for a minimum of 24 h observation and it is useful to have high dependency unit available for nursing care if necessary. Appropriate analgesic agents and oxygen supplementation are given as and when necessary. In general, a soft diet is recommended for the first couple of days. The patient is advised to swallow slightly slower than normal as in the earlier post-operative phase, they may experience laryngeal penetration or mild aspiration. Once patients have made adequate post-operative recovery, they are discharged on oral antibiotics for a week and a small dose of dexamethasone (2 mg twice or thrice daily for three further days). Analgesic agents (usually codeine and/or non-steroidal anti-inflammatory agents such as diclofenac) and mouth wash are also recommended for a few days. Most of our patients recover fully after 2–3 weeks with normal swallowing without any problems with aspiration.

19.6 Discussion

DISE has enabled more accurate evaluation of the upper airway collapse and the role of the epiglottis collapse has been better recognised [5, 12]. Epiglottic surgery may be conducted as a sole procedure or as part of multi-level surgery [7, 13, 14] with favourable outcomes reported by all. Golz et al. [15] reported good objective improvement in the sleep study parameters in 27 patients who underwent laser epiglottectomy. In their group, the improvement in overall oxygen saturation was significant from the preoperative levels recorded at 66% +/−17.6% to postoperative levels of 95% +/− 13.2%. Similarly, they found the RDI (respiratory distress index) reduced from 45 +/−14.6 per hour to 14 +/− 5.1 per hour. Babademez et al. [9] reported a statistically significant improvement in the mean apnea-hypopnea index (AHI) from 27.89/h preoperatively to 10.58/h postoperatively in their group of 21 patients with inward curling of the epiglottis. An important point made in this study was regarding stabilisation of the epiglottis remnant in that excessive medial trimming should be avoided and they suggest to use an imaginary line through the arytenoid cartilage as a possible landmark. Catalfumo et al. [16] reported an improved cure rate in their group of OSA patients from 50% to 65% when partial epiglottectomy was performed with other surgical procedures such as palatal surgery.

Literature on epiglottic surgery is somewhat sparse compared to that of palatal surgery and based on this, the complications encountered following epiglottic surgery do not appear to be frequently listed. However, surgeons have to be extremely aware of the potential serious complications of epiglottic surgery. This being said, our own experience in terms of persistent dysphagia or any aspiration has been negligible [7]. Recognising that the epiglottis is causing the issue in upper airway obstruction and understanding the nature of the problem is crucial before embarking on any specific surgical epiglottic resection and further research is needed to better appreciate this [17].

References

1. De Vito A, Carrasco-Llatas M, Ravesloot MJ, Kotecha B, de Vries N, et al. European position paper on drug-induced sleep endoscopy: 2017 update. Clin Otolaryngol. 2018;43:1541–52.
2. Lechner M, Wilkins D, Kotecha B. A review on drug induced sedation endoscopy – technique, grading systems and controversies. Sleep Med Rev. 2018;41:141–8.
3. Virk JS, Kotecha BT. When continuous positive airway pressure (CPAP) fails. J Thoracic Dis. 2016;8(10):E1112–21.
4. Lan MC, Liu SY, Lan MY, Modi R, Capasso R. Lateral pharyngeal wall collapse associated with hypoxaemia in obstructive sleep apnea. Laryngoscope. 2015;125:2408–12.
5. Koutsourelakis I, Safiruddin F, Ravesloot M, Zakynthinos S, de Vries N. Surgery for obstructive sleep apnea: sleep endoscopy determinants of outcome. Laryngoscope. 2012;122:2587–91.
6. Leder SB, Burrell MI, Van Daele DJ. Epiglottis is not essential for successful swallowing in humans. Ann of Otol Rhinol Laryngol. 2010;119(12):795–8.
7. Arora A, Chaidas K, Garas G, et al. Outcome of TORS to tongue base and epiglottis in patients with OSA intolerant of conventional treatment. Sleep Breath. 2016;20(2):739–47.
8. Delakorda M, Ovsenik N. Epiglottis shape as a predictor of obstructive level in patients with sleep apnea. Sleep Breath. 2019;23(1):311–7.
9. Babademez MA, Gul F, Bulut KS, Sancak M, Atalay SK. Robotic modification of epiglottis trimming in the treatment of obstructive sleep apnea. Otolaryngol head neck Surg; 2021. p. 1–7.
10. Oluwasanmi AF, Mal RK. Diathermy epiglottectomy: endoscopic technique. J Laryngol Otol. 2001;115:289–92.
11. Cassano M. Endoscopic coblator-assisted epiglottoplasty in "obstructive sleep apnoea syndrome" patients. Clin Otolaryngol. 2015;42:1112–4.
12. Bosco G, Morato M, Perez-Martin N, Navarro A, Racionero MA, et al. One-stage multilevel surgery for treatment of obstructive sleep apnea syndrome. J Clin Med. 2021;10(4822):1–9.
13. Mickelson SA, Rosenthal L. Midline glossectomy and epiglotticdectomy for obstructive sleep apnea syndrome. Laryngoscope. 1997;107:614–9.
14. Toh ST, Han HJ, Tay HN, Kiong KL. Transoral robotic surgery for obstructive sleep apnea in Asian patients: a Singapore sleep Centre experience. JAMA Otolaryngol Head Neck Surg. 2014;140:624–9.
15. Golz A, Goldenberg D, Westerman ST, et al. Laser partial epiglotticdectomy as a treatment for obstructive sleep apnea and laryngomalacia. Ann Otol Rhinol Laryngol. 2000;109:1140–5.
16. Catalfumo FJ, Golz A, Westerman ST, Gilbert LM, Joachims HZ, Goldenberg D. The epiglottis and obstructive sleep apnoea syndrome. J Laryngol Otol. 1998;112:940–3.
17. Torre C, Camacho M, Liu SY-C, Huon L-K, Capasso R. Epiglottis collapse in adult obstructive sleep apnea: a systematic review. Laryngoscope. 2016;126:515–23.

Epiglottis Stiffening Operation (ESO) 20

Fabrizio Salamanca and Federico Leone

20.1 Introduction

The identification of upper respiratory tract obstruction site(s) in obstructive sleep apnea/hypopnea syndrome (OSAHS) patients is important in order to select the best therapeutic strategy. Nowadays, among different diagnostic tools, drug-induced sleep endoscopy (DISE), although not ideal, plays a key role in the decision making process [1]. The introduction of routinely use of DISE studies in OSAHS patients demonstrated that the upper airway (UA) obstruction results from the collapse of one or more pharyngeal and/or laryngeal structures [2–4].

In the large majority of patients, laryngeal involvement consists of epiglottis collapse; this may be primary (in which case it is described as "floppy epiglottis") or secondary, when a bulky tongue base pushes the epiglottis backwards. Primary epiglottis collapse (EC) in patients with obstructive sleep apnea/hypopnea syndrome (OSAHS) still represents a challenge in terms of conservative treatments, such as oral appliances [5, 6] and CPAP [7]; therefore, its identification has important implications for surgical treatment. In order to approach EC, we got inspired by the

Supplementary Information The online version contains supplementary material available at https://doi.org/10.1007/978-3-031-34992-8_20. The videos can be accessed individually by clicking the DOI link in the accompanying figure caption or by scanning this link with the SN More Media App.

F. Salamanca
Unit of Otorhinolaryngology – Head and Neck Surgery – Snoring and OSA Research Centre, Humanitas San Pio X, Milan, Italy

Department of Biomedical Sciences, Humanitas University, Milan, Italy

F. Leone (✉)
Unit of Otorhinolaryngology – Head and Neck Surgery – Snoring and OSA Research Centre, Humanitas San Pio X, Milan, Italy

M. Delakorda, N. de Vries (eds.), *The Role of Epiglottis in Obstructive Sleep Apnea*, https://doi.org/10.1007/978-3-031-34992-8_20

CAPSO (Cautery Assisted Palate Stiffening Operation) described by Pang et al. [8] It consists of the removal of an area of palatal mucosa with an electric scalpel inducing scar retraction without sutures, so that stiffening of the soft palate is obtained, decreasing snoring and palatal prolapse. Similarly, we applied this principle at the lingual surface of the epiglottis, naming our procedure "Epiglottis Stiffening Operation" (ESO) [9].

20.2 Indications

The presence of a primary epiglottic collapse at DISE evaluation is the main indication for this type of procedure.

20.3 Preoperative Work-Up

The preoperative diagnostic work-up includes complete physical examination, endoscopic evaluation, polysomnographic study (PSG), and DISE. Treatment was planned taking into account clinical features and preferences of every single patient.

20.4 Surgical Technique

Exposition of the epiglottis in direct microlaryngoscopy is performed. The working area is identified as a rectangular area extended 1/3 in the upper half and 2/3 in the lower half of the epiglottis, between the lateral glosso-epiglottic folds (including the median glosso-epiglottic fold) (Fig. 20.1).

The lingual side of the epiglottis within the working area is cauterized using a suction cautery avoiding reaching the free margin of the epiglottis itself (Fig. 20.2a–d). In this phase, it's important to reach the perichondrium in order to induce stiffening and scar retraction of the tissues as a result of healing by secondary intention (Fig. 20.2e).

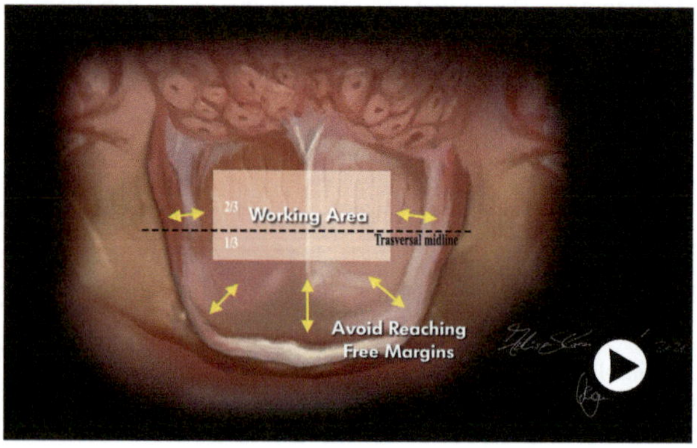

Fig. 20.1 (Video 20.1) ESO working area: a rectangular area extended 1/3 in the upper half and 2/3 in the lower half of the epiglottis (▶ https://doi.org/10.1007/000-bfn)

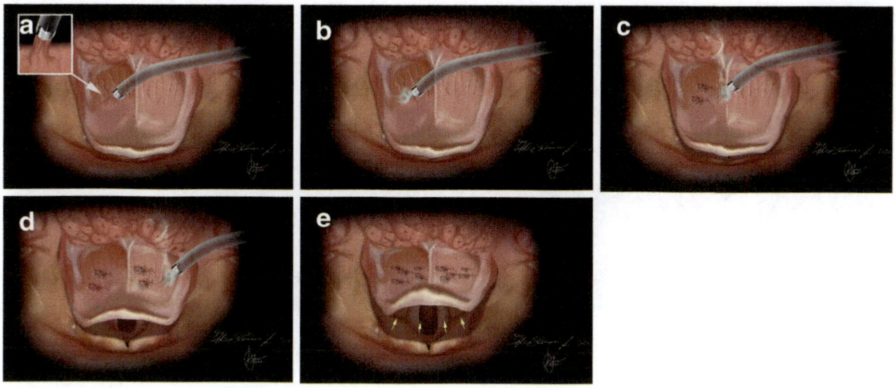

Fig. 20.2 Step by step procedure. The excessive mucosa of the lingual side of the epiglottis within the work area is raised (**a**) and cauterized (**b**–**d**) using a suction cautery causing an immediate and visible retraction of the epiglottis (**e**)

20.5 Tips and Tricks

Some tips and tricks must be taken into account performing ESO: a) the scarification is made using a suction cautery in order to cauterize and at the same time removing the excess of lax tissues; b) it's important to reach the perichondrium of the lingual side of epiglottis, especially on the midline, in order to induce an effective stiffening in the direction of median tiroepiglottic ligament; c) it is necessary to leave a rim of healthy tissue along the free border of the epiglottis to preserve sensitive receptors allowing the activation of reflexes; d) using a small endotracheal tube allows a good and complete visualization of the epiglottis; e) very low cauterization power avoids heat transmission, reducing the chance of healing problems or even loss of substance of the epiglottis; f) postoperative antibiotic administration is strongly recommended.

20.6 Postoperative Management

After surgery, at the first postoperative day, a verbal Numerical Rating Scale 11 (vNRS-11) and an Eating Assessment Tool 10 (Italian version)(I-EAT-10) [10] is administered; patients are discharged afterwards. Patients are followed for at least 3 months postoperatively according to our protocol that includes endoscopic evaluation on seventh and 30th postoperative day and PSG at about 3 months (Fig. 20.3).

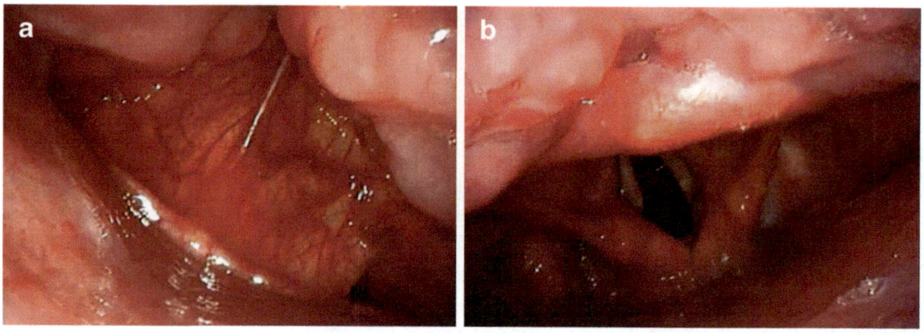

Fig. 20.3 Preoperative DISE with primary epiglottis collapse (**a**); postoperative DISE with outcome after ESO (**b**)

20.7 Contraindications

Body mass index (BMI) >35 and factors making laryngeal exposure difficult (e.g., presence of trismus, mandibular prognatism, etc.) [11] should be considered as restrictions precluding the use of our technique.

20.8 Complications

In our experience, this procedure is devoid of major complications. No patient had dysphagia, aspiration, or dysphonia. Some minor complications are mainly due to postoperative infections which can be managed with oral antibiotics.

20.9 Our Experience

Between 1 January 2016 and 31 December 2020, we have performed 536 surgical procedures for OSAHS and a total of 87 patients who underwent ESO exclusively. A strong predominance of male was found, since only 10 patients were female (11,5%), while 77 were male (88,5%); the mean age was 53,1 years (SD ± 11,1). The mean BMI was 26.8 kg/m^2 (SD ± 3,1). Fourteen (16,1%) patients were affected by simple snoring; 73 (83,9%) patients were affected by OSAHS with a mean AHI of 30/h (SD ± 20,3). The postoperative course of all patients was uneventful substantially without pain (vNRS-11 range from 0 to 3) with discharge in the first post-op day. Moreover, no patient had dysphagia, aspiration (I-EAT 10 range from 0 to 2), or dysphonia. Two patients affected by diabetes mellitus had postoperative epiglottitis treated with oral antibiotics and subsided within 6 days. Postoperative fibronasolaryngoscopy on seventh and 30th postoperative day showed good results in terms of retraction of epiglottis in all patients. Follow-up ranged between 6 and 68 months (mean, 18 months; SD ± 13,4).

20.10 Summary

The epiglottis is an important anatomical structure that was largely ignored and/or underestimated in the early research on obstructive breathing disorders [12]. Recent studies, however, have shown that it plays an important role, either on its own or in combination with other pharyngeal structures. [13, 14] Primary collapse of the epiglottis represents a challenging situation because CPAP treatment may sometimes aggravate airway obstruction by further pushing the epiglottis down into the laryngeal aditus. [7, 15] Furthermore, an epiglottis collapse can in some cases persist even while performing a mandibular protrusion during the DISE, making it difficult to treat exclusively with an oral appliance application. [6, 16] For all these reasons, surgical treatment could represent a good option when dealing with EC, though up to now no standardized surgical protocol has been described.

It's important to remember that the epiglottis plays a role in preventing aspirations thanks to its sensitive receptors (distributed on the laryngeal surface, ariepiglottic folds, arytenoids, and posterior commissure) that stimulate the so-called "glottis closure reflex".[16] For this reason, we stopped to perform "partial epiglottectomy"[17] for the treatment of primary epiglottis collapse, developing the surgical procedure we are actually reporting about.

Since its advent as a tool for the treatment of OSAHS, the scope of surgery has evolved to address multiple areas of obstruction simultaneously [18, 19]. The treatment of EC is generally part of multi-site procedures, explaining why we currently lack enough scientific evidence to support any surgical treatment that is intended to address this specific site of obstruction. To date, different surgical approaches [16, 17, 20] were described with the aim of treating this peculiar region, but some of these are technically complex and eventually associated with complications, such as bleeding, edema, persistent dysphagia, dysgeusia, etc. [20].

Our experience allows us to affirm that our ESO is a safe procedure, devoid of complications, easy to perform, and effective to treat EC that presents itself as a single or coexistent site of UA obstruction without altering epiglottis fundamental functions. The short healing time and the lack of discomfort for the patients allow surgeons to approach this surgery alone or in association with other techniques in a multimodal approach or multilevel surgical treatment.

References

1. Delakorda M, Ovsenik N. Epiglottis shape as a predictor of obstruction level in patients with sleep apnea. Sleep Breath. 2018;149:1–7. https://doi.org/10.1007/s11325-018-1763-y.
2. Azarbarzin A, Marques M, Sands SA, et al. Predicting epiglottic collapse in patients with obstructive sleep apnoea. Eur Respir J. 2017;50:1700345–20. https://doi.org/10.1183/13993003.00345-2017.
3. Campanini A, Canzi P, De Vito A, et al. Awake versus sleep endoscopy: personal experience in 250 OSAHS patients. Acta Otorhinolaryngol Ital. 2010;30:73–7.
4. Salamanca F, Costantini F, Bianchi A, et al. Identification of obstructive sites and patterns in obstructive sleep apnoea syndrome by sleep endoscopy in 614 patients. Acta Otorhinolaryngol Ital. 2013;33:261–6.

5. Giarda M, Brucoli M, Arcuri F, et al. Efficacy and safety of maxillomandibular advancement in treatment of obstructive sleep apnoea syndrome. Acta Otorhinolaryngol Ital. 2013;33:43–6.
6. Kent DT, Rogers R, Soose RJ. Drug-induced sedation endoscopy in the evaluation of OSA patients with incomplete Oral appliance therapy response. Otolaryngol Head Neck Surg. 2015;153:302–7. https://doi.org/10.1177/0194599815586978.
7. Verse T, Pirsig W. Age-related changes in the epiglottis causing failure of nasal continuous positive airway pressure therapy. J Laryngol Otol. 2007;113:1022. https://doi.org/10.1017/S0022215100145888.
8. Pang KP, Terris DJ. Modified cautery-assisted palatal stiffening operation: new method for treating snoring and mild obstructive sleep apnea. Otolaryngol Head Neck Surg. 2016;136:823–6. https://doi.org/10.1016/j.otohns.2006.11.014.
9. Salamanca F, Leone F, Bianchi A, et al. Surgical treatment of epiglottis collapse in obstructive sleep apnoea syndrome: epiglottis stiffening operation. Acta Otorhinolaryngol Ital. 2019;39:404–8. https://doi.org/10.14639/0392-100X-N0287.
10. Schindler A, Mozzanica F, Monzani A, et al. Reliability and validity of the Italian eating assessment tool. Ann Otol Rhinol Laryngol. 2013;122:717–24. https://doi.org/10.1177/000348941312201109.
11. Incandela F, Paderno A, Missale F, et al. Glottic exposure for transoral laser microsurgery: proposal of a mini-version of the laryngoscore. Laryngoscope. 2018;24:135–7. https://doi.org/10.1002/lary.27525.
12. Catalfumo FJ, Golz A, Westerman ST, et al. The epiglottis and obstructive sleep apnoea syndrome. J Laryngol Otol. 2007;112:940. https://doi.org/10.1017/S0022215100142136.
13. Kwon OE, Jung SY, Al-Dilaijan K, et al. Is epiglottis surgery necessary for obstructive sleep apnea patients with epiglottis obstruction? Laryngoscope. 2019;115:538–6. https://doi.org/10.1002/lary.27808.
14. Torre C, Camacho M, Liu SY-C, et al. Epiglottis collapse in adult obstructive sleep apnea: a systematic review. Laryngoscope. 2015;126:515–23. https://doi.org/10.1002/lary.25589.
15. Dedhia RC, Rosen CA, Soose RJ. What is the role of the larynx in adult obstructive sleep apnea? Laryngoscope. 2013;124:1029–34. https://doi.org/10.1002/lary.24494.
16. Roustan V, Barbieri M, Incandela F, et al. Transoral glossoepiglottopexy in the treatment of adult obstructive sleep apnoea: a surgical approach. Acta Otorhinolaryngol Ital. 2018;38:38–44. https://doi.org/10.14639/0392-100X-1857.
17. Oluwasanmi AF, Mal RK. Diathermy epiglottectomy: endoscopic technique. J Laryngol Otol. 2006;115:289–92. https://doi.org/10.1258/0022215011907479.
18. Lin H-C, Friedman M, Chang H-W, Gurpinar B. The efficacy of multilevel surgery of the upper airway in adults with obstructive sleep apnea/hypopnea syndrome. Laryngoscope. 2008;118:902–8. https://doi.org/10.1097/MLG.0b013e31816422ea.
19. Montevecchi F, Meccariello G, Firinu E, et al. Prospective multicentre study on barbed reposition pharyngoplasty standing alone or as a part of multilevel surgery for sleep apnoea. Clin Otolaryngol. 2017;43:483–8. https://doi.org/10.1111/coa.13001.
20. Bourolias C, Hajiioannou J, Sobol E, et al. Epiglottis reshaping using CO2 laser: a minimally invasive technique and its potent applications. Head Face Med. 2008;4:539–4. https://doi.org/10.1186/1746-160X-4-15.

Glossoepiglottopexy

21

Marco Barbieri, Marco Fragale, and Davide Mocellin

21.1 Introduction

The role of the epiglottis collapse regarding the hypopharyngeal obstruction in OSA patients is become more relevant in the last years. Although it is well known that the gold standard's treatment of OSA syndrome is the CPAP therapy, some patients show a non-responsiveness or even a worsening of the apnea-hypopnea index during administration of CPAP. In fact, in case of primary epiglottis collapse, it is believed that continuous positive pressure may further push the epiglottis down in the laryngeal aditus. The importance of epiglottis is also underlined by the evidence that many patients who are adult affected by sleep apnea syndrome are affected by multilevel obstruction in upper airways and among these, the epiglottis collapse shows a prevalence of 15% [1].

Primary epiglottis collapse is not properly evaluable during office-based endoscopy. Consequently, it is strongly suggested to perform Drug Induced Sleep Endoscopy (DISE) in patients that are intolerant to CPAP or have an incomplete response to medical device therapy. Nevertheless, the sleep endoscopy is possible to evaluate anatomical changes after previous surgical treatment.

Supplementary Information The online version contains supplementary material available at https://doi.org/10.1007/978-3-031-34992-8_21. The videos can be accessed individually by clicking the DOI link in the accompanying figure caption or by scanning this link with the SN More Media App.

M. Barbieri (✉)
ENT Dept., IRCCS Ospedale Policlinico San Martino, Genoa, Italy

M. Fragale
Department of Medical and Surgical Sciences and Advanced Technologies "GF Ingrassia", ENT Section, University of Catania, Catania, Italy

D. Mocellin
ENT Dept., Ospedale S.Paolo, Savona, Italy

M. Delakorda, N. de Vries (eds.), *The Role of Epiglottis in Obstructive Sleep Apnea*, https://doi.org/10.1007/978-3-031-34992-8_21

In the year 2018, Roustan and colleagues developed a surgical technique called glossoepiglottopexy (GEP) [2]. This procedure was borrowed from that conceived by Monnier for children affected by laryngomalacia [3] and modified to ensure a stabilization of the epiglottis in adult patients. This surgical technique is performed by a transoral approach to perform a scarification of lingual surface of epiglottis and part of the tongue base to afford a scarring between these two structures helped by a transcervical suture that fortifies the adhesion; the suture has to be maintained for about 3 weeks.

When approaching to this surgical technique, it deserves to remember the importance of glottic closure reflex mediated by stimulation of the superior laryngeal nerve. The correct function of this reflex guarantees a successful sphincteric protection of laryngeal inlet. To afford this, performing the GEP is mandatory to spare the free margin of the epiglottis and to avoid injury of the numerous sensitive receptors that are represented. Therefore, this procedure provides a stable support to the epiglottis without influencing its function during swallowing while preserving laryngeal anatomy and physiology.

Roustan et al. analysed a group of 20 patients who underwent GEP and pharyngoplasty between January 2015 and September 2016 [2]. ESS scores, AHI, ODI and T90 values showed a significant decrease after 6 months from surgery, and the mean oxygen saturation showed a significant increase of its value at the polysomnographic study. Those findings demonstrated the safety and effectiveness of the GEP and allow us to consider this technique as a valid and safe choice to treat adults who suffer from sleep apnoeas with primary epiglottis collapse.

21.2 Indications and Contraindications

The main indication for this surgical technique is the primary epiglottis collapse that can be seen and better detected during drug-induced sleep endoscopy. Every patient with a suspicion of epiglottis collapse needs to be scheduled for a DISE to confirm the correct indication of the surgical procedure. The retrodisplacement can principally be due to the laxity of the glossoepiglottic ligament, but recent studies have underlined the importance of the shape of the epiglottis. Delakorda and colleagues described three different shapes of the epiglottis: type 1, omega-shaped epiglottis; type 2, normal concave epiglottis shape; type 3, flat epiglottis. Among these three types, the latter appears to be the most associated with obstruction [4]. The GEP affords to reduce the retrodisplacement stitching together the epiglottis and the base of the tongue; additionally, the suture embracing the suprahyoid epiglottis provides a more significative convexity to the epiglottis itself.

Individual parameters of the patient could make the laryngeal exposure harder; among them, a low grade of extension of the neck, trismus, macroglossia, high BMI index, or others can be found. To help to better stratify the different types of patients during operative microlaryngoscopy, a clinical predictor score for difficult laryngeal exposure (DLE) as the Laryngoscore described by Piazza et al. can be used [5].

Contraindication of primary importance is the presence of major comorbidities as cardiovascular, pulmonary, or neurologic disease. Moreover, the presence of cranio-facial malformations either isolated or syndromic could be avoid to execution of this surgical procedure properly. For example, the presence of micrognathia can make very challenging the microlaryngoscopic exposition of the larynx; moreover, these patients often present an epiglottis collapse secondary to a severe retroposition of the tongue base, the hyoid bone or the mandible itself and take more advantage from mandibular advancement devices, mandibular distraction or maxillomandibular advancement surgery.

Finally, among the contraindications deserve to be mentioned those patients affected by neurological dysfunction which determine dysphagia where the swallowing function is already impaired preoperatively.

21.3 Surgical Technique

The surgery is performed under general anesthesia. The patient lies supine in the Boyce-Jackson's position. The eyes are protected with wet gauze and the superior teeth with a silicone mouthguard.

For the transoral intubation, a smallest endotracheal tube is needed to be chosen to provide the adequate ventilation for the patient (Laser Shield II Endotracheal Tube, Medtronic Xomed, Jacksonville, FL, USA). The first goal for the surgeon is to expose the base of the tongue, the epiglottic vallecula, and the epiglottis with a Sataloff laryngoscope (MicroFrance Sataloff Laryngoscopes 124, Medtronic ENT, Jacksonville, FL, USA) (Fig. 21.1). The hyoid bone is identified and marked on the skin as a reference point. The CO_2 laser is set on the ultra-pulse mode and 3 W of power are delivered, working with the microscope at 400 mm of distance from the surgical field.

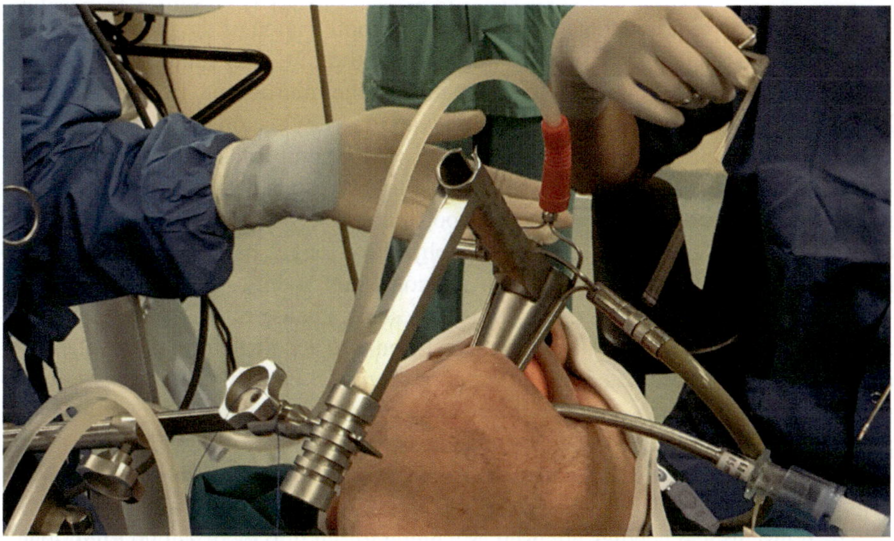

Fig. 21.1 The setting of the surgical procedure of glossoepiglottopexy. The patient can be seen in the Boyce-Jackson's position after intubation and the positioning of the laryngoscope

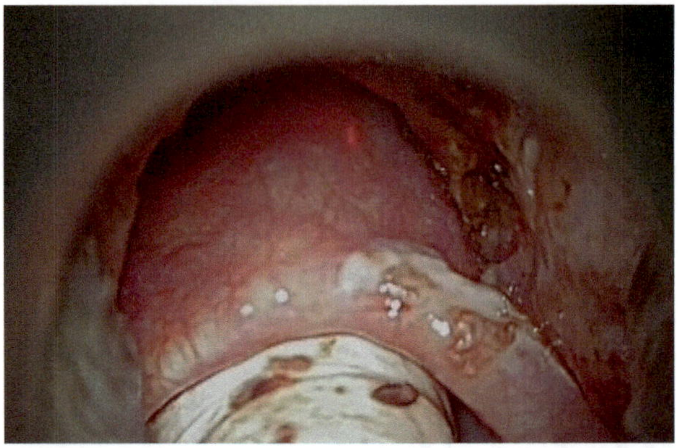

Fig. 21.2 The microlaryngoscopic view of the lingual surface of epiglottis before starting the vaporization of its mucosa where the *red spot* of the CO_2 laser can be seen. The mucosa of the tongue base had been already vaporizated

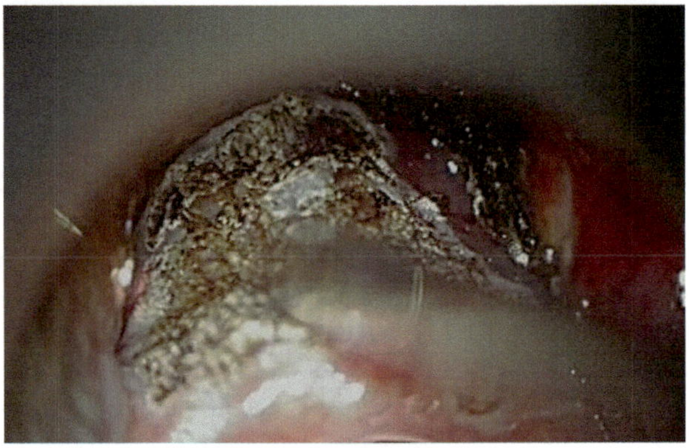

Fig. 21.3 The microlaryngoscopic view during the vaporization of the mucosa. Out of focus, it can be seen the surgical aspirator used to pull the epiglottis to expose the entire mucosa of the lingual surface

The next step requires the switch to a microscopic vision of the pharynx and the larynx through the laryngoscope (Fig. 21.2). With the CO_2 laser (Ultrapulse Dualpro Laser CO_2, Lumenis, Yokneam, Israel), paired to the microscope, the mucosa overlying the vallecula and the tongue base are vaporized by the operator (Fig. 21.3).

The surgical field is always blood-free, thanks to the ability of the CO_2 laser to coagulate vessels with a diameter less than 0.5 mm. For the vessels with a higher diameter, it needs to be used as an electrocautery monopolar and, if necessary, surgical clips. If present a moderate to severe degree of hypertrophy of the tongue base, the resection of the lymphatic tissue may be combined as an additional step of this technique.

Surgical tip: Even when the epiglottis represents a cause of obstruction, its function in protecting the upper airway must be taken into account. To maintain the glottic closure reflex coordinated by the superior laryngeal branch of the vagal nerve, it is necessary to leave a 3–4 mm rim of healthy cartilage and mucosa along the entire profile of the epiglottis with the aim of address food to the piriform sinuses.

From the outside side of the neck, two 16-gauge needles are inserted through the skin, the tongue base and the vallecula to pierce the epiglottis (Figs. 21.4 and 21.5).

The transcervical needles are used as a guide to run into them as two Premilene® sutures: number 1 (Premilene, Braun, Melsungen, Germany): the first wire is inserted in the first needle (Fig. 21.6); then, the second wire is inserted in the second

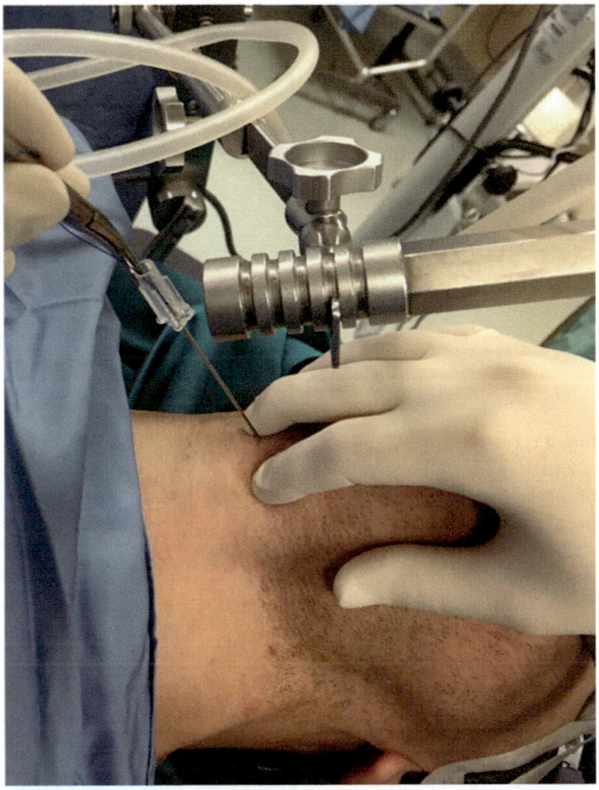

Fig. 21.4 The insertion of the needle through the skin above the hyoid bone. The wire of Premilene® running inside the needle can be seen

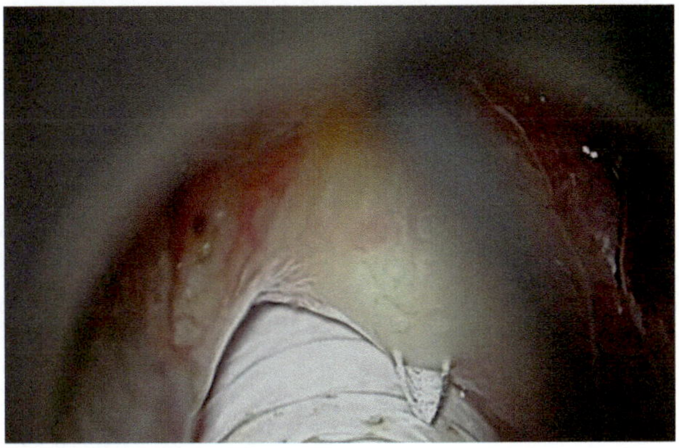

Fig. 21.5 Microlaryngoscopic view of the first needle piercing the epiglottis after its transcervical insertion

needle forming a loop (Fig. 21.7) and subsequently the first wire is passed through the loop outside of the laryngoscope.

The transcervical stitch must be tied up embracing the epiglottis so to keep together its lingual surface to the base of the tongue (Figs. 21.8 and 21.9); then, it is tied outside of the neck, anteriorly to the larynx, using a silicone surgical sheet to protect the skin from local trauma (Fig. 21.10).

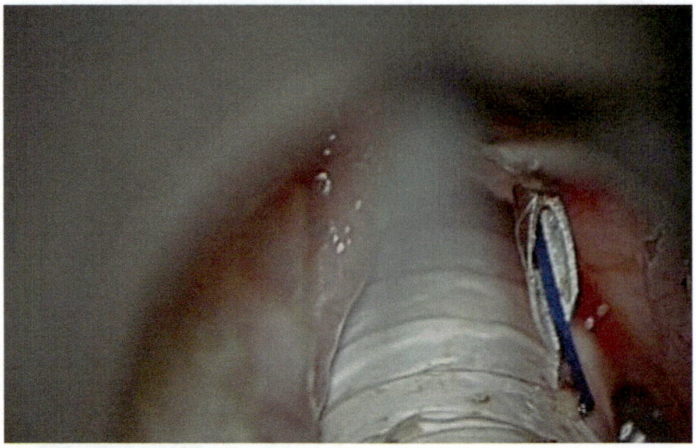

Fig. 21.6 Microlaryngoscopic view of the wire of Premilene® running inside the needle. In the next step, the surgeon has to catch the wire and pull it out from the laryngoscope

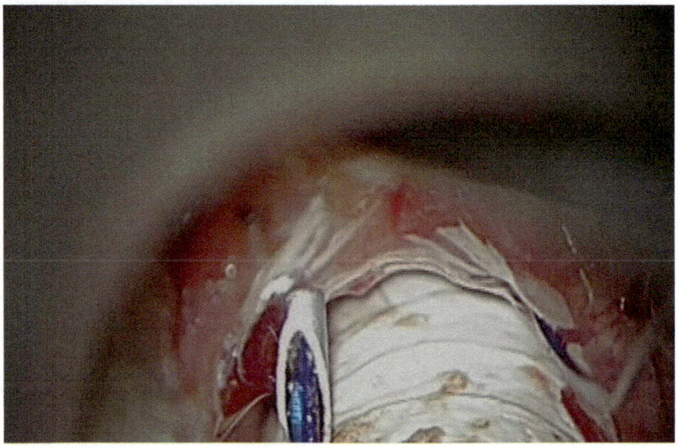

Fig. 21.7 Microlaryngoscopic view of the second 16-gauge needle after its transcervical insertion. The wire inside the needle is folded to create a loop and it will be pulled out from the laryngoscope by the operator

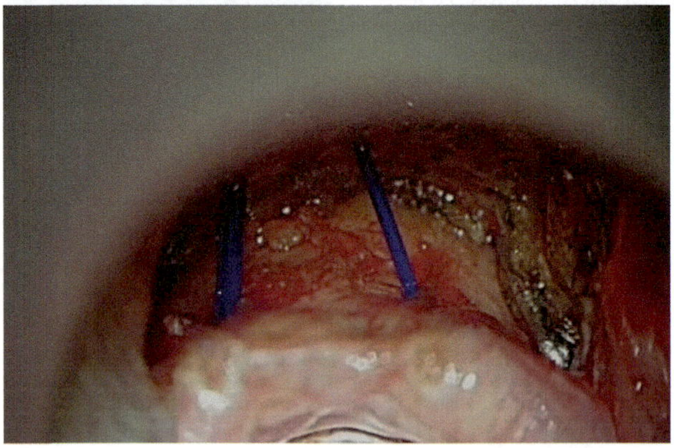

Fig. 21.8 Microlaryngoscopic view of the vallecula and the wires previously inserted because the needles had been removed. Now the wires can be knotted

The wires need to be placed both superiorly or inferiorly to the hyoid bone. If one is placed superiorly and the other inferiorly, the risk of injury of the epiglottis is too high because of the excessive tension created. Before tying the suture, a small

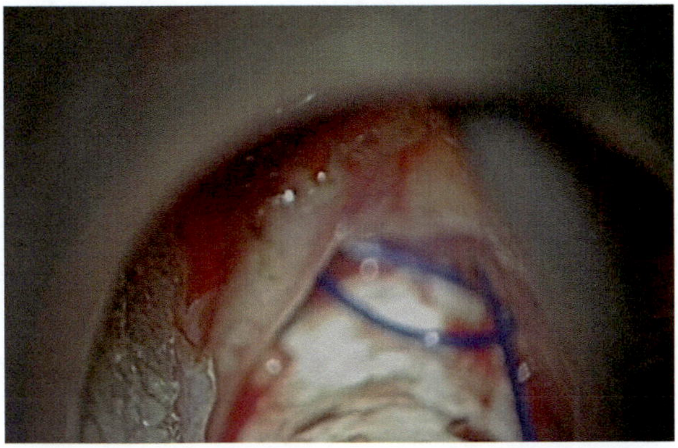

Fig. 21.9 The first wire passing through the loop of the second wire (this step needs to be done outside of the laryngoscope). The loop of the wire is used to take out the inner side of the other wire outside of the neck

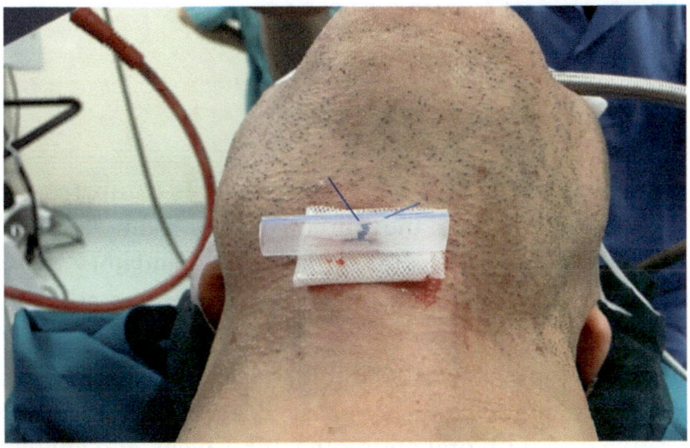

Fig. 21.10 The stitch of the transcervical wire at the end of the surgical procedure. A silastic sheet is positioned to avoid the decubitus of the knot on the skin

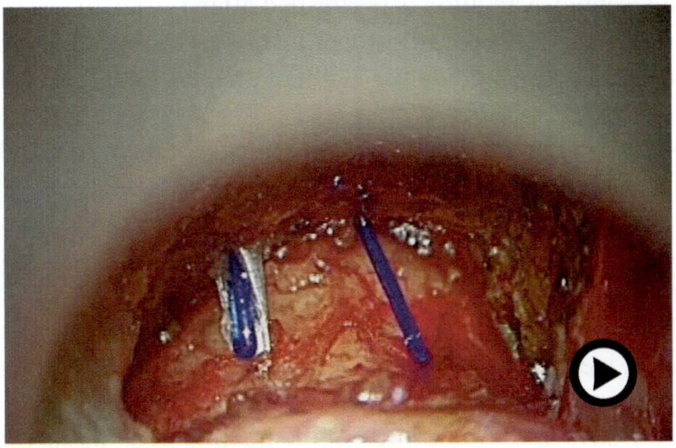

Fig. 21.11 (Video 21.1) Epiglottic vallecula during performing the GEP (▶ https://doi.org/10.1007/000-bfq)

amount of Tisseel® (Baxter, Westlake Village, CA, USA) is spread in the epiglottic vallecula using a Duplocath® (Baxter, Westlake Village, CA, USA) catheter (Figs. 21.11 and 21.12).

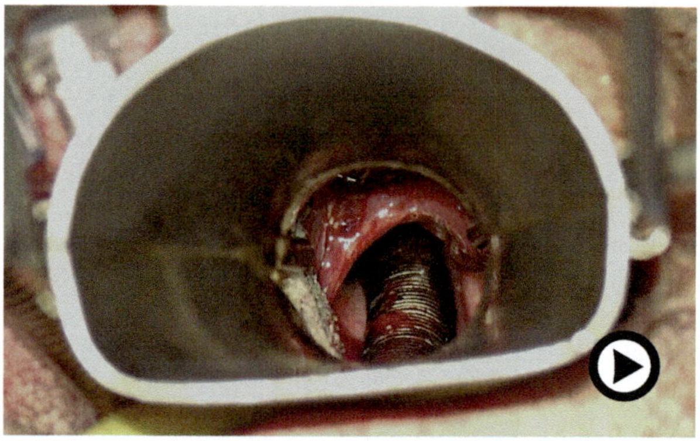

Fig. 21.12 (Video 21.2) Microlaryngoscopic view of the epiglottis at the end of the GEP procedure (▶ https://doi.org/10.1007/000-bfp)

21.4 Postoperative Care

At the end of the procedure, the patient is extubated and transferred to the recovery room for 30 min and then directly to his room.

On the first postoperative day, it is mandatory to evaluate the swallowing function with water and soft foods. If no disorders are detected, the patient can start to drink and to eat a soft diet for 7 days. During hospitalization time, intravenous antibiotics are generally administrated.

If no complications are observed, the patient is discharged in the second postoperative day, with oral antibiotics for 1 week and analgesics if required.

Video laryngoscopic evaluation is performed after 1 week to test the penetration-aspiration scale. After 3 weeks, postoperatively it is repeated and the stich is removed under endoscopic guidance without the necessity of general or local anesthesia.

Six months after the procedure, every patient is submitted to an additional polysomnography test to evaluate the efficacy of surgery.

21.5 Complications

In our experience, we treated 49 patients affected by OSA with primary collapse of epiglottic. Complications occurred only in 2 out of 49 procedures. One patient had suture breakage 7 days after procedure but the flexible trans-nasal video endoscopy revealed a stability of the GEP.

The second complication was observed in a patient that developed a laceration of the epiglottis by the sutures: the reason of that was the wire placed involving the hyoid bone, because of the excessive tension created. Anyway, in this last case, we did not observe bleeding, dysphagia, or aspiration and postoperative AHI improved from 66 to 10.

A potential complication is a slight bleeding during surgery that can be routinely controlled with bipolar clamp. Theoretically, oedema of supraglottic region of the larynx, dysphagia, or dysgeusia could be developed but the surgical technique described herein is able to preserve laryngeal anatomy and physiology. Moreover, it provides stable support to the epiglottis without interfering with its function during swallowing and reinforcing the wall of the airway by creating a kind of "landslide barrier" to prevent the falling down of the tongue base posteriorly.

References

1. Torre C, Camacho M, Liu SYC, Huon LK, Capasso R. Epiglottis collapse in adult obstructive sleep apnea: a systematic review. Laryngoscope. 2016;126:515–23. https://doi.org/10.1002/lary.25589.
2. Roustan V, Barbieri M, Incandela F, Missale F, Camera H, Braido F, et al. Glossoepiglottoplastica con approccio trans-orale nel trattamento delle apnee ostruttive notturne nell'adulto. Acta Otorhinolaryngol Ital. 2018;38:38–44. https://doi.org/10.14639/0392-100X-1857.
3. Monnier P. Pediatric airway surgery: management of laryngotracheal stenosis in infants and children. Berlin: Springer; 2010.
4. Delakorda M, Ovsenik N. Epiglottis shape as a predictor of obstruction level in patients with sleep apnea. Sleep Breath. 2019;23:311–7. https://doi.org/10.1007/s11325-018-1763-y.
5. Piazza C, Mangili S, Del Bon F, Paderno A, Grazioli P, Barbieri D, et al. Preoperative clinical predictors of difficult laryngeal exposure for microlaryngoscopy: the laryngoscore. Laryngoscope. 2014;124:2561–7. https://doi.org/10.1002/lary.24803.

22 Upper Airway Stimulation

Clemens Heiser

22.1 Introduction

Hypoglossal nerve stimulation (HNS) or also called as upper airway stimulation (UAS) has rapidly become a powerful and useful therapy option for patients, who are suffering from obstructive sleep apnea (OSA) and who are non-adherent or non-compliant to the standard treatment positive airway pressure (PAP) therapy [1]. In 1978, John Remmers et al. described the main upper airway opener "the genioglossus muscle", which is also the main target during HNS [2]. Further trials from different research groups showed that the stimulation of this muscle opens the pharyngeal airway during sleep [3–5]. That was the cornerstone for the further development of the different upper airway stimulation systems of the hypoglossal nerve. Since more than 10 years, multiple, international, prospective trails have shown the effectiveness of this therapy [6–9].

22.2 Available Technologies

Nowadays, three technologies, in different stages of development with regard to clinical data, are available in Europe and the United States with different clinical data: Inspire, LivaNova (former: ImThera) and Nyxoah [1, 10]. These three devices differ from each other mainly in two points such as (Table 22.1):

Supplementary Information The online version contains supplementary material available at https://doi.org/10.1007/978-3-031-34992-8_22. The videos can be accessed individually by clicking the DOI link in the accompanying figure caption or by scanning this link with the SN More Media App.

C. Heiser (✉)
Department of Otorhinolaryngology, Head and Neck Surgery, Klinikum Rechts der Isar, Technical University of Munich, Munich, Germany

Translational Neurosciences, University of Antwerp, Antwerp, Belgium
e-mail: clemens.heiser@tum.de

M. Delakorda, N. de Vries (eds.), *The Role of Epiglottis in Obstructive Sleep Apnea*, https://doi.org/10.1007/978-3-031-34992-8_22

Table 22.1 Different systems for upper airway stimulation and their differences regarding the anatomical location on the hypoglossal nerve and stimulation dependence regarding the breathing cycle

Anatomical location on the hypoglossal nerve	Unilateral distal selective placement of the stimulation cuff	Unilateral main trunk placement of the stimulation cuff	Bilateral distal selective placement of the stimulation paddles
Breathing cycle	Breathing cycle dependent	Non-dependent	Duty cycle dependent

1. Anatomical location of the stimulation side on the hypoglossal nerve.
2. Breathing cycle dependency.

22.3 The Anatomy of the Hypoglossal Nerve and its Anatomical Stimulations Sides

The hypoglossal nerve and its terminating branches can be divided into two main groups such as [11, 12]:

- Lateral branches: supplying the main retractors of the tongue (styloglossus muscle and hyoglossus muscle).
- Medial branches: supplying the main protrusions of the tongue: horizontal and oblique part of the genioglossus muscle.

The Genio and Inspire system, which are placed selectively at the protruding fibers of the tongue, actively open the upper airway during stimulation [13–15]. The Aura6000 system, which also includes the lateral fibers of the nerve, is placed at the main trunk of the HN. The system has multiple contacts with the opportunity to increase the permutations for selective activation of the nerve fibers [16]. The effect of stimulation is not an active upper airway opening; its mode of action is more a stiffening and re-shaping of the tongue, with only a small amount of protrusion.

22.4 Active Hyoid Suspension

Active opening of the lower upper airway can be achieved by an "active hyoid suspension" [17–19]. Moving the hyoid bone actively forward helps to open obstructions on the lower hypopharyngeal levels. Pengo et al. could show that stimulation of the genioglossus and geniohyoid muscle reduces the resistance of the upper airway [20]. The epiglottis is the upper part of the larynx and attaches to the hyoid bone via the hyoepiglottic ligament, which is an elastic-like band (Fig. 22.1). The petiolus of the epiglottis is attached to the thyroid cartilage through the thyroepiglottic ligament. The hyoid bone can be moved forward by the contraction of the geniohyoid muscle (Fig. 22.2) [21, 22].

Pulling the hyoid bone forward is normally needed during deglutition. The geniohyoid muscle is narrow, and its insertion is to the medial border of the mylohyoid muscle. This muscle originates from the inferior mental spine on the inner side of the mandible and runs slightly downwards to its insertion at the anterior part of the hyoid bone.

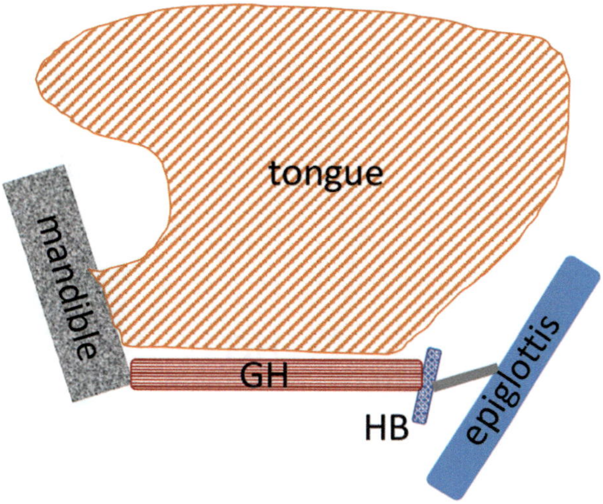

Fig. 22.1 The geniohyoid muscle is attached to the mental spine on the inner side of the mandible and runs to the anterior part of the hyoid bone. The hyoid bone is connected through the hyoepiglottic ligament (*grey bar*) to the epiglottis. *GH* geniohyoid muscle, *HB* hyoid bone

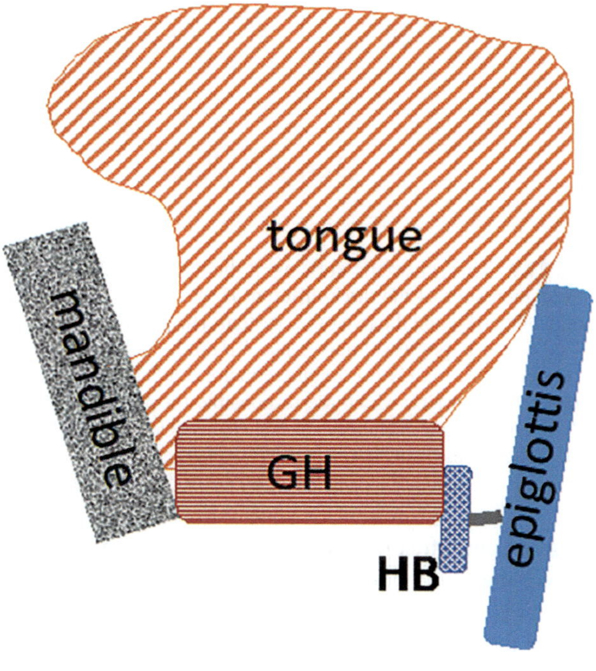

Fig. 22.2 Active contraction of the geniohyoid muscle moves the hyoid bone forward and puts the epiglottis in a more perpendicular position (compare with Fig. 22.1). *Grey bar* hyoepiglottic ligament, *GH* geniohyoid muscle, *HB* hyoid bone

22.5 Anatomical Variations of the First Cervical Nerve (C1)

The innervation of this muscle is done by the first cervical nerve (C1), which is running next to the HN and leaves the main trunk at its distal branches (Fig. 22.3) [21]. During selective HN surgery, this fiber should be carefully identified [23–25]. Heiser et al. were the first to describe this anatomical diversity and developed a new

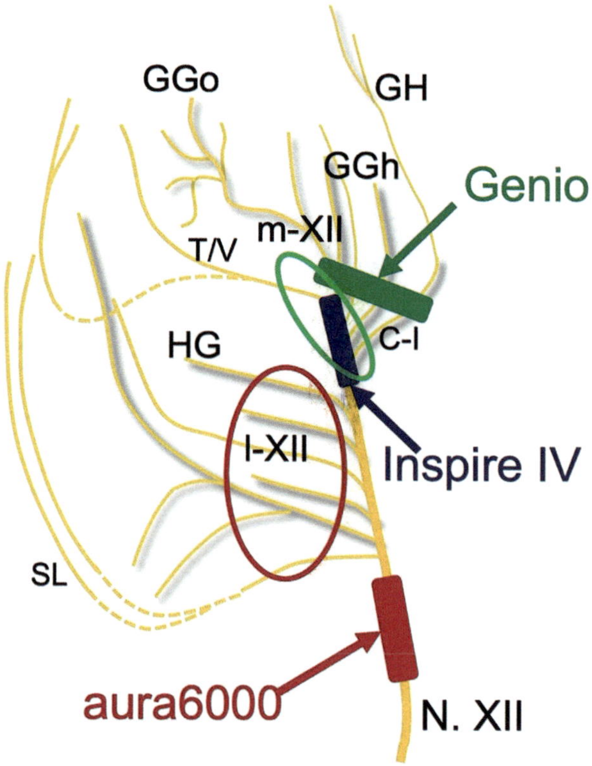

Fig. 22.3 This schematic drawing of the hypoglossal nerve (HN) shows the different anatomical stimulation sites of the three different HNS systems. Aura6000 (LivaNova) is placed at the main trunk of the HN and the two other systems (Inspire & Genio system Nyxoah) are placed selectively distal on the hypoglossal nerve. The *red circle* includes all the lateral branches of the HN, which are responsible mainly for tongue retractors and elevators. The *green circle* includes all the medial branches of the HN, which are responsible for protruding the tongue. *N.XII* nervus hypoglossus, *SL* superior longitudinal nerve fibers, *HG* hyoglossus muscle nerve fibers, *T/V* intrinsic transversal and vertical muscle nerve fibers, *l-XII* lateral nerve fibers, *m-XII* medial nerve fibers, *C1* first cervical nerve, *GGo* genioglossus (*oblique*) nerve fibers, *GGh* genioglossus (*horizontal*) nerve fibers

surgical classification system [12]. Three different types of C1 have been established, mainly depending on the point where C1 leaves the main trunk. In 60% of the cases (type a, Fig. 22.4a), C1 runs parallel to the main trunk of the HN and leaves the trunk in an acute sharp angle. In 10% of the cases, C1 leaves the main trunk very proximal and in a blunt angle (type b, Fig. 22.4b). Leaving the main trunk very distally and late in a blunt angle occurs in 30% of the cases (type c, Fig. 22.4c).

The importance of C1 and hyoid movement could be shown during an ultrasound study from Hofauer et al. [17]. A video of active and passive contractions of the geniohyoid muscle and hyoid bone movement during stimulation is attached to this chapter (Fig. 22.5a, b).

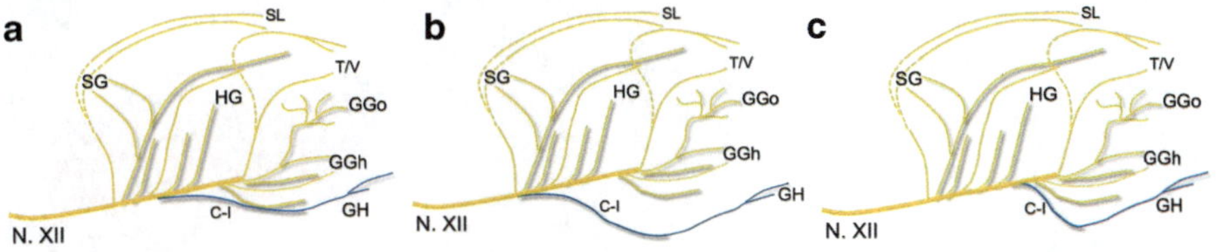

Fig. 22.4 (**a–c**) Different anatomical variations of the first cervical nerve (*C-1*, *blue line*) leaving the main trunk of the hypoglossal nerve at different anatomical sides. *N.XII* nervus hypoglossus, *SL* superior longitudinal nerve fibers, *HG* hyoglossus muscle nerve fibers, *T/V* intrinsic transversal and vertical muscle nerve fibers, *C-1* first cervical nerve, *GGo* genioglossus (*oblique*) nerve fibers, *GGh* genioglossus (*horizontal*) nerve fibers

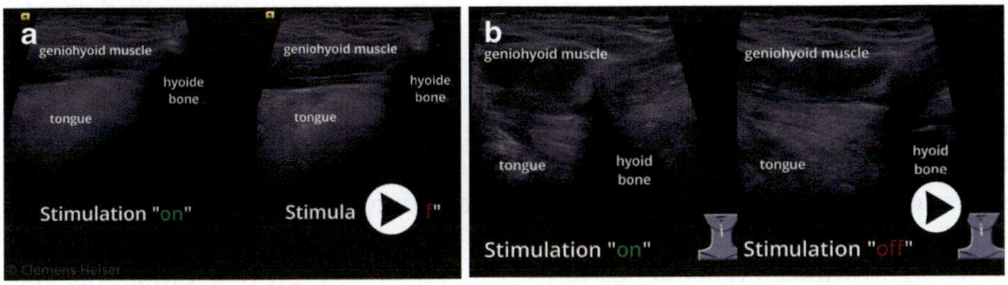

Fig. 22.5 (Video 22.1) (**a**) Passive contractions of the geniohyoid muscle (GH) and hyoid bone during stimulation of the hypoglossal nerve visualized with an ultrasound. The tongue is contracting but not the GH muscle. (**b**) Active contractions of the geniohyoid muscle (GH) and hyoid bone during stimulation of the hypoglossal nerve visualized with an ultrasound. The tongue and the GH is contracting and moving the hyoid actively forward (▶ https://doi.org/10.1007/000-bfs)

22.6 Scientific Evidence of Activating C1

Sixteen patients, who received an implantation of Inspire II Upper Airway Stimulation System (Maple Grove, USA), were examined with ultrasound (US) after the initiation of therapy [17]. Different planes for US were used, and hyoid protrusion was measured and correlated to the reduction of the apnea hypopnea index (AHI). The extent of the hyoid protrusion did not correlate with the improvement of AHI or oxygen desaturation index (ODI). One major limitation of the study was that non-responders to HNS therapy were NOT included. Just patients with significant improvements in objective parameters were asked to participate in this study [17]. In addition, the US examinations were performed 2 months after surgery while already using the effective stimulation amplitude that was defined in an overnight titration polysomnography in the sleep laboratory. In another retrospective study in 114 patients, Kumar et al. examined whether C1 had been included or not during implantation [26]. In 87 patients, C1 seemed to be included in the stimulation cuff, while 27 patients did not have C1 included. No objective measurement such as ultrasound was performed to check the inclusion of this nerve fiber. The authors could not find any correlation between C1 inclusion and non-inclusion regarding the AHI and

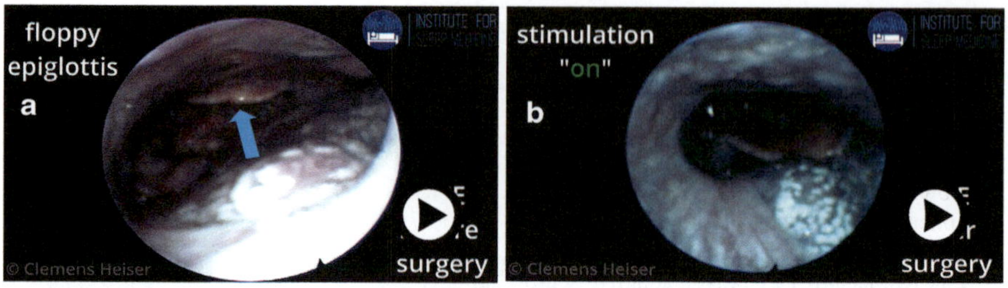

Fig. 22.6 (Video 22.2) (**a**) Floppy epiglottis during drug induced sleep endoscopy (DISE). The *blue arrow* marks how the epiglottis gets sucked to the pharyngeal wall. (**b**) The floppy epiglottis during drug induced sleep endoscopy (DISE) is solved by upper airway stimulation (▶ https://doi.org/10.1007/000-bfr)

summarized that inclusion of C1 may not provide any additional benefit [26]. The major limitations of this study were the retrospective study design, no objective measurement of C1 inclusion and using a titrated AHI during a titration night. Heiser et al. responded in a letter to the editor to take exception to an overreaching claim that C1 is not influencing clinical outcomes [19]. The major problem is that the C1 branch is sometimes difficult to detect during surgery due to its high variable branching patterns (Fig. 22.4a–c) [12]. In addition, in some cases, the intraoperative neuromonitoring (NIM), which is used during implantation, can be misleading [12, 24]. Furthermore, intraoperative muscle contractions, which can be seen during stimulation with the NIM, can be weak and obviously tongue motions do not reveal if C1 is included or not. One solution to answer these questions could be to perform an electromyogram (EMG) of the geniohyoid muscle during surgery, or as already mentioned, to perform an ultrasound in a larger cohort trial. Hofauer et al. have done this in a pilot study [17]. Heiser showed in a case report how a floppy epiglottis can be treated with advanced titration (Fig. 22.6a, b) [18].

In sum, inclusion of the small C1 fiber can be challenging. In some cases, surgeons may miss this part of the wider hypoglossal nerve. Changing stimulation settings from unipolar to monopolar for example could result in a broader and deeper field of electrical activation [18].

22.7 Conclusion

Moving the hyoid bone forward helps to solve obstruction at the level of the epiglottis. An "active hyoid suspension" can be achieved by the activation of the associated geniohyoid muscle, which is innervated by C1. In combination with the active opening of the upper airway at the level of the tongue base by stimulating the horizontal fibers of the genioglossus muscle, additional forces on the whole lower pharyngeal/hypopharyngeal level are released. Therefore, to obtain optimal clinical outcome, precise and selective cuff placement is necessary during surgery and identifying of all nerve structures by NIM, muscle contractions and tongue motions are needed. C1 should always be included in selective HNS.

References

1. Heiser C, Hofauer B. Addressing the tone and synchrony issue during sleep: pacing the hypoglossal nerve. Sleep Med Clin. 2019;14(1):91–7.
2. Remmers JE, et al. Pathogenesis of upper airway occlusion during sleep. J Appl Physiol Respir Environ Exerc Physiol. 1978;44(6):931–8.
3. Miki H, et al. Effect of electrical stimulation of genioglossus muscle on upper airway resistance in anesthetized dogs. Tohoku J Exp Med. 1987;153(4):397–8.
4. Miki H, et al. Effects of submental electrical stimulation during sleep on upper airway patency in patients with obstructive sleep apnea. Am Rev Respir Dis. 1989;140(5):1285–9.
5. Hida W, et al. Submental stimulation and supraglottic resistance during mouth breathing. Respir Physiol. 1995;101(1):79–85.
6. Heiser C, et al. Outcomes of upper airway stimulation for obstructive sleep apnea in a Multicenter German Postmarket Study. Otolaryngol Head Neck Surg. 2017;156(2):378–84.
7. Heiser C, et al. Post-approval upper airway stimulation predictors of treatment effectiveness in the ADHERE registry. Eur Respir J. 2019;53(1):1801405.
8. Thaler E, et al. Results of the ADHERE upper airway stimulation registry and predictors of therapy efficacy. Laryngoscope. 2019;130:1333.
9. Steffen A, et al. Long-term follow-up of the German post-market study for upper airway stimulation for obstructive sleep apnea. Sleep Breath. 2020;24(3):979–84.
10. Hofauer B, Heiser C. The use of selective upper airway stimulation therapy in Germany. Somnologie. 2018;22(2):98–105.
11. Heiser C, Knopf A, Hofauer B. The terminal hypoglossal nerve and its anatomical variability. HNO. 2019;67(4):242–50.
12. Heiser C, Knopf A, Hofauer B. Surgical anatomy of the hypoglossal nerve: a new classification system for selective upper airway stimulation. Head Neck. 2017;39(12):2371–80.
13. Safiruddin F, et al. Effect of upper-airway stimulation for obstructive sleep apnoea on airway dimensions. Eur Respir J. 2015;45(1):129–38.
14. Heiser C, et al. Cross motor innervation of the hypoglossal nerve-a pilot study of predictors for successful opening of the soft palate. Sleep Breath. 2021;25(1):425–31.
15. Heiser C, et al. Palatoglossus coupling in selective upper airway stimulation. Laryngoscope. 2017;127(10):E378–83.
16. Meadows PM, Whitehead MC, Zaidi FN. Effects of targeted activation of tongue muscles on oropharyngeal patency in the rat. J Neurol Sci. 2014;346(1–2):178–93.
17. Hofauer B, et al. Sonographic evaluation of tongue motions during upper airway stimulation for obstructive sleep apnea-a pilot study. Sleep Breath. 2017;21(1):101–7.
18. Heiser C. Advanced titration to treat a floppy epiglottis in selective upper airway stimulation. Laryngoscope. 2016;126(Suppl 7):S22–4.
19. Heiser C, Hofauer B. In reference to inclusion of the first cervical nerve does not influence outcomes in upper airway stimulation for treatment of obstructive sleep apnea. Laryngoscope. 2020;130(7):E454.
20. Pengo MF, Steier J. Emerging technology: electrical stimulation in obstructive sleep apnoea. J Thorac Dis. 2015;7(8):1286–97.
21. Mu L, Sanders I. Human tongue neuroanatomy: nerve supply and motor endplates. Clin Anat. 2010;23(7):777–91.
22. Sanders I, Mu L. A three-dimensional atlas of human tongue muscles. Anat Rec (Hoboken). 2013;296(7):1102–14.
23. Heiser C, et al. Updates of operative techniques for upper airway stimulation. Laryngoscope. 2016;126(Suppl 7):S12–6.
24. Heiser C, et al. Nerve monitoring-guided selective hypoglossal nerve stimulation in obstructive sleep apnea patients. Laryngoscope. 2016;126(12):2852–8.
25. Heiser C, et al. Technical tips during implantation of selective upper airway stimulation. Laryngoscope. 2018;128(3):756–62.
26. Kumar AT, et al. Inclusion of the first cervical nerve does not influence outcomes in upper airway stimulation for treatment of obstructive sleep apnea. Laryngoscope. 2020 May;130(5):E382–5. https://doi.org/10.1002/lary.28256.

Tongue Base Surgery

23

Vikas Agrawal, Vijaya Krishnan, and Srinivas Kishore

23.1 Introduction

Obstructive sleep apnea (OSA) is a disorder caused by repetitive collapse of the upper airway during sleep, resulting in either partial or complete airflow obstruction [1, 2]. In the adult population, the prevalence of OSA is 22% in men and 17% in women [3]. The morphology of upper-airway structures plays a major role in the pathogenesis of OSA.

Treatment of OSA with continuous positive airway pressure (CPAP) is still considered as the "gold standard"; however, despite its proven efficacy, a significant number of patients cannot tolerate the device and require therapeutic alternatives such as surgery, oral appliances, and/or positional devices.

In the past, the prevalence of epiglottis collapse evaluated by clinical examination was estimated to be 12% in OSAS patients, although nowadays, it is possible to show that the prevalence of epiglottis collapse in determining the airway obstruction is actually much higher, thanks to the introduction of drug-induced sedation endoscopy (DISE) [4–6].

DISE has been previously described in the adult and pediatric populations for the purpose of evaluating the dynamic airway in the supine position during a sleep-like state [7–9]. It is an increasingly useful tool in the evaluation of children with

V. Agrawal (✉)
Speciality ENT Hospital, Mumbai, Maharashtra, India
e-mail: doctor@enthospital.com

V. Krishnan
Department of Snoring & Sleep Disorders, Madras ENT Research Foundation, Chennai, Tamil Nadu, India

S. Kishore
AIG Hospitals, Hyderabad, Telangana, India

M. Delakorda, N. de Vries (eds.), *The Role of Epiglottis in Obstructive Sleep Apnea*, https://doi.org/10.1007/978-3-031-34992-8_23

persistent OSA after initial therapy, children with OSA without tonsil or adenoid hypertrophy, or children with significant craniofacial anomalies.

Sleep surgery is considered as one of the important treatment strategies for patients who cannot tolerate CPAP [10], and the success rates of uvulopalatopharyngoplasty (UPPP) in moderate and severe OSA patient groups were 42.5% and 26.5%, respectively [11]. However, the UPPP success rate is unsatisfactory in patients with small tonsils and a bulky tongue base. Additional therapy for the tongue base is recommended, particularly for patients with anatomical tongue-base obstruction during sleep [12]. At the same time, failure to recognize epiglottic collapse along with tongue base collapse is one of the most common reasons for the failure of OSA surgery and poor CPAP compliance.

Various surgical methods have been adopted for bulky tongue base treatment, including transoral robotic surgery, coblation endoscopic lingual reduction, submucosal minimally invasive lingual excision, tongue base radiofrequency reduction, and tongue base suspension [13, 14]. In all the above-described procedures, the epiglottic collapse has to be addressed according to the type and pattern of collapse along with the tongue base surgery. When base of the tongue collapses onto the epiglottis and obstructs the airway, it is called secondary epiglottic collapse and in these cases, tongue base surgery helps to prevent airway obstruction by the epiglottis.

23.2 Relevant Surgical Anatomy of the Tongue Base

In the vast majority of OSA cases, the soft tissue in the middle part of the tongue base causes collapses on the epiglottis to cause airway obstruction, though in a few cases, the lateral part of the tongue also contributes to the obstruction.

The tongue base is made up of intrinsic muscles and is covered by a layer of lymphoid tissue. Accordingly, the obstruction can be caused by either lymphoid hypertrophy (lingual tonsils) or hypertrophic muscular tongue base. In a few subjects with OSA, a high amount of fat also accumulates in the tongue base, which adds to the volume.

The neurovascular bundle, which consists of the lingual vessels and the hypoglossal nerve (HLNVB), is situated at a distance of 1.5–2 cm from the midline and 1.5–2 cm deep from the surface (Fig. 23.1). The lingual artery is an important component in tongue base surgery and care is to be taken for the lingual artery due to the susceptibility of damage during surgery. Injury to the lingual artery during surgery can lead to a life-threatening hemorrhage, and if both lingual arteries are damaged, necrosis of the tongue can occur [15]. Ten cadaver heads were dissected to determine the position of the HLNVB with respect to soft tissue and bony landmarks at the tongue base [16]. The results indicate the position of the HLNVB in the base of tongue is significantly inferior and lateral, that is, 2.7 cm inferior and 1.6 cm lateral to the foramen caecum, 0.9 cm superior to the hyoid bone, and 2.2 cm medial to the mandible. This inferolateral location allows the potential for aggressive tongue base

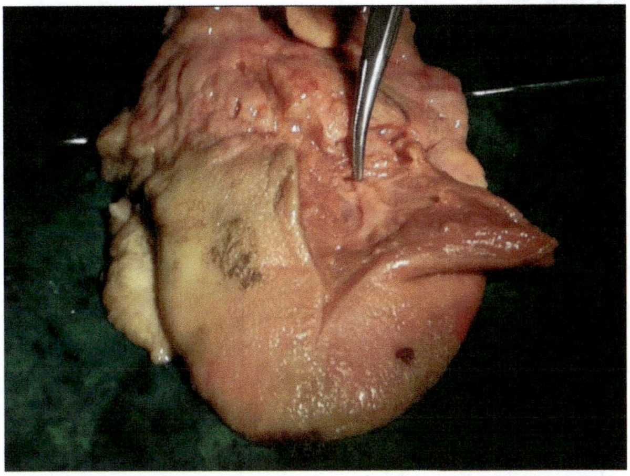

Fig. 23.1 Cadaver dissection of the tongue showing the Neurovascular bundle and its relation to the midline

resection without neurovascular compromise. Cohen et al. [17] have measured the distance of the neurovascular bundle from the foramen caecum in surgical simulated positions. Measurements from foramen cecum to palatoglossus muscle ($P < 0.042$) were significantly different when comparing anatomical to surgically simulated positions. Importantly, the location of the lingual artery in reference to the surface landmarks measured was dramatically altered with tongue retraction. With retraction, the branches of the dorsal lingual artery were not encountered posterior to a horizontal line between midway circumvallate papilla (mCVP). This explains that the HLNVB surface landmarks in the base of tongue differs significantly between resting and a surgically simulated tongue position. Also the dorsal branch of the lingual artery seems more superficial in the base of tongue than previously described. A safe zone may exist posterior to an imaginary horizontal line between mCVP.

23.3 Addressing Secondary Epiglottic Collapse with Tongue Base Surgery

23.3.1 Patient Selection

Patients are selected based on the findings of DISE, as discussed in the previous chapters, or by dynamic MRI.

However, an assessment of the type of obstruction, whether it is lymphoid tissues of the tongue base (lingual tonsils) or by hypertrophic muscular tissue in the tongue base, is of paramount importance, as the technique of surgery, intraoperative and postoperative monitoring, and possible complications are different in the two subsets of patients.

23.3.2 Technology

Trans Oral Robotic Surgery (TORS) and coblation-assisted tongue base ablation are the two major technologies being used for base tongue resection, besides others. The coblation technology (Smith & Nephew, USA) involves the creation of a plasma field with bipolar radiofrequency that leads to soft tissue dissolution at a lower temperature with simultaneous hemostasis.

23.4 Surgical Technique

Under general anesthesia with nasotracheal intubation, the patient is positioned supine with the surgeon sitting on the head end with a mild extension of the neck. The authors' preference is the Trendelenburg position by 5–10°, which helps for the saline used in the coblation technology to accumulate in the nasopharynx and not to pool in the hypopharynx.

A FK retractor or Boyle Davis mouth gag with appropriate size tongue blade is applied in order to visualize the base of tongue. However, 1–0 silk stay suture is placed in the middle of the dorsum of the tongue to retract for proper visualization of the surgical site (Fig. 23.2).

Angled endoscopes preferably 30 or 70° rigid Hopkins endoscopes have been used. The authors prefer to use 45° endoscopes.

Procise max or Evac 70 extra HP coblation wand is being used. For better access to the surgical site, the wand is bent 30–40° gently without making a sharp angle which may block the suction and irrigation flow (Fig. 23.3). The generator settings are kept at 7–9 for ablation and 3–4 for coagulation, depending on the surgeon's preference.

The extent of dissection is marked, starting from the midline at foramen caecum and lateral limits are marked 1.5 cm on each side. Anteriorly, it is limited to the imaginary line drawn at the level of foramen caecum and posteroinferiorly up to the level of the median glossoepiglottic ligament. The wedge-shaped ablation is performed layer by layer under direct visualization with a 45° endoscope starting from the surface of the tongue base down in the midline up to a depth of 1–1.5 cm and laterally up to 1.25–1.5 cm on each side where a depth of 0.5–0.75 cm is maintained (Figs. 23.4 and 23.5).

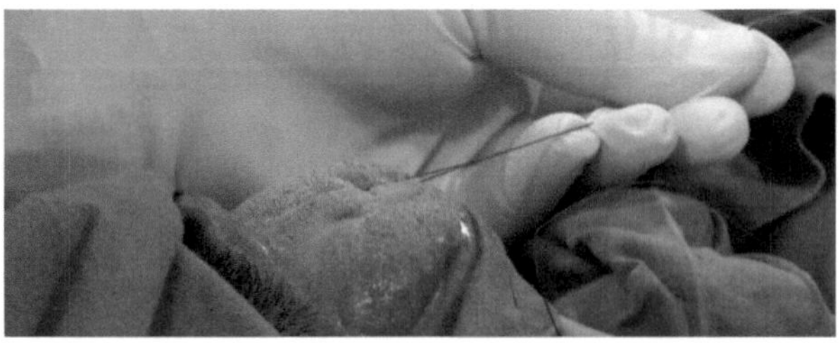

Fig. 23.2 Silk suture is in place on the dorsum of the tongue in the midline to pull the tongue out for proper exposure of tongue base

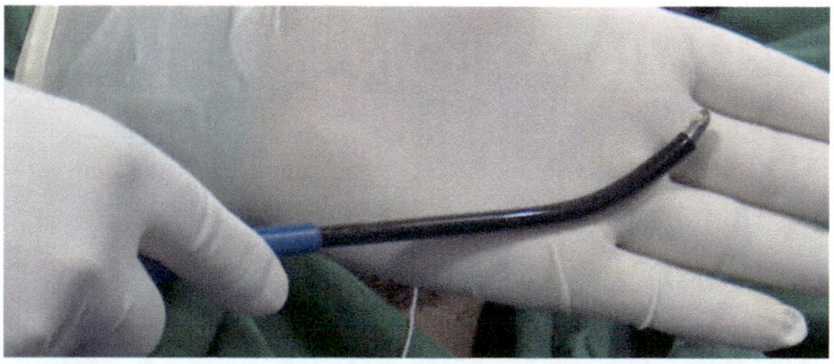

Fig. 23.3 The coblation wand is bent 30–40° gently without making a sharp angle

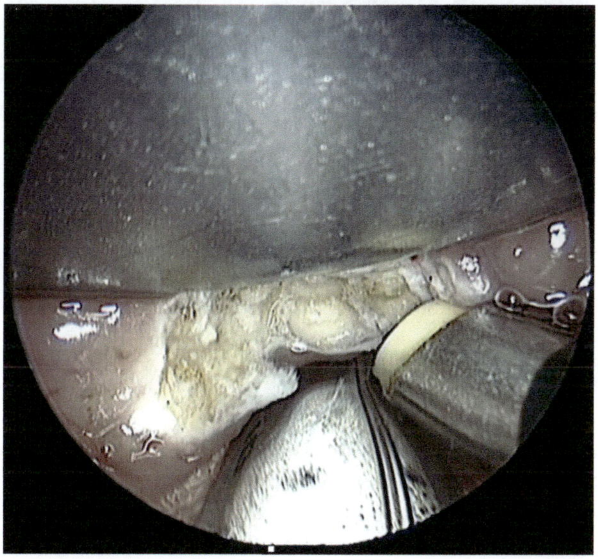

Fig. 23.4 The hypertrophied tongue base being ablated using coblation at the beginning of the procedure

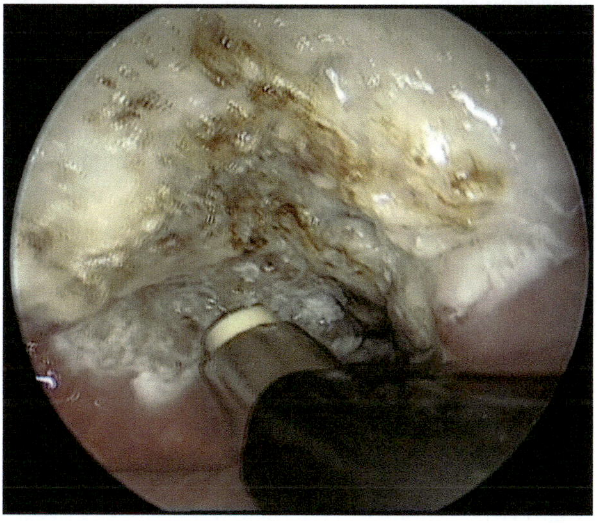

Fig. 23.5 The resected tongue base down to the level of median glossoepiglottic ligament using coblation at the end of the procedure

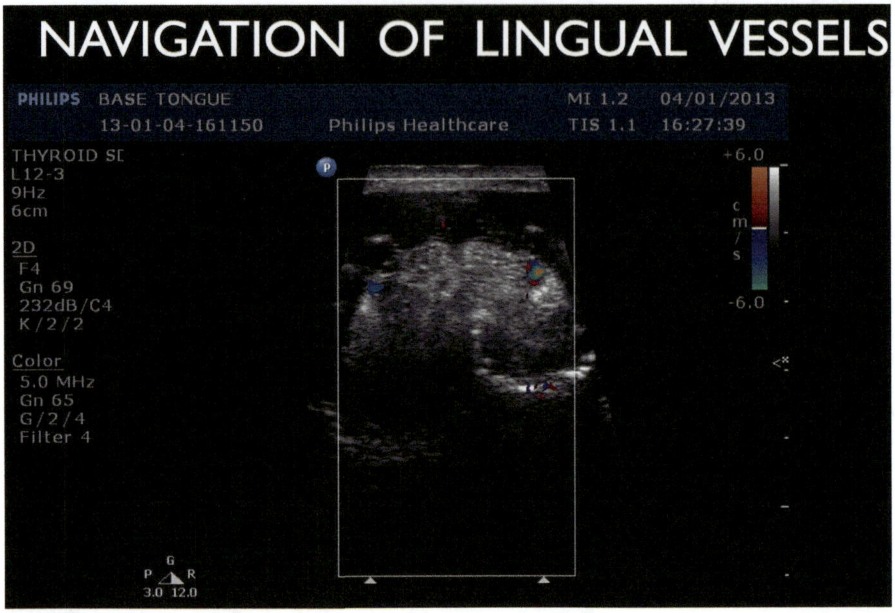

Fig. 23.6 The position of the lingual vessels in relation to the dissecting instruments monitored in real-time intraoperatively by the use of color doppler ultrasonography imaging

The position of the lingual vessels in relation to the dissecting instruments and the extent of the dissection are monitored in real-time intraoperatively by the use of color doppler ultrasonography imaging (Fig. 23.6).

The volumetric reduction of the base of the tongue is calculated by measuring the thickness of tongue at the start of the procedure using ultrasonography and again measuring at the end of the procedure (Figs. 23.7 and 23.8). The volumetric reduction achieved by the excision of the obstructing tongue base indirectly prevents the epiglottic collapse.

The above-described procedure is mainly used for excising hypertrophic lingual tonsils, but can also be performed to address muscular hypertrophy of the tongue base. The other commonly performed techniques are radiofrequency or coblation channelling of the tongue base and various submucosal approaches to the tongue base have been described.

Radiofrequency channelling of the tongue base for patients with macroglossia can be performed with monopolar or bipolar radiofrequency, or with coblation. A series of patients who underwent a combination of coblation tongue channelling and modified uvulopalatopharyngoplasty demonstrated that patients with Friedman stage III (Friedman tongue position III and IV, tonsil sizes 0, 1 or 2, BMI <40) showed more encouraging response, with 71% surgical success, compared to the reported 8% surgical success in Friedman stage III patients who underwent UPPP alone as shown by Friedman et al. [18].

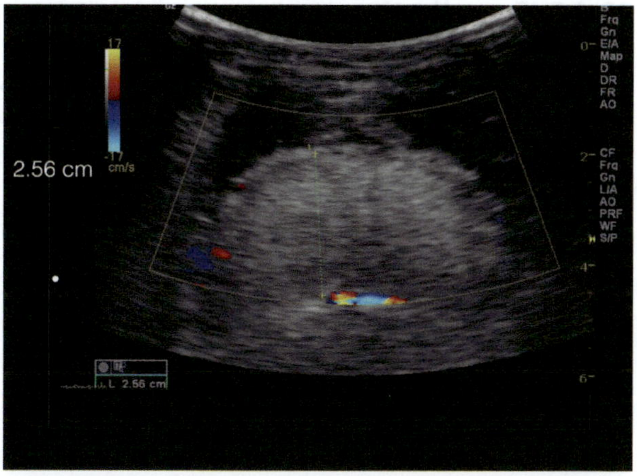

Fig. 23.7 The thickness of the base of the tongue at the level of foramen caecum at the start of the procedure is 2.56 cm

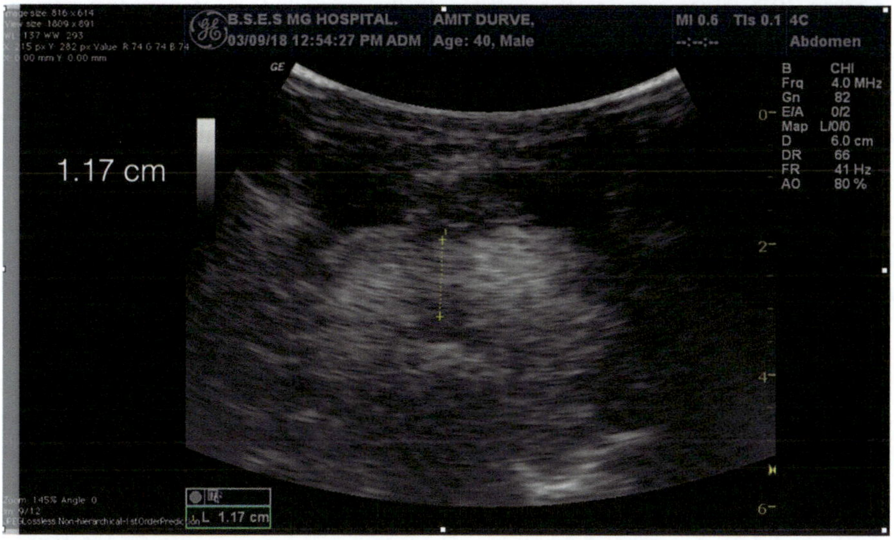

Fig. 23.8 The thickness of the base of the tongue at the level of foramen caecum at the end of the procedure is 1.17 cm, thereby denoting that the reduction was 1.39 cm

23.4.1 Intubation and Extubation

Nasal intubation is preferred as it provides space at the tongue base area for better exposure and dissection. Patients with grade 2 and 3 lingual tonsil hypertrophy and/or minimal muscular hypertrophy with incomplete collapse during DISE can be extubated on the table. Gross muscular hypertrophy cases are kept in intensive care unit with nasal intubation for 24 h and then extubated after visualising the surgical site with flexible laryngoscopy and making sure there is no edema or bleeding. The patient has to be fully awake and extubation is done in a sitting position.

23.4.2 Complications

Minor complications are not uncommon in these airway procedures. However, they can be sometimes potentially severe, causing hemorrhage and airway compromise requiring reintubation or tracheostomy [19–21]. Primary bleeding within 24 h from the lingual artery or one of its branches can occur if dissection is done in-depth beyond 1.5 cm and 1.25–1.5 cm lateral to the midline. Bleeding from the dorsal lingual artery is more common since it is more superficial. In between the 7th and 14th postoperative day, secondary bleeding can occur at the surgical site, because of infection which can lead to granulations.

23.4.3 Post-Operative Management

An intravenous antibiotic like second-generation cephalosporin along with steroids is given 30 minutes prior to the surgery. In the immediate post-operative period, intravenous fluids are to be continued and vitals to be monitored. Intravenous antibiotic, pain killers and steroids to be given for the next 2 days, then switched to oral medications except for steroids. Cold clear fluids and ice cream to be started after 6–8 h of extubation. Soft diet after 24–48 h till 2 weeks. A normal diet can be started after 2–3 weeks.

23.5 Conclusion

Tongue base ablation surgery with coblation for secondary epiglottic collapse is a successful surgical treatment option for patients with OSA. In our experience increased total sleep time, reduced daytime sleepiness, and improved sleep efficiency along with a significant reduction in respiratory arousal index were observed in the successful surgery group. Though the procedure has limited but dreadful complications like secondary bleeding into the airway, proper technique and hospital setting can be a life-saving.

References

1. Torre C, Camacho M, Liu SY, et al. Epiglottis collapse in adult obstructive sleep apnea: a systematic review. Laryngoscope. 2016;126:515–23.
2. Ma MA, Kumar R, Macey PM, et al. Epiglottis cross-sectional area and oropharyngeal airway length in male and female obstructive sleep apnea patients. Nat Sci Sleep. 2016;8:297–304.
3. Franklin KA, Lindberg E. Obstructive sleep apnea is a common disorder in the population-a review on the epidemiology of sleep apnea. J Thorac Dis. 2015;7:1311–22.
4. Cavaliere M, Russo F, Iemma M. Awake versus drug-induced sleep endoscopy: evaluation of airway obstruction in obstructive sleep apnea/hypopnoea syndrome. Laryngoscope. 2013;123:2315–8.

5. Fernández-Julián E, García-Pérez MÁ, García-Callejo J, et al. Surgical planning after sleep versus awake techniques in patients with obstructive sleep apnea. Laryngoscope. 2014;124:1970–4.
6. Koutsourelakis I, Safiruddin F, Ravesloot M, et al. Surgery for obstructive sleep apnea: sleep endoscopy determinants of outcome. Laryngoscope. 2012;122:2587–91.
7. Myatt HM, Beckenham EJ. The use of diagnostic sleep nasendoscopy in the management of children with complex upper airway obstruction. Clin Otolaryngol Allied Sci. 2000;25(3):200–8.
8. Croft CB, Pringle M. Sleep nasendoscopy: a technique of assessment in snoring and obstructive sleep apnoea. Clin Otolaryngol Allied Sci. 1991;16(5):504–9.
9. Abdullah VJ, Wing YK, van Hasselt CA. Video sleep nasendoscopy: the Hong Kong experience. Otolaryngol Clin North Am. 2003;36(3):461–71.
10. Woods CM, et al. Long-term quality-of-life outcomes following treatment for adult obstructive sleep apnoea: comparison of upper airway surgery, continuous positive airway pressure and mandibular advancement splints. Clin Otolaryngol. 2016;41:762–70.
11. Friedman M, Vidyasagar R, Bliznikas D, Joseph N. Does severity of obstructive sleep apnea/hypopnea syndrome predict uvulopalatopharyngoplasty outcome? Laryngoscope. 2005;115:2109–13.
12. Li HY, Lee LA, Kezirian EJ. Efficacy of coblation endoscopic lingual lightening in multilevel surgery for obstructive sleep apnea. JAMA Otolaryngol Head Neck Surg. 2016;142:438–43.
13. Lin HS, et al. Transoral robotic surgery for treatment of obstructive sleep apnea-hypopnea syndrome. Laryngoscope. 2013;123:1811–6.
14. Babademez MA, et al. Comparison of minimally invasive techniques in tongue base surgery in patients with obstructive sleep apnea. Otolaryngol Head Neck Surg. 2011;145:858–64.
15. Mun MJ, Lee CH, Lee BJ, Lee JC, Jang JY, Jung SH, Wang SG. Histopathologic evaluations of the lingual artery in healthy tongue of adult cadaver. Clin Exp Otorhinolaryngol. 2016;9(3):257–62.
16. Lauretano AM, Li KK, Caradonna DS, Khosta RK, M P Fried MP. Anatomic location of the tongue base neurovascular bundle. Laryngoscope. 1997;107(8):1057–9. https://doi.org/10.1097/00005537-199708000-00010.
17. Cohen DS, Low GM, Melkane AE, Mutchnick SA, Waxman JA, Patel S, Shkoukani MA, Lin HS. Establishing a danger zone: an anatomic study of the lingual artery in base of tongue surgery. Laryngoscope. 2017;127(1):110–5. https://doi.org/10.1002/lary.26048.
18. Friedman M, Ibrahim H, Bass L. Clinical staging for sleep-disordered breathing. Otolaryngol Head Neck Surg. 2002;127:13–21.
19. Wee JH, Tan K, et al. Evaluation of coblation lingual tonsil removal technique for obstructive sleep apnea in Asians: preliminary results of surgical morbidity and prognosticators. Eur Arch Otorhinolaryngol. 2015;272(9):2327–33.
20. Leitzbach SU, Bodlaj R, et al. Safety of cold ablation (coblation) in the treatment of tonsillar hypertrophy of the tongue base. Eur Arch Otorhinolaryngol. 2014;271(6):1635–9.
21. Zhang Q, Zhou W, et al. Preliminary study on treatment of lingual tonsil hypertrophy by endoscopic assisted coblation. Lin Chuang Er Bi Yan Hou Tou Jing Wai Ke Za Zhi. 2013;27(14):787–9.

Transoral Robotic Surgery (TORS) 24

Filippo Montevecchi and Claudio Vicini

24.1 Introduction

Transoral robotic surgery (TORS) for obstructive sleep apnea (OSA) is just one more of the many applications of robotic surgery in the otolaryngology literature. The first case of TORS used in humans for cancer resection was described by Weinstein in 2006. The first TORS for OSA was carried out in 2008 in Forlì by Vicini & Montevecchi. It was performed after more than one year of training in Italy, France (IRCAD, Strasbourg), and the US (PENN University, Philadelphia). Transoral robotic tongue base reduction and supraglottoplasty have been deeply inspired by Chabolle's tongue base reduction with a hyoid-epiglottoplasty procedure [1] and by Weinstein-O'Malley's transoral robotic tongue base and supraglottic cancer resection [2, 3]. The first pilot series of TORS for OSA was reported in 2010. At that time, the most effective tongue base (TB) procedure for moderate to severe OSA in Europe was Chabolle's operation, while in the US the most popular approaches to TB reduction were either transoral endoscopic Coblation® resection or radiofrequency ablation. In less than 10 years, TORS for OSA has spread over the world and this diffusion is illustrated by an increasing number of published papers in the literature. Nowadays, there are three meta-analyses and a multicentric study about the efficacy and safety of TORS for OSA [4–7]. The unsurpassed

Supplementary Information The online version contains supplementary material available at https://doi.org/10.1007/978-3-031-34992-8_24. The videos can be accessed individually by clicking the DOI link in the accompanying figure caption or by scanning this link with the SN More Media App.

F. Montevecchi (✉)
Forlì Private Hospitals, Forlì, Italy

C. Vicini
Department of Otolaryngology and Head-Neck Surgery, Morgagni-Pierantoni Hospital, Forlì, Italy

M. Delakorda, N. de Vries (eds.), *The Role of Epiglottis in Obstructive Sleep Apnea*, https://doi.org/10.1007/978-3-031-34992-8_24

visualization, dexterity, and control provided by the Da Vinci Surgical System® offers the following benefits for the surgeon: superior exposure and 3D HD visualization of the target anatomy inside the pharynx, more precise dissection and improved preservation of intra-lingual vessels and nerves, shorter learning curve, shorter operating time, and a more reproducible approach as compared to traditional open as well as endoscopic techniques. It also offers significant patient benefits: excellent cosmetic outcomes, no neck scars (except for tracheostomy, if necessary), reduced likelihood of iatrogenic injury to vessels and nerves, better and faster functional recovery compared to the trans-cervical approach, reduced operating room time, and shortened length of hospital stay.

24.2 Indications

Endoscopic findings are essential to guide surgical decision-making. During awake endoscopy, it is possible to evaluate an unstable/floppy epiglottis by asking the patient to breathe fast and assess the movement of epiglottis. It has to be acknowledged that awake endoscopy may frequently underestimate the degree of the hypopharyngeal and laryngeal obstruction. Drug-induced sleep endoscopy (DISE) is a fiberoptic examination of the upper airway under controlled sedation to determine the exact site(s) of upper airway collapse in patients with sleep disordered breathing. Quantifying the location and mechanism of upper airway collapse with DISE in OSA patient can be used to tailor surgical treatments and improve surgical outcomes. In 2010, a retrospective study on 250 consecutive patients was published making a comparison between awake and DISE findings [8]. In this study, significant differences were found between hypopharyngeal degree and pattern of obstruction (59% and 49%, respectively), while up to 30% of cases demonstrated laryngeal obstruction by DISE. Laryngeal obstruction was classified as primary if the collapse was produced by intrinsic instability of the larynx, or secondary if the tongue base or the lateral pharyngeal walls were responsible for the supraglottic collapse. As observed in the larynx, we have also seen retropalatal obstruction during DISE, that either was primary or secondary.

24.3 Surgical Technique

24.3.1 Exposure

The patient is always in supine position with neck flexed and head extended in order to achieve the best exposure. If needed external laryngeal compression is allowed during the dissection (e.g., hyoid compression or other maneuvers). Tongue base exposure is achieved by using a tongue tip traction (with a 0-0 silk horizontal mattress suture) (Fig. 24.1) and tongue body displacement by Davis Meyer® mouth gag under direct visualization. Tongue blades of different sizes with integrated suction tubes (for smoke and blood) are important during the procedure. A combination of tongue base traction and the right mouth gag blade length is the key for exposure. Usually, the short or the medium blade (such as Storz blade number 1 and 2) is very

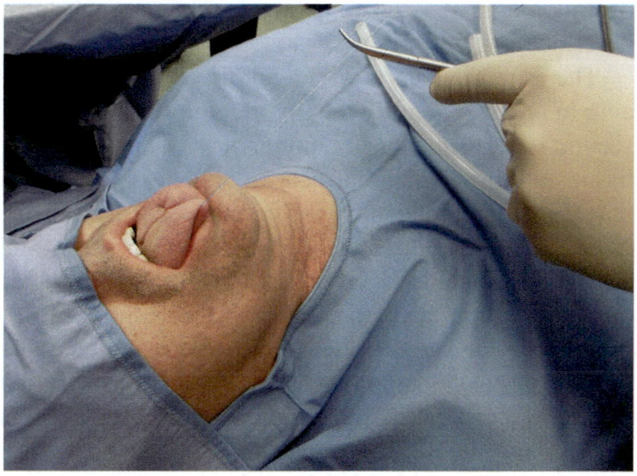

Fig. 24.1 Tongue base exposure is achieved in the standard TORS approach with a combination of tongue tip traction (0 silk stitch horizontal mattress suture) and tongue body displacement by mouth gag

effective for completing tongue base as well epiglottis procedures. If a second blade is to be inserted after the initial resection, the new position must be carefully verified in order to avoid the loss of proper orientation. The 30° scope (upward facing) is our preferred choice. If available, an 8 mm scope may be very helpful in particular cases (minimal inter-incisive distance, extreme macroglossia, etc.). Only two robotic 5 mm instruments are routinely used for each patient: A Maryland Dissector for grasping and dissecting tissue and a monopolar cautery with a spatula tip for dissection and coagulation. Hemostasis could be performed by using clips or by using a coagulation-suction tube. Bipolar forceps are important for safe coagulation. The forceps must be insulated from the tip to the handle, in order to avoid burns of the oral commissure. A bipolar Dessi® (Microfrance) coagulating device originally designed for sinus surgery may be helpful as well. The bedside assistant helps the first operator with two additional suction devices (Lawton suction® Cat. 160274 and/or Medicon suction® Cat.098508). These instruments can be used for retraction and for smoke and blood.

Usually, the TORS approach for OSA includes two different surgical steps, tongue base reduction (TBR) and supraglottoplasty (SGP), frequently performed in the same procedure according to the patient's features [9–11]. They will be described in detail.

24.3.2 Tongue Base Reduction

The goal of TBR is to enlarge the oropharyngeal space by removing the tissue from tongue base. The end point of TBR is achieved when the surgical view improves from a Cormack & Lehane grade IV or III to a grade II or I [12]. In many cases, the lymphoid tissue as well as the tongue base muscle must be removed in order to clear the retrolingual space. In case of huge lymphoid hyperplasia, less muscular tissue needs to be removed. If the lingual tonsil is not enlarged, a more aggressive muscular reduction is required in order to obtain Cormack & Lehane Grade II or I. The mean volume of the tissue removed is typically 10 mL, but in some cases, the overall volume may be up to 50 mL. The surgical steps are standardized and will be described in detail.

The procedure starts with a midline split of the lingual tonsil from foramen caecum in order to identify the tip of epiglottis and the valleculae (Fig. 24.2). The dissection is performed using monopolar cautery until the junction between lymphatic tissue and muscle is identified. In patients with huge lingual tonsil hypertrophy, it may be difficult to identify the foramen caecum and circumvallate papillae. In these cases, debulking of the midline lymphoid tissue may help the surgeon to identify the essential surgical landmarks. At the beginning of the dissection, it is recommended that the surgeon positions the tip of the scope far from the tongue base in order to provide a wide surgical view under low magnification. At the end of this first step, the lingual tonsils are completely divided in the midline. Dissection is performed using the tip of the spatula, by dissecting layer by layer through the tissue in order to maintain direct visualization of the tip of the instrument. In order to grasp the adequate tissue with Maryland forceps, a deep cut must be created, otherwise repeated grasping attempts will produce tedious, excessive bleeding (Fig. 24.3). After midline dissection, the superior (sulcus terminalis), lateral (glosso-tonsillar sulcus), and inferior (glosso-epiglottic sulcus) borders of the right lingual tonsil are identified and marked by cautery. The right lingual tonsillectomy is performed "en block" superiorly to inferiorly maintaining the dissection plane close to the lympho-muscular junction. During this step, the scope is positioned closer to the surgical field for better identification of neurovascular structures. After completing right lingual tonsillectomy (Fig. 24.4), left lingual tonsillectomy is completed in the same way after side inversion of the robotic arms and tools (Fig. 24.5).

The surgical field is now inspected in order to evaluate the residual degree of obstruction (Fig. 24.6). If Cormack & Lehane Grade is greater than II, additional resection in the muscle layer is required. Additional information is provided by the volume of tissue resected and measured using a graduated syringe filled with saline.

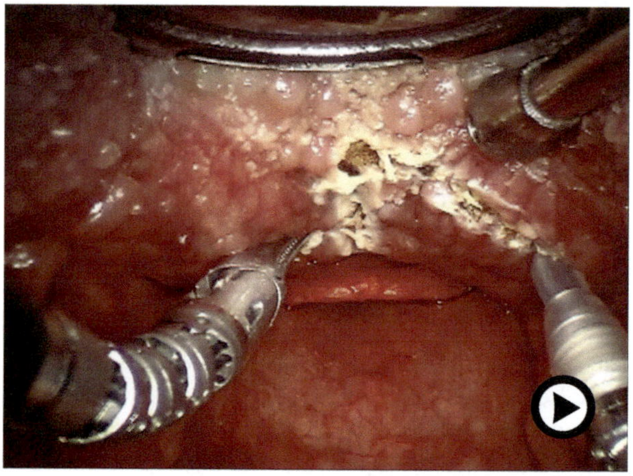

Fig. 24.2 (Video 24.1) The procedure starts with a midline split of the two lingual tonsils from foramen caecum in order to identify the tip of epiglottis and vallecular. Initial dissection of the right tongue base posteriorly to the circumvallate papilla (▶ https://doi.org/10.1007/000-bft)

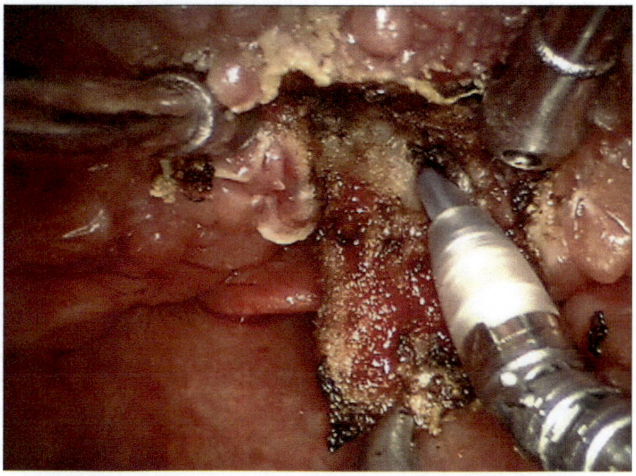

Fig. 24.3 Bed-side assistant maintains counter-traction in order to assist the surgeon during dissection; increasing the tension allows more precise and quicker dissection

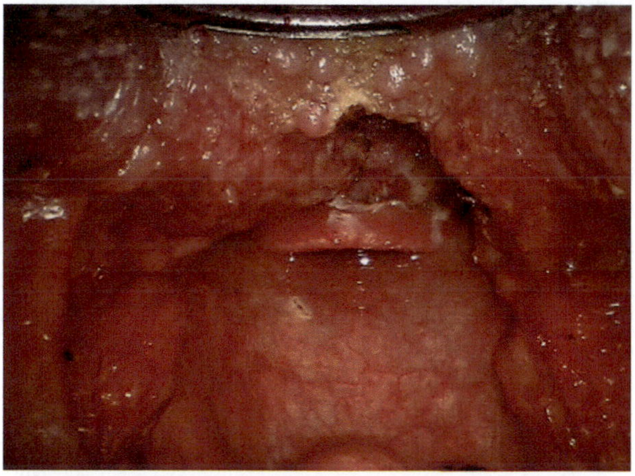

Fig. 24.4 Surgical field after right lingual tonsillectomy

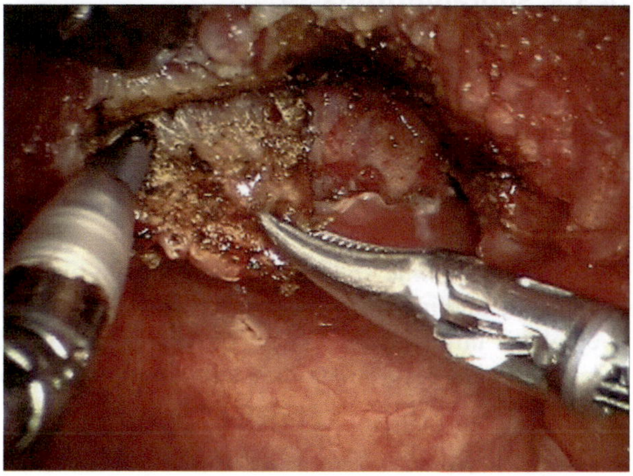

Fig. 24.5 Left lingual tonsillectomy is completed in the same way of the right after side inversion of the robotic arms and tools. Dissection of deeper layers

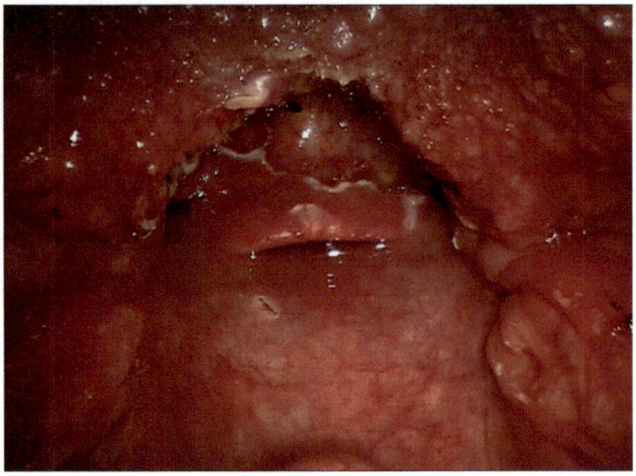

Fig. 24.6 Surgical field at the end of the lingual tonsillectomy. At this step, a view of the epiglottis is possible

If the overall volume of resected tissue is less than 7 mL, additional resection may be recommended [13, 14].

In some cases, it may be necessary to remove muscle in addition to lymphoid tissue. When entering the muscular layer, it is important to avoid injury to the neurovascular structures including the dorsal branches of the lingual arteries and hypoglossal nerve. Some surgeons have published interesting cadaveric dissections [15–17] describing practical anatomical landmarks in this area. Woodson stresses the importance of intraoperative mapping of the tongue vasculature using ultrasound if available. Most authors would agree that anatomical landmarks are unreliable due to great individual anatomic variability and to the extreme mobility of the active tongue. In addition, the tongue shape is modified in the surgical setting due to retraction and positioning. The overall time required for TBR is about 30 min.

24.3.3 Supraglottoplasty

SGP may be carried out concurrent with TBR in patient with primary and in some cases secondary epiglottic collapse. The role of SGP is to prevent inward collapse of the floppy epiglottis and/or redundant supraglottic tissue. The additional time required for SPG is usually less than 15 min. The most common procedure in supraglottic area includes the following steps:

- A vertical midline splitting of supra-hyoid epiglottis; this step is carried out along the midline, following the medial glosso-epiglottic fold, from the tip of the epiglottis inferiorly, preserving at least 5 mm of epiglottis above the deep vallecular plane (a sufficient remnant of epiglottic cartilage is left to avoid aspirations) (Fig. 24.7).

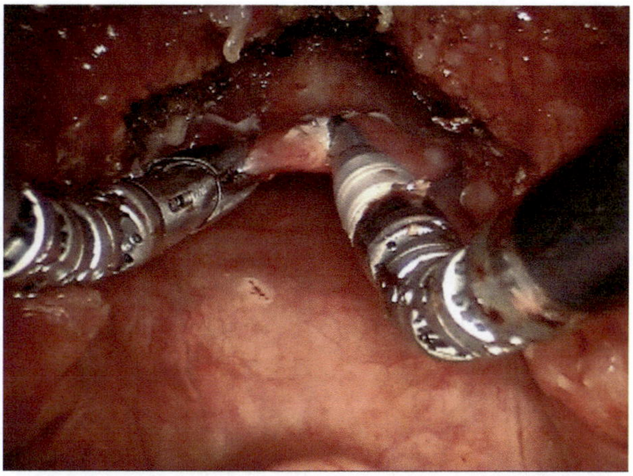

Fig. 24.7 Vertical midline splitting of supra-hyoid epiglottis

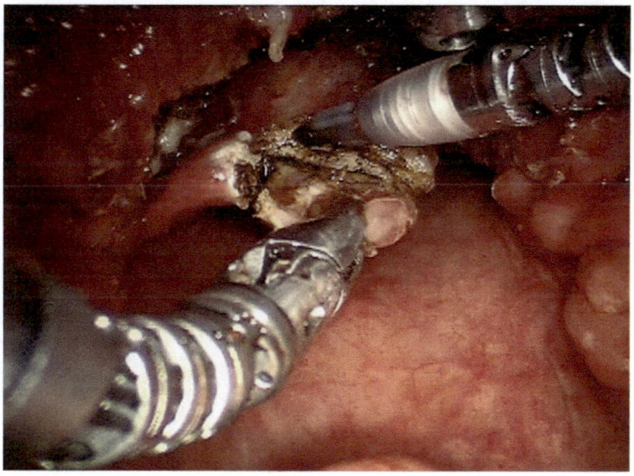

Fig. 24.8 Right lateral dissection of the epiglottis immediately over the pharyngo-epiglottic fold

- A horizontal section is performed bilaterally in a plane joining the vertical section in the midline and running laterally immediately over the pharyngo-epiglottic fold, in order to leave a lateral fold preventing aspirations, and to avoid possible bleeding from the superior laryngeal vessels (Figs. 24.8, 24.9, 24.10, and 24.11). Scarring of the vallecular and perivallecular area leads to progressive adhesion and stabilization of the residual epiglottis to the tongue base.
- A modification of the previously described procedure as described by Magnuson (unpublished data) is the "V-shape" epiglottoplasty". A V-shaped wedge is removed from the central upper border of the epiglottis. This technique is probably safer to prevent aspirations and the superior laryngeal vascular bundle damage.

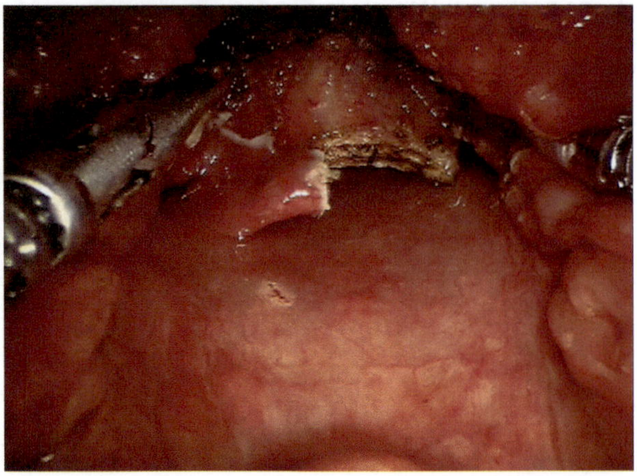

Fig. 24.9 Surgical field at the end of the right epiglottoplasty

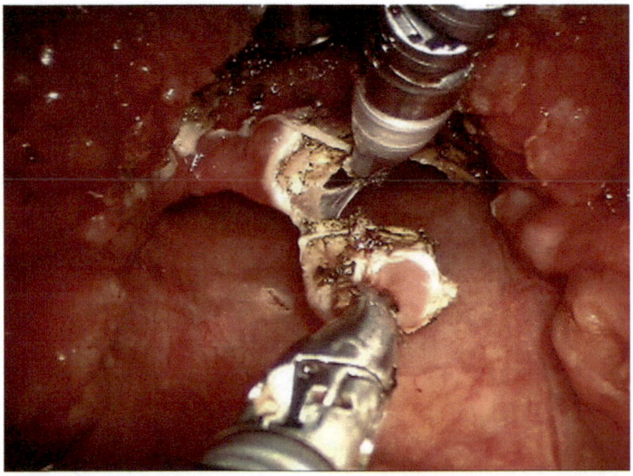

Fig. 24.10 Left lateral dissection of the epiglottis immediately over the pharyngo-epiglottic fold

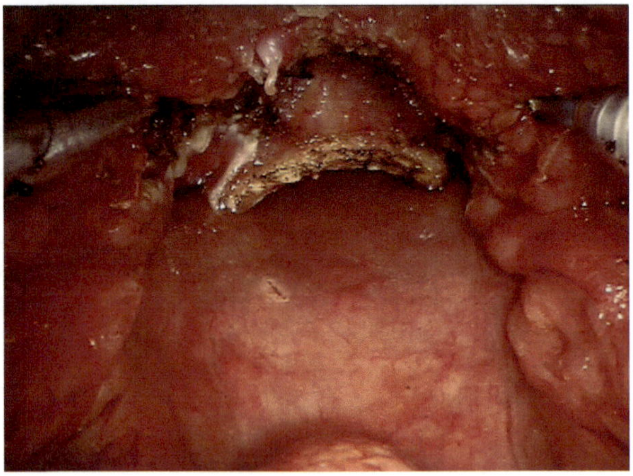

Fig. 24.11 Surgical field at the end of the epiglottoplasty

Tracheostomy is not performed routinely for patients undergoing TORS, but is performed in certain circumstances: in patients who were found to have a difficult intubation, or in situations in which emergent reintubation is anticipated to be difficult [18, 19]. It is important to understand that tracheostomy is not performed solely due to an enlarged tongue base. In most cases, surgeon preference dictates either trans-nasal or trans-oral intubation for benign base of the tongue TORS procedures. Discussing with the anesthesist about the possibility of tracheostomy both before and after intubation might be indicated. Although unplanned tracheostomy is rare, patients should be aware and consented for this possibility.

24.4 Post-operative Care Management

The postoperative analgesia in OSA patients is always a critical point. Major opioids (e.g., morphine, buprenorphine, and oxycodone) should be reduced. If morphine is indispensable, additive drugs must be used (e.g., ketamine and ketorolac) to reduce the dose in a multimodal analgesia strategy. The use of nonsteroidal anti-inflammatory drugs (NSAIDs) and paracetamol (acetaminophen) should be performed at regular times rather than "as needed". An elastomeric infusion pump with low dose morphine and ketorolac for 24–36 h is used in our institution, and we have no serious adverse events. In other western countries, most patients are discharged after 24 h; at home, patients use a combinations of narcotics (oxycodone elixir, dilaudid, and hydrocodone) as well as topical analgesics (viscous lidocaine) and in some cases gabapentin, steroids and COX-2 inhibitors.

24.5 Complication Management

24.5.1 Intraoperative Bleeding/Hemostasis

During the TORS procedure, a vessel clip applier and an insulated bipolar forceps should be readily available throughout the surgery. The bipolar forceps need to have an angled tip to achieve adequate access. This can allow the bedside assistant to manage intra-operative bleeding. As a 30° upward facing scope is utilized during the procedure, all the non-robotic instruments should be angled, especially the suction devices that are used to suction smoke, blood, and provide counter-traction.

At the end of the procedure, the wound is inspected carefully for hemostasis, and cautery, or vessel clips that are used as needed for persistent bleeding. The tongue and airway are inspected for edema at the end of the procedure to assess the possibility of an early tube removal or the necessity of a prolonged intubation or tracheostomy.

24.5.2 Post-operative Complications

The immediate post-operative period is crucial to avoid serious complications and the patient should be monitored carefully in a high acuity nursing setting. Intravenous steroids are given to minimize lingual edema and nausea. Intravenous broad-spectrum antibiotics are infused pre- and post-operatively as per hospital protocol or surgeon preference to avoid possible infections.

If the patient did not undergo tracheostomy as the initial step in the operative procedure, the patient should have a prolonged post-operative intubation either in recovery or in an intensive care setting. This is done to avoid laryngospasm that may result from aspiration of saliva or blood. In an already difficult airway, re-intubation is made even more difficult due to post-operative edema, bleeding and modified anatomy. Prior to removal of the endotracheal tube, we check the airway with a flexible endoscope. This optimizes the timing of tube removal and is usually a few hours after the surgery. In the US, patients are usually extubated in the operating room and observed overnight in the ICU or in a setting with cardiopulmonary monitoring and skilled nursing.

As detailed previously, at our institution, for patients with severe OSA, severe comorbid conditions, a narrow mouth opening or other anatomical features suggesting a difficult intubation and reintubation a planned tracheostomy is recommended for post-operative ventilation assistance, especially if multi-level surgery is scheduled. Among the above-quoted reasons for a preventive tracheostomy, the key one is the degree of difficulty for re-intubation in case of post-surgical airway edema or post-operative bleeding.

During the first post-operative night, patients should be monitored in a high-acuity setting. In most institutions, this would be in an intensive care or high dependency unit rather than the typical postoperative hospital ward. The patient should have continuous pulse-oximetry and suction should be available at all times by the bedside. The patient should be watched closely for bleeding and respiratory depression.

We find that many patients can swallow liquids comfortably without aspiration within a day of surgery, but this can vary considerably between patients [20]. At our institution, we routinely do not insert a feeding tube, while a liquid diet is started on postoperative day 1. We also continue oral steroids post-discharge on a tapering dose. Narcotics are used as needed, but this must be in the context of close observation of respiratory rate and level of consciousness, as recommended postoperatively for other OSA surgical procedures.

The length of stay can vary considerably depending upon a number of variables and surgeon comfort level. Tracheostomy by itself necessitates a multi-day hospital stay. Other determinants include the extent of surgery, comorbidities, pain control, and swallowing ability. In the US, the patient is discharged on the first post-operative day. However, in Europe, a longer hospitalization of 3–5 days is usually followed.

In case of delayed post-operative bleeding, if conservative measures fail, a suspension laryngoscope should be used to achieve an operative view of the base of tongue. It is unlikely that a view of the bleeding area will be achieved with a tonsil gag. Typically, a suction-monopolar diathermy device is then used for hemostasis.

Another important and difficult to manage long-term complication is that of a synechia formation or stenosis of the oro-hypopharynx following TORS. If adequate exposure is not achieved at the time of TORS, and there is no sufficient space between tongue base-epiglottis and the posterior pharyngeal wall, it is possible to injure the mucosa of the posterior and lateral oropharyngeal walls with monopolar cautery. This circumferential damage could produce a concentric scar in the first months after surgery. This complication may necessitate long-term tracheostomy and nasogastric feeding tube. In order to avoid a concentric scar, especially in patients in which palate surgery is also performed, a 1–2 cm strip of intact mucosa should be preserved between the palatine tonsil fossa and the tongue base. Pharyngeal stenosis is a devastating complication, so prevention is the best strategy.

24.6 Conclusion

While many patients benefit from the use of ventilation therapy, non-compliant patients require a surgical procedure to eliminate the obstruction. TORS for OSA allows the surgeon to address the base of tongue and epiglottis obstruction with several advantages. The procedure is well tolerated by the patient and outcomes have already been proved in the literature [7]. Since the tongue base surgical approach and epiglottoplasty by using TORS requires high-tech instrumentation and sleep apnea patients are difficult to manage during the operative and postoperative period, it is crucial to perform an accurate diagnosis and indication for such treatment to avoid failures and complications and to achieve the best results.

References

1. Chabolle F, Wagner I, Blumen MB, et al. Tongue base reduction with hyoepigottoplasty: a treatment for severe obstructive sleep apnea. Laryngoscope. 1999;109(8):1273–80.
2. O'Malley BW Jr, Weinstein GS, Snyder W, Hockstein NG. Transoral robotic surgery (TORS) for base of tongue neoplasms. Laryngoscope. 2006;116(8):1465–72.
3. Weinstein GS, O'Malley BW Jr, Snyder W, Hockstein NG. Transoral robotic surgery: supraglottic partial laryngectomy. Ann Otol Rhinol Laryngol. 2007;116(1):19–23.
4. Meccariello G, Cammaroto G, Montevecchi F, Hoff PT, Spector ME, Negm H, Shams M, Bellini C, Zeccardo E, Vicini C. Transoral robotic surgery for the management of obstructive sleep apnea: a systematic review and meta-analysis. Eur Arch Otorhinolaryngol. 2017;274(2):647–53.
5. Lee JA, Byun YJ, Nguyen SA, Lentsch EJ, Gillespie MB. Transoral robotic surgery versus plasma ablation for tongue base reduction in obstructive sleep apnea: meta-analysis. Otolaryngol Head Neck Surg. 2020;162(6):839–52.
6. Lechien JR, Chiesa-Estomba CM, Fakhry N, Saussez S, Badr I, Ayad T, Chekkoury-Idrissi Y, Melkane AE, Bahgat A, Crevier-Buchman L, Blumen M, Cammaroto G, Vicini C, Hans S. Surgical, clinical, and functional outcomes of transoral robotic surgery used in sleep surgery for obstructive sleep apnea syndrome: a systematic review and meta-analysis. Head Neck. 2021;43(7):2216–39.

7. Vicini C, Montevecchi F, Campanini A, Dallan I, Hoff PT, Spector ME, Thaler E, Ahn J, Baptista P, Remacle M, Lawson G, Benazzo M, Canzi P. Clinical outcomes and complications associated with TORS for OSAHS: a benchmark for evaluating an emerging surgical technology in a targeted application for benign disease. ORL J Otorhinolaryngol Relat Spec. 2014;76(2):63–9.
8. Campanini A, Canzi P, De Vito A, et al. Awake versus sleep endoscopy: personal experience in 250 OSAHS patients. Acta Otorhinolaryngol Ital. 2010;30(2):73–7.
9. Vicini C, Dallan I, Canzi P, Frassineti S, La Pietra MG, Montevecchi F. Transoral robotic tongue base resection in obstructive sleep apnoea-hypopnoea syndrome: a preliminary report. ORL J Otorhinolaryngol Relat Spec. 2010;72(1):22–7.
10. Vicini C, Montevecchi F, Tenti G, Canzi P, Dallan I, Huntley TC. Transoral robotic surgery: tongue base reduction and supraglottoplasty for obstructive sleep apnea. Otolaryngol Head Neck Surg. 2012;23(1):45–7.
11. Vicini C, Dallan I, Canzi P, et al. Transoral robotic surgery of the tongue base in obstructive sleep apnea-hypopnea syndrome: anatomic considerations and clinical experience. Head Neck. 2012;34:15–22.
12. Cormack RS, Lehane J. Difficult tracheal intubation in obstetrics. Anaesthesia. 1984;39(11):1105–11.
13. Vicini C, Hoff PT, Montevecchi F. Transoral robotic surgery for obstructive sleep apnea. Cham: Springer; 2016.
14. Vicini C, Montevecchi F. Transoral robotic surgery for obstructive sleep apnea. Sleep Med Clin. 2019;14(1):67–72.
15. Sequert C, Lestang P, Baglin AC, Wagner I, Ferron JM, Chabolle F. Hypoglossal nerve in its intralingual trajectory: anatomy and clinical implications. Ann Otolaryngol Chir Cervicofac. 1999;116(4):207–17.
16. Lauretano AM, Li KK, Caradonna DS, Khosta RK, Fried MP. Anatomic location of the tongue base neurovascular bundle. Laryngoscope. 1997;107(8):1057–9.
17. Wu D, Qin J, Guo X, Li S. Analysis of the difference in the course of the lingual arteries caused by tongue position change. Laryngoscope. 2015;125(3):762–6.
18. Campanini A, De Vito A, Frassineti S, Vicini C. Temporary tracheotomy in the surgical treatment of obstructive sleep apnea syndrome: personal experience. Acta Otorhinolaryngol Ital. 2003;23(6):474–8.
19. Sun H, Lou W, Wang L, Wu Y. Clinical significance of preoperative tracheotomy in preventing perioperative OSAHS severe complications. Lin Chuang Er Bi Yan Hou Ke Za Zhi. 2005;19(9):394–5.
20. Eesa M, Montevecchi F, Hendawy E, D'Agostino G, Meccariello G, Vicini C. Swallowing outcome after TORS for sleep apnea: short- and long-term evaluation. Eur Arch Otorhinolaryngol. 2015;272(6):1537–41.

Maxillomandibular Advancement

25

Ning Zhou, Jean-Pierre T.F. Ho, and Jan de Lange

25.1 Introduction

Obstructive sleep apnea (OSA) is the most common sleep-related breathing disorder. It is characterized by recurrent upper airway collapse during sleep, leading to intermittent hypoxemia, hypercapnia, and frequent cortical arousals [1]. Continuous positive airway pressure (CPAP) is generally regarded as the gold standard therapy for patients with moderate to severe OSA [1, 2]. However, its efficacy is often hampered by the low tolerance and poor compliance, promoting OSA patients to seek alternatives to CPAP, such as a mandibular advancement device or surgical therapy [2, 3].

Supplementary Information The online version contains supplementary material available at https://doi.org/10.1007/978-3-031-34992-8_25. The videos can be accessed individually by clicking the DOI link in the accompanying figure caption or by scanning this link with the SN More Media App.

N. Zhou
Department of Oral and Maxillofacial Surgery, Amsterdam UMC and Academic Centre for Dentistry Amsterdam (ACTA), University of Amsterdam, Amsterdam, The Netherlands

Department of Orofacial Pain and Dysfunction, Academic Center for Dentistry Amsterdam (ACTA), University of Amsterdam and Vrije Universiteit Amsterdam, Amsterdam, The Netherlands

J.-P. T.F. Ho (✉)
Department of Oral and Maxillofacial Surgery, Amsterdam UMC and Academic Centre for Dentistry Amsterdam (ACTA), University of Amsterdam, Amsterdam, The Netherlands

Department of Oral and Maxillofacial Surgery, Northwest Clinics, Alkmaar, The Netherlands
e-mail: j.p.ho@amsterdamumc.nl

J. de Lange
Department of Oral and Maxillofacial Surgery, Amsterdam UMC and Academic Centre for Dentistry Amsterdam (ACTA), University of Amsterdam, Amsterdam, The Netherlands

M. Delakorda, N. de Vries (eds.), *The Role of Epiglottis in Obstructive Sleep Apnea*, https://doi.org/10.1007/978-3-031-34992-8_25

Of the surgical options for OSA, MMA has been widely demonstrated to be the most effective treatment (apart from tracheotomy) [4, 5]. MMA involves simultaneous advancement and rotation of the maxilla and mandible through a Le Fort I osteotomy of the maxilla and bilateral sagittal split osteotomy (BSSO) of the mandible [6]. It has been suggested that by altering the skeletal framework, MMA can enlarge the entire retropalatal and retrolingual airway and stabilize the pharyngeal dilator muscles, thereby reducing upper airway collapsibility [7, 8].

Upper airway collapse may occur at the level of one or multiple pharyngeal structures, usually the soft palate, the oropharynx, the base of tongue, and the epiglottis [9, 10]. Identifying the collapse site(s) is crucial to determine the appropriate therapeutic strategy for patients with OSA, especially when non-CPAP therapy is considered [11, 12]. Nowadays, drug-induced sleep endoscopy (DISE) plays a key role in facilitating the decision-making process, through visualizing the upper airway obstruction during sedated sleep. With the use of DISE, epiglottis collapse has been found to occur more frequently than previously described [13]. While the role of the epiglottis in contributing to OSA has been underestimated in early research, the importance of this anatomical site and the management of epiglottis collapse have begun to gain more and more attention [13–15].

In this chapter, we firstly present some general information regarding MMA surgery for OSA treatment, and secondly, we provide a review of the current evidence on the role of MMA for epiglottis collapse.

25.2 Indication and Contraindication

Despite there being several different protocols for MMA surgery in the OSA management, the precise indications and staging protocols (primary and secondary MMA) remain undefined. The most current American Academy of Sleep Medicine (AASM) practice guidelines recommend that "MMA is indicated for surgical treatment of severe OSA in patients who cannot tolerate or who are unwilling to adhere to positive airway pressure therapy, or in whom oral appliances, which are more often appropriate in mild and moderate OSA patients, have been considered and found ineffective or undesirable (Option)" [16]. Of note, this practice recommendation is given as an "Option" instead of a "Guideline", as it is drawn from the relatively low quality of evidence. Most recently, Liu et al. [17] adopted a protocol at Stanford, in which MMA surgery is considered as a first-line treatment in OSA patients with preexisting dentofacial deformity, severe OSA, and specific airway collapse pattern (complete centric collapse at velum, and complete collapse at lateral pharyngeal wall) during DISE. The relative contraindications for MMA mainly include medical comorbidities (e.g., severe or unstable cardiopulmonary disease, uncontrolled diabetes, immune compromise), morbid obesity, older age, active alcohol/illicit drug abuse, and unstable psychological problems [18, 19].

25.3 Surgical Technique

25.3.1 Preoperative Planning

During the last decade, virtual surgical planning (VSP) has been utilized to plan and perform MMA accurately [20]. VSP for MMA begins with the clinical data gathering phase, mainly involving medical and sleep history, polysomnography (PSG), head and neck physical examination, radiographs, and facial analysis. Next, with the use of proprietary virtual planning software, three-dimensional (3D) computed tomography (CT) or cone beam computed tomography (CBCT) data and dental model are integrated as a 3D virtual model of the patient, which is used to precisely plan the operation based on surgeons' expertise (Fig. 25.1). Three-dimensional printed surgical splints allow for accurate translation of the virtual surgical plan to the surgical procedure in the operating room (Fig. 25.2).

25.3.2 Surgical Procedure

25.3.2.1 Bilateral Sagittal Split Osteotomy

The patient is in a supine position with a neutral head position. General anesthesia is administered through nasotracheal intubation. Local anesthesia is then injected to help with hemostasis. The surgery can be performed through either a maxilla-first or mandible-first protocol [21] (Fig. 25.3). When the mandible-first protocol is used, a mucosal incision is made along the anterior border of the ramus which continues inferiorly, along the sulcus of the

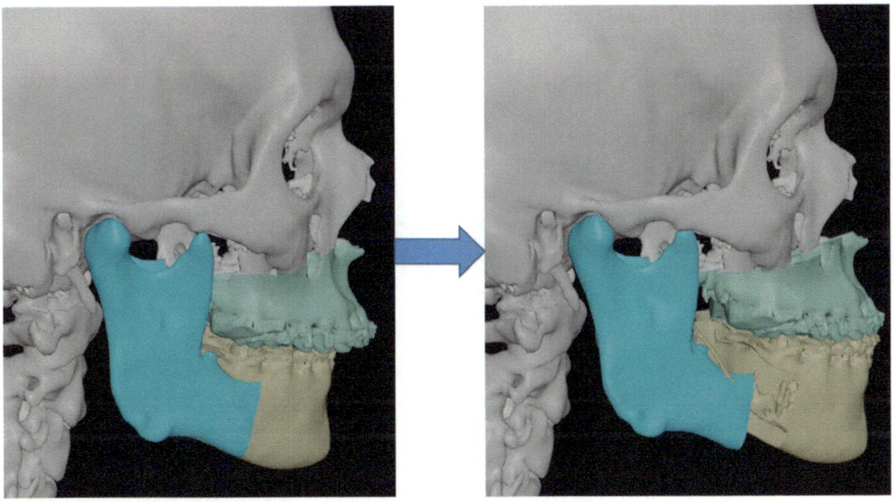

Fig. 25.1 Virtual surgical planning for maxillomandibular advancement (*left panel*, before MMA; *right panel*, after MMA)

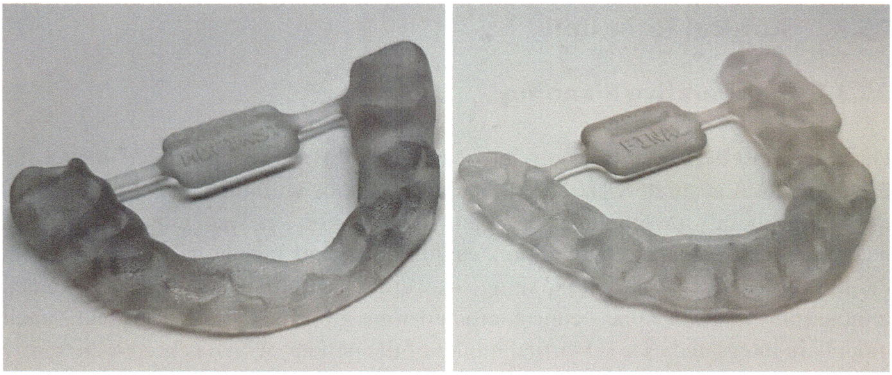

Fig. 25.2 Three-dimensional printed surgical splints (*left side*, intermediate splint; *right side*, final splint)

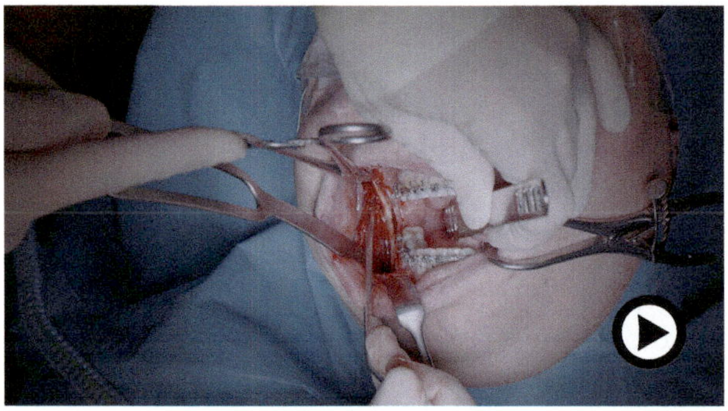

Fig. 25.3 (Video 25.1) Surgical technique of maxillomandibular advancement (▶ https://doi.org/10.1007/000-bfv)

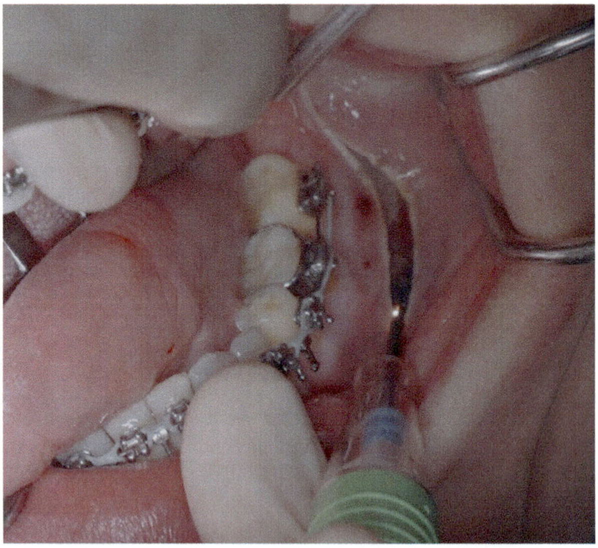

Fig. 25.4 Mucosal incision for bilateral sagittal split osteotomy for the *left side* of the mandible

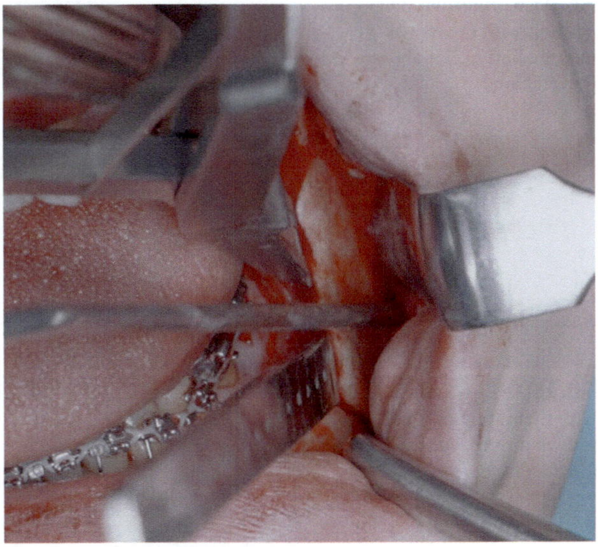

Fig. 25.5 Separation of bone segments of the mandible with osteotome and bone spreader

mandible till the first molar (Fig. 25.4). Subperiosteal dissection is performed to expose the lateral aspect of the mandible, the anterior ramus, and the medial ramus above the inferior alveolar nerve. The Hunsuck modification of the Obwegeser and Dal Pont BSSO technique is applied [22]. Using a bur or saw, a horizontal osteotomy is made just above the lingula, parallel to the occlusal plane. The osteotomy continues inferiorly along the oblique line of the ramus to the level of the first molar (remaining approximately 5 mm lateral to the teeth). Then, a vertical osteotomy is made along the buccal surface of the mandibular body, to the inferior border which is extended from the lateral to medial of the inferior border. Thin osteotomes are placed through the entire length of the cuts to begin separation of bone segments (Fig. 25.5). The completion of osteotomy is confirmed using a bone spreader. At this point, the distal tooth bearing segment can be moved three dimensionally. The inferior alveolar nerve is then identified, and if it is present in the buccal cortex, it is then completely dissected from the buccal cortex and positioned toward the lingual side. Once completing the osteotomies on both sides, the mobile distal tooth bearing segment is repositioned in the virtual planned desired position with guidance of the intermediate surgical splint. After intermaxillary fixation (IMF) is applied (Fig. 25.6), rigid fixation is utilized with screws alone or a combination of titanium plates and screws on both sides [23, 24] (Fig. 25.7). IMF is then released and the mandible is mobilized to verify the planned occlusion. In cases where there are large gaps between osteotomy segments, one may choose to augment the mandible with autogenous and/or alloplastic bone.

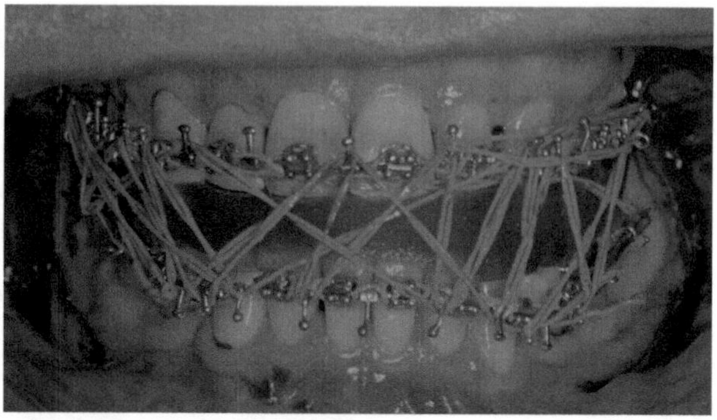

Fig. 25.6 Intermaxillary fixation with the use of the intermediate splint and powerchains

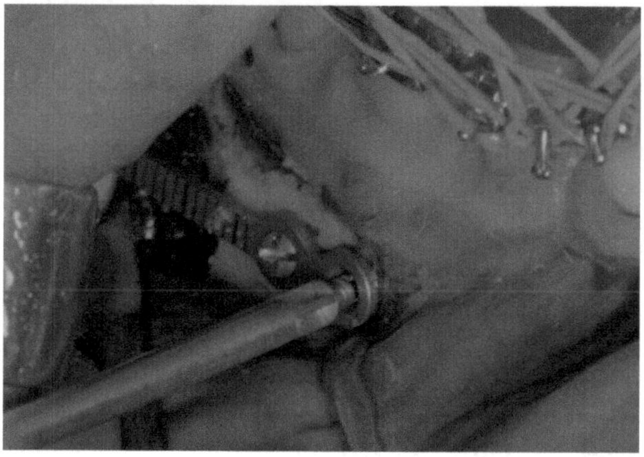

Fig. 25.7 Rigid fixation with titanium plates and screws for the *right side* of the mandible

25.3.2.2 Le Fort I Osteotomy

Access to the Le Fort I osteotomy begins with a maxillary gingivobuccal incision, which is made from the first molar on one site to the first molar on the opposite site to expose both the lateral and medial buttresses of the maxilla. Subperiosteal dissection is performed to expose the anterior and lateral surface of the maxilla (from the piriform rims to the pterygoid processes) (Fig. 25.8). The nasal mucosa is dissected and released. A fixed skeletal marker (K-wire or screw) is placed in the glabella region. This will allow vertical measurements before and after the osteotomy, to ensure the correct maxillary planned height is achieved (Fig. 25.9). Then, a maxillary osteotomy is made with a fissure bur or saw from the ipsilateral piriform rim to the pterygomaxillary fissures bilaterally. A U-shaped or V-shaped osteotome is used to separate the nasal septum from the maxilla (Fig. 25.10). The posterior maxillary wall and lateral nasal wall is then fractured with an osteotome. A curved osteotome is then used to separate the pterygomaxillary junction. Once the osteotomies are completed, the down-fracture is performed with digital pressure or a bone-hook (Fig. 25.11). After completing down-fracture and mobilization with Rowes forceps, a final surgical splint is used to position the maxilla accurately by IMF. The surgical

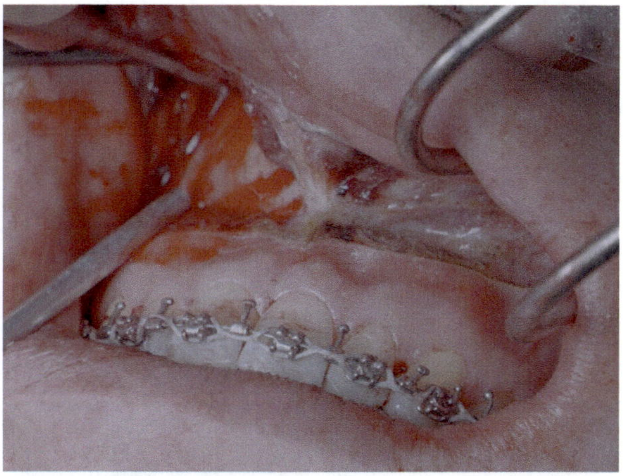

Fig. 25.8 Subperiosteal dissection for Le Fort I osteotomy of the maxilla

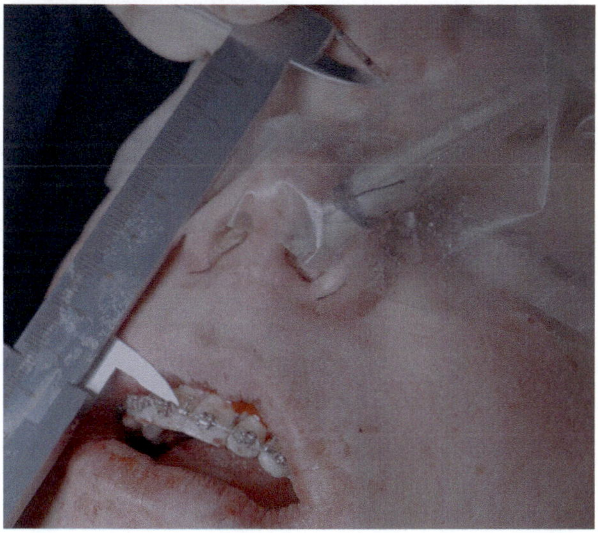

Fig. 25.9 K-wire in the glabella region for vertical measurement

splint ensures that the virtual plan is translated in all dimensions except for the cranial-caudal dimension. The planned movement in this dimension achieved by is maxillary impaction, which is often due to a planned counterclockwise rotation. The impaction requires appropriate reduction of anterior maxillary bone, septum, and/or vomer. Rigid fixation is then accomplished utilizing four titanium miniplates and mono-cortical screws [17, 25] (Fig. 25.12). Following fixation, IMF is released and the mandible is mobilized to verify the planned occlusion. After confirming proper occlusion, the incisions are closed with absorbable sutures. Orthodontic elastics may be used for postoperative guidance of the occlusion on orthodontic appliances or arch bars if present [17].

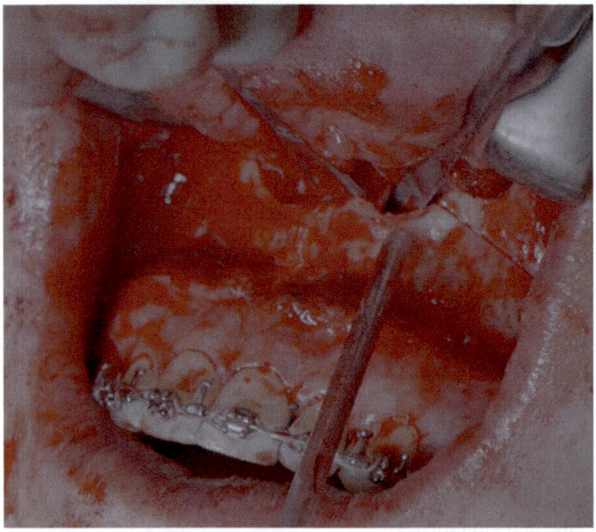

Fig. 25.10 Separation of the nasal septum from the maxilla with a U-shaped osteotome

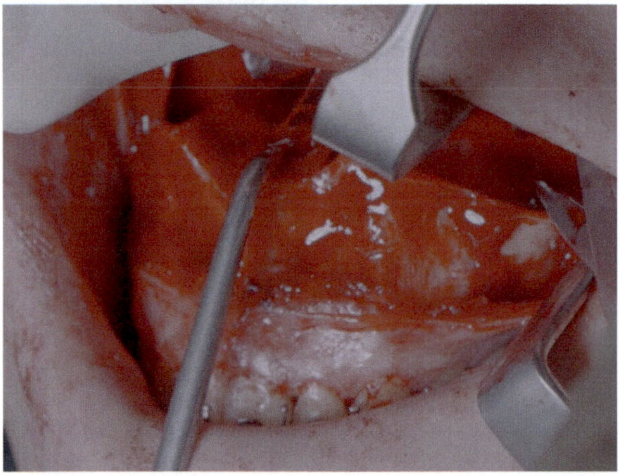

Fig. 25.11 Down-fracture of the maxilla with a bone-hook

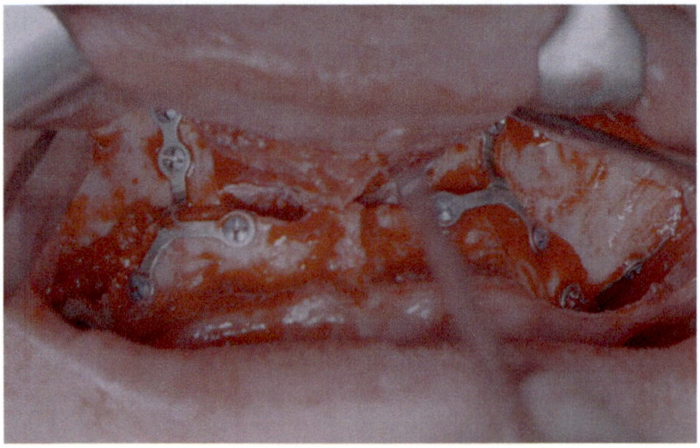

Fig. 25.12 Rigid fixation with titanium plates and screws for the maxilla

25.4 Postoperative Care

Following MMA, patients are often carefully monitored overnight in an intensive care unit (ICU) [26]. Usually, the patients are transferred out of the ICU to a regular ward with continuous airway monitoring on the first postoperative day. The average length of hospitalization is 3.5 days [4]. Postoperative medications include antibiotics, analgesics, and steroids. Applying a light pressure dressing and ice is recommended for the first 48 hours to help minimize the swelling. Rinses of the oral cavity and gentle toothbrushing should start on the first postoperative day to maintain proper oral hygiene. Patients' diet is adapted with a clear liquid diet for the first week, followed by a strict non-chew diet for approximately 1 month. The patients can return to normal activities with physical restriction 1 or 2 weeks after surgery [27].

The frequency of follow-up generally depends on surgeons' preference and patients' recovery. Usually, postoperatively radiographs and/or CT or CBCT are made. An overnight PSG is necessary, typically 3–6 months after MMA, to evaluate therapeutic efficacy.

25.5 Complications

No death has been reported for the MMA procedure. Reoperation is likely required for hardware removal, malunion, nonunion, and severe malocclusion. Previously reported rates of reoperation range from 0 to 40% [16, 28, 29]. The most common complication of MMA is facial paresthesia caused by impairment of the inferior alveolar nerve and/or maxillary nerve. Our recent systematic review shows that facial paresthesia was transient in 76.9% cases and persistent in 18.5% of cases following MMA [4]. Patients' age, addition of genioplasty, and large degree of mandibular advancement may increase the risk of paresthesia of the lower lip and chin [30]. Malocclusion can happen in some patients following MMA, which requires orthodontic treatment or surgical correction. The reported risk of malocclusion ranges from 0 to 24% [6, 31, 32]. Other less frequently reported complications mainly include temporomandibular joint disorder, local infection, and velopharyngeal insufficiency in patients with previous or concurrent soft palate surgery, dyspnea, palatal perforation, and transient deviation of angle of mouth [4].

Additionally, there are some concerns about aesthetic alterations resulting from MMA, such as excessive maxillomandibular protrusion, increase of the alar base, and nasal tip elevation. However, it has been suggested that a majority of patients perceived the facial changes as positive or neutral [4, 31]. Various surgical techniques, such as counterclockwise rotation of the maxillomandibular complex and recontouring of the anterior nasal spine, have been applied into MMA to limit the potential negative aesthetic effect.

25.6 Outcome of MMA

MMA has been suggested to be the most successful surgical therapy for OSA (apart from tracheostomy), with a therapeutic efficacy comparable to CPAP. As reported in our recent meta-analysis, 19 MMA studies, describing 393 subjects with mean preoperative apnea hypopnea index (AHI) of 57.3 ± 26.6/h, showed a statistical improvement in AHI of 46.2/h, lowest oxygen saturation (LSAT) of 13.5%, oxygen desaturation index (ODI) of −30.3/h, and Epworth Sleepiness Scale (ESS) of −8.5. The pooled rates of surgical success and cure for MMA were 85.0% and 46.3%, respectively [4]. The predictors of increased surgical success include younger age, lower preoperative weight and AHI, and greater degree of maxillary advancement [5].

The efficacy of MMA can persist for most patients on a long-term basis. A meta-analysis by Camacho et al. demonstrated that the improvements in AHI, LSAT, and daytime sleepiness for patients who underwent MMA for OSA maintained in the long term (4 to <8 years), while the mean AHI increased to moderate OSA in the very long term (≥8 years) [33]. Vigneron et al. demonstrated that the success rate of MMA was 41.4% at 12.5 years after MMA, and the success rate was 100% in young patients (age <45 years old) with BMI <25 kg/m^2, AHI <45/h, SNB <75°, narrow retrolingual space (<8 mm), and preoperative orthodontics (success was defined as an AHI of <10/h and almost a 50% reduction in AHI following MMA) [28]. Marked weight gain, significant skeletal relapse, and aging may counteract the benefit of MMA in the long term [34, 35]. To maintain the therapeutic efficacy, long-term follow-up is needed for OSA patients.

Several studies have also evaluated the impact of MMA on quality of life. Pottel et al. reported the OSA quality of life (OSA QoL) questionnaire score at 19-year follow-up in nine MMA patients [34]. They reported immediately postoperative improvements in symptoms of headache, blood pressure, daytime sleepiness, concentration, insomnia, nocturia, snoring, and sexual performance. At approximately 19 years after MMA, the improvements in all previously reported symptoms persisted, except for blood pressure, nocturia, and sexual activity. Boyd et al. investigated the QoL for 14 patients who underwent MMA for OSA using the Functional Outcomes of Sleep Questionnaire (FOSQ) [31]. The patients reported a significant improvement in mean FOSQ scores of 4.7 at 2 years after MMA. It is suggested that the short-term improvements in QoL after MMA may be maintained in a long term.

25.7 Role of MMA for Epiglottis Collapse

To date, there is limited evidence on the role of MMA for epiglottis collapse [7, 36]. In 2016, Liu et al. used DISE to study dynamic changes of the upper airway following MMA [7]. In their study, MMA was performed in 20 patients. Four out of 20 patients showed baseline anteroposterior epiglottis collapse (complete collapse: $n = 2$; partial collapse: $n = 2$). After MMA, this collapse pattern persisted in two patients (partial collapse: $n = 1$; complete collapse: $n = 1$). Two out of 20 patients had complete lateral epiglottis collapse preoperatively, and one patient had partial lateral epiglottis collapse postoperatively. Due to the small numbers of events for epiglottis collapse, their study cannot be an indicative of the role of MMA on epiglottis collapse.

The upper airway collapse patterns during DISE before and after MMA were also evaluated by Kastoer et al. in 2020 [36]. Eight out of 14 patients had anteroposterior epiglottis collapse at baseline (partial collapse: $n = 5$; complete collapse: $n = 3$). Residual epiglottis collapse after MMA was present in six patients (partial collapse: $n = 3$; complete collapse: $n = 3$), two of which exhibited a floppy epiglottis. No significant difference was found in distribution of epiglottis collapse before and after MMA. They assumed that MMA surgery may not be an effective therapeutic option for epiglottis collapse. However, due to the small number of patients, conclusions must be taken with care.

In our previous study consisting of 64 OSA patients who underwent baseline DISE followed by MMA, the association between airway collapse patterns in DISE findings and MMA surgery outcome was investigated [10]. It was found that complete anteroposterior epiglottis collapse was independently related to non-response to MMA after correction for confounders (i.e., age, gender, BMI, baseline AHI, degree of maxillary advancement, and degree of mandibular advancement). This finding is supported by the study did by Kastoer et al. [36].

Of note, several mechanisms have been proposed to explain the epiglottis collapse: (1) secondary to an anteroposterior collapse of the tongue base that pushes the epiglottis backwards; (2) a complete isolated anteroposterior epiglottis collapse, also known as floppy epiglottis or trapdoor phenomenon; and (3) lateral epiglottis collapse due to underdevelopment of the epiglottis [37]. The role of MMA for different types of epiglottis collapse may be different. The lack of studies on this topic should be addressed in the future.

25.8 Conclusions

According to the current evidence, MMA could be less effective in addressing epiglottis collapse, especially complete anteroposterior epiglottis collapse. For OSA patients with epiglottis collapse, subsequent therapy may be needed to treat this collapse when MMA surgery fails and residual epiglottis collapse is present. Given the limited availability of data, further investigation is essential to fully understand the role of MMA for epiglottis collapse, and in which the type of epiglottis collapse it is indicated.

References

1. Mannarino MR, Di Filippo F, Pirro M. Obstructive sleep apnea syndrome. Eur J Intern Med. 2012;23(7):586–93.
2. Gottlieb DJ, Punjabi NM. Diagnosis and management of obstructive sleep apnea: a review. JAMA. 2020;323(14):1389–400.
3. Rotenberg BW, Vicini C, Pang EB, Pang KP. Reconsidering first-line treatment for obstructive sleep apnea: a systematic review of the literature. J Otolaryngol Head Neck Surg. 2016;45(1):1–9.
4. Zhou N, Ho J-PT, Huang Z, et al. Maxillomandibular advancement versus multilevel surgery for treatment of obstructive sleep apnea: a systematic review and meta-analysis. Sleep Med Rev. 2021;57:101471.
5. Holty J-EC, Guilleminault C. Maxillomandibular advancement for the treatment of obstructive sleep apnea: a systematic review and meta-analysis. Sleep Med Rev. 2010;14(5):287–97.
6. Li KK, Riley RW, Powell NB, Troell R, Guilleminault C. Overview of phase II surgery for obstructive sleep apnea syndrome. Ear Nose Throat J. 1999;78(11):851–7.
7. Liu SY, Huon LK, Iwasaki T, et al. Efficacy of maxillomandibular advancement examined with drug-induced sleep endoscopy and computational fluid dynamics airflow modeling. Otolaryngol Head Neck Surg. 2016;154(1):189–95.
8. Hsieh Y-J, Liao Y-F, Chen N-H, Chen Y-R. Changes in the calibre of the upper airway and the surrounding structures after maxillomandibular advancement for obstructive sleep apnoea. Br J Oral Maxillofac Surg. 2014;52(5):445–51.
9. Kezirian EJ, Hohenhorst W, de Vries N. Drug-induced sleep endoscopy: the VOTE classification. Eur Arch Otorhinolaryngol. 2011;268(8):1233–6.
10. Zhou N, Ho JTF, de Vries N, Bosschieter PFN, Ravesloot MJL, de Lange J. Evaluation of drug-induced sleep endoscopy as a tool for selecting patients with obstructive sleep apnea for maxillomandibular advancement. J Clin Sleep Med. 2021;18:1073.
11. Vanderveken OM, Maurer JT, Hohenhorst W, et al. Evaluation of drug-induced sleep endoscopy as a patient selection tool for implanted upper airway stimulation for obstructive sleep apnea. J Clin Sleep Med. 2013;9(5):433–8.
12. Op de Beeck S, Dieltjens M, Verbruggen AE, et al. Phenotypic labelling using drug-induced sleep endoscopy improves patient selection for mandibular advancement device outcome: a prospective study. J Clin Sleep Med. 2019;15(8):1089–99.
13. Torre C, Camacho M, Liu SYC, Huon LK, Capasso R. Epiglottis collapse in adult obstructive sleep apnea: a systematic review. Laryngoscope. 2016;126(2):515–23.
14. Vonk P, Ravesloot M, Kasius K, van Maanen J, de Vries N. Floppy epiglottis during drug-induced sleep endoscopy: an almost complete resolution by adopting the lateral posture. Sleep Breath. 2020;24(1):103–9.
15. Kim H-Y, Sung C-M, Jang H-B, Kim HC, Lim SC, Yang HC. Patients with epiglottic collapse showed less severe obstructive sleep apnea and good response to treatment other than continuous positive airway pressure: a case-control study of 224 patients. J Clin Sleep Med. 2021;17(3):413–9.
16. Aurora RN, Casey KR, Kristo D, et al. Practice parameters for the surgical modifications of the upper airway for obstructive sleep apnea in adults. Sleep. 2010;33(10):1408–13.
17. Liu S, Awad M, Riley RW. Maxillomandibular advancement: contemporary approach at Stanford. Atlas Oral Maxillofac Surg Clin North Am. 2019;27(1):29–36.
18. Prinsell JR. Maxillomandibular advancement (MMA) in a site-specific treatment approach for obstructive sleep apnea: a surgical algorithm. Sleep Breath. 2000;4(4):147–54.
19. Holty JE, Guilleminault C. Surgical options for the treatment of obstructive sleep apnea. Med Clin North Am. 2010;94(3):479–515.
20. Barrera JE. Virtual surgical planning improves surgical outcome measures in obstructive sleep apnea surgery. Laryngoscope. 2014;124(5):1259–66.

21. Stokbro K, Liebregts J, Baan F, et al. Does mandible-first sequencing increase maxillary surgical accuracy in bimaxillary procedures? J Oral Maxillofac Surg. 2019;77(9):1882–93.
22. Hunsuck E. A modified intraoral sagittal splitting technic for correction of mandibular prognathism. J Oral Surg. 1968;26(4):250–3.
23. van Ewijk LJ, van Riet TCT, van der Tol IGH, Ho J, Becking AG. Power chains as an alternative to steel-wire ligatures in temporary maxillomandibular fixation: a pilot study. Int J Oral Maxillofac Surg. 2021;S0901-5027(21):00317-9.
24. Kuik K, Ho J, de Ruiter MHT, et al. Stability of fixation methods in large mandibular advancements after sagittal split ramus osteotomy: an in vitro biomechanical study. Br J Oral Maxillofac Surg. 2021;59(4):466–71.
25. Buchanan EP, Hyman CH. LeFort I osteotomy. Semin Plast Surg. 2013;27:149–54.
26. Ravesloot MJL, de Raaff CAL, van de Beek MJ, et al. Perioperative care of patients with obstructive sleep apnea undergoing upper airway surgery: a review and consensus recommendations. JAMA Otolaryngol Head Neck Surg. 2019;145(8):751–60.
27. Otero JJ, Detriche O, Mommaerts MY. Fast-track orthognathic surgery: an evidence-based review. Ann Maxillofac Surg. 2017;7(2):166–75.
28. Vigneron A, Tamisier R, Orset E, Pepin J-L, Bettega G. Maxillomandibular advancement for obstructive sleep apnea syndrome treatment: long-term results. J Craniomaxillofac Surg. 2017;45(2):183–91.
29. De Ruiter M, Apperloo R, Milstein D, De Lange J. Assessment of obstructive sleep apnoea treatment success or failure after maxillomandibular advancement. Int J Oral Maxillofac Surg. 2017;46(11):1357–62.
30. Van Sickels JE, Hatch JP, Dolce C, Bays RA, Rugh JD. Effects of age, amount of advancement, and genioplasty on neurosensory disturbance after a bilateral sagittal split osteotomy. J Oral Maxillofac Surg. 2002;60(9):1012–7.
31. Boyd SB, Walters AS, Waite P, Harding SM, Song Y. Long-term effectiveness and safety of maxillomandibular advancement for treatment of obstructive sleep apnea. J Clin Sleep Med. 2015;11(7):699–708.
32. Vicini C, Dallan I, Campanini A, et al. Surgery vs ventilation in adult severe obstructive sleep apnea syndrome. Am J Otolaryngol. 2010;31(1):14–20.
33. Camacho M, Noller MW, Del Do M, et al. Long-term results for maxillomandibular advancement to treat obstructive sleep apnea: a meta-analysis. Otolaryngol Head Neck Surg. 2019;160(4):580–93.
34. Pottel L, Neyt N, Hertegonne K, et al. Long-term quality of life outcomes of maxillomandibular advancement osteotomy in patients with obstructive sleep apnoea syndrome. Int J Oral Maxillofac Surg. 2019;48(3):332–40.
35. Riley RW, Powell NB, Li KK, Troell RJ, Guilleminault C. Surgery and obstructive sleep apnea: long-term clinical outcomes. Otolaryngol Head Neck Surg. 2000;122(3):415–20.
36. Kastoer C, Op de Beeck S, Dom M, et al. Drug-induced sleep endoscopy upper airway collapse patterns and maxillomandibular advancement. Laryngoscope. 2020;130(4):E268–e274.
37. Vonk PE, Ravesloot MJL, Kasius KM, van Maanen JP, de Vries N. Floppy epiglottis during drug-induced sleep endoscopy: an almost complete resolution by adopting the lateral posture. Sleep Breath. 2020;24(1):103–9.

Anesthesia Management in OSA Patient 26

Abdulrahman Dardeer, Muhammad Firas Alhammad, and Nabil A. Shallik

26.1 Introduction

Obstructive sleep apnea (OSA) is a disorder involving frequent breathing pauses during sleep. According to the International Classification of Sleep Disorders (ICSD-3) in adults without associated symptoms or comorbidities, it is classified according to Apnea Hypopnea Index (AHI) into mild OSA (5–15 AHI), moderate OSA (15–30 AHI), and sever OSA (> 30 AHI). In a patient with associated medical or psychiatric disorders, the clinical signs and symptoms will be more exaggerated. Common signs and symptoms of OSA include snoring (frequently noted by other family members rather than the patient himself) and sleepiness or feeling tired during the daytime [1]. The estimated OSA prevalence rate in recent studies was around 14% in men and 5% in women aged 30 to 70 years, and it may increase to 20–30% in elderly or obese population [2]. The risk factors for OSA include obesity [3, 4], family history of sleep apnea [5], and allergy [6, 7]. Some studies suggested that occupational stress could be a possible risk factor for OSA [8, 9]. The focus of this chapter is on perioperative management of OSA patients, with special attention to OSA caused by the epiglottis. Those patients are a small in number but challenging group. A more detailed overview of OSA will be discussed in other chapters of this book.

A. Dardeer · M. F. Alhammad
Department of Anaesthesia, ICU and Perioperative Medicine, Hamad Medical Corporation, Doha, Qatar

N. A. Shallik (✉)
Department of Anaesthesia, ICU and Perioperative Medicine, Hamad Medical Corporation, Doha, Qatar

Department of Clinical Anesthesiology, Weill Cornell Medical College in Qatar, Al Rayyan, Qatar

Department of Clinical Anesthesiology, Qatar University, Doha, Qatar
e-mail: nshallik@hamad.qa

M. Delakorda, N. de Vries (eds.), *The Role of Epiglottis in Obstructive Sleep Apnea*, https://doi.org/10.1007/978-3-031-34992-8_26

Epiglottis pathology is an uncommon cause of OSA and may be very challenging to both anesthetists and surgeons in terms of diagnosis and management and is usually overlooked and ignored [10]. Epiglottis prolapse during inspiration is an unusual cause of airway obstruction and a rare cause of OSA [11]. Closing door epiglottis or floppy epiglottis (Fig. 26.1) is a collapsible epiglottis that blocks the airway and is one of the most challenging situations that a sleep surgeon can encounter. Omega-shaped epiglottis (or pipe-line epiglottis) which is another anatomic variation that can cause dynamic obstruction of the airway (Fig. 26.2). Epiglottic collapse should be identified as it may cause treatment failure, either by CPAP or surgically. Misidentification of the condition may even lead to worsening of OSA symptoms with CPAP, or may lead to non-compliance by patients as the treatment becomes suboptimal [11–14]. Schwannoma of the epiglottis is a rare condition [15] and usually a solitary incident rather than being part of a more systemic condition, like neurofibromatosis, either type 1 or 2 [16]. While these conditions are more

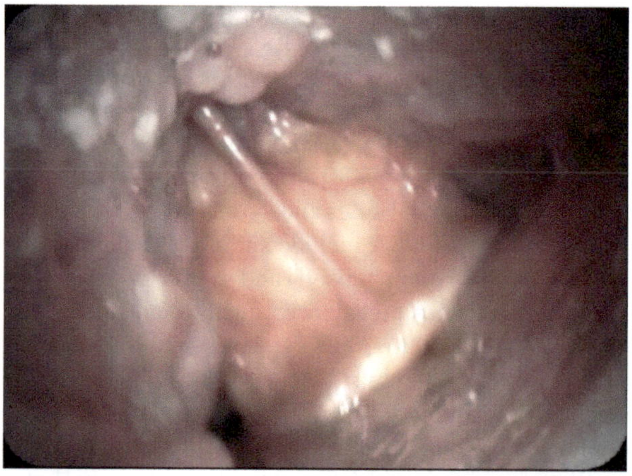

Fig. 26.1 Closing door epiglottis

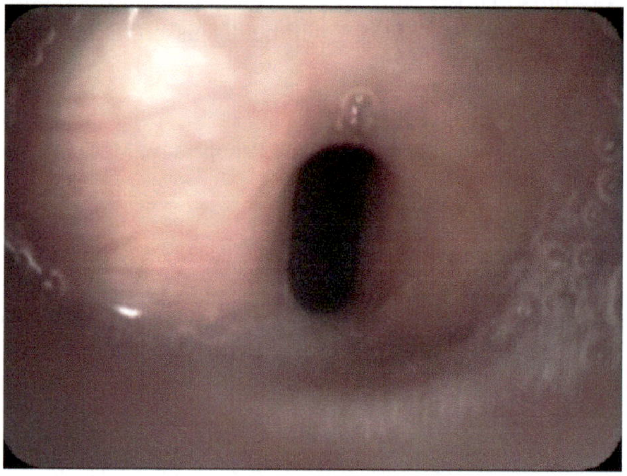

Fig. 26.2 Pipe-line epiglottis

chronic in nature, some acute conditions related to epiglottis can also cause airway obstruction, with more devastating outcomes if improperly managed. Acute epiglottitis and epiglottic abscess are life-threatening situations with serious implications because of the potential for laryngospasm and irrevocable loss of the airway. There is inflammatory edema of the arytenoids, aryepiglottic folds, and epiglottis. The term supraglottitis may be used instead of or preferred to the term acute epiglottitis [17]. In children, epiglottitis is more challenging as the apprehensive child might make it difficult for the anesthetists to manage his airway. There is always a risk of impending airway obstruction and difficult bag-mask ventilation and of course, difficult intubation (DI). It is crucial not to upset the child or manipulate the airway to keep it patent. The anesthesia considerations in such patients are increased risk of aspiration, little or almost no time to airway stabilization, and associated sepsis, in addition to other usual pediatric considerations (e.g., difficult cannulation, apprehensive parents, etc.).

26.2 Preoperative Assessment and Optimization

Preoperative evaluation is a powerful tool that defines the safe practice of anesthesia from unsafe, especially in patients with OSA. It helps formulate a sound perioperative plan that ensure maximum safety and the least risk possible to the patient. A proper preoperative assessment should ensure sufficient time for any possible optimization of the patient's condition to decrease his perioperative risk. Every preoperative evaluation should include the following:

1. The detailed history of all medical conditions and prior surgical procedures and anesthesia received before, and if the patient had any reaction or difficulty during the conduct of previous anesthetics. The history should include the STOP-BANG survey or Berlin Questionnaire. Patients should be referred for Sleep study if they score high to categorize the severity of OSA.
2. American Society of Anesthesiologists (ASA) physical status score.
3. Routine investigations, and additionally any further investigations indicated by patient's condition (e.g., Pulmonary Function Test, Arterial Blood Gases, etc.).
4. Anesthesia plan (e.g., General Anesthesia, Monitored Anesthesia Care, Regional Anesthesia [RA]). It is advisable to plan for RA if feasible, especially if OSA is severe.
5. Airway management strategy (awake fiberoptic intubation [AFOI], video laryngoscopy [VL], direct laryngoscopy [DL], tracheostomy, etc.).
6. Indication for special monitoring (e.g., arterial catheter, central line, advance cardiac output monitoring, etc.).
7. Probability for the need of blood and blood derived products substituting.
8. Patient disposition postoperatively.

9. Airway evaluation in more detail in Difficult Airway Clinic (DAC) to include the following, if possible:
   (a) Routine airway assessment.
   (b) Naso-endoscopy or naso-laryngoscopy: this proved to be the most important office-based diagnostic tool of upper airway pathologies and would recognize epiglottis pathologies and guide further investigations or management plan.
   (c) Ultrasound (US) assessment of the upper airway.
   (d) Dynamic documentation in electronic health system.
   (e) Difficult Airway Alert Card (DAAC).
   (f) Virtual Endoscopy (VE) and 3D-CT reconstruction of the upper airway.

26.2.1 The Role of 3D Reconstruction and Virtual Endoscopy (VE)

Studies have demonstrated that inadequate assessment and planning contribute to airway complications and that current airway assessment strategies have poor diagnostic accuracy in predicting DI in the general population [18]. Virtual endoscopy (VE) can simulate endoscopic intraluminal views like those obtained by the conventional fiberoptic bronchoscopy (FOB). It is non-invasive and easily obtained by postprocessing a routinely acquired high-resolution computed tomography (CT) data set using simple computer software. Multi-plane CT scanning is often performed for patients with head and neck disease [18, 19]. Compared with FOB, which is limited for the evaluation of intraluminal pathologies, VE in a single examination which can depict intraluminal manifestations of different diseases, along with a bird-eye-like demonstration of surrounding anatomy, giving a more holistic view of the airway. Preprocedural VE information with precise mapping of location and extent of airway pathologies helps in proper planning of anesthesia [20]. Evidence indicates that multi-slice detector CT imaging with a 3D reconstruction of the images can significantly increase the diagnostic accuracy of the procedure up to 94–100% [21]. VE can be very helpful in detecting epiglottis pathologies. Though not able to detect dynamic pathologies, it can detect other pathologies like morphological anomalies or misplaced epiglottis. This would save the patient discomfort of naso-endoscopy in some instances. For example, one can find the epiglottitis in adult patient with VE after CT-3D reconstruction (Fig. 26.3a) and with the bronchoscopic exam in the same patient (Fig. 26.3b). There are now some trials to get 3D images from MRI scans to better visualize the soft tissue [22, 23].

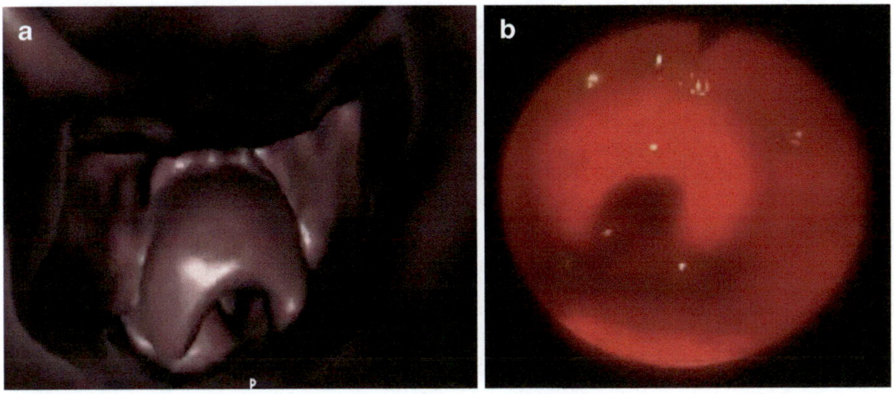

Fig. 26.3 **(a)** VE of epiglottitis and **(b)** bronchoscopic view of epiglottitis

26.3 Airway Management

Difficult airway, either difficult mask ventilation (DMV) or DI, may be common in OSA patients [24, 25]. According to the most recent ASA practice guidelines, a difficult airway includes the clinical situation in which anticipated or unanticipated difficulty or failure is experienced by a physician trained in anesthesia care, including but not limited to one or more of the following: face-mask ventilation, laryngoscopy, ventilation using a supraglottic airway, tracheal intubation, extubation, or invasive airway [26].

26.3.1 Optimizing Preoxygenation, Positioning (Safety Apnea Rescue Time)

It cannot be stressed enough how the bed position, such a simple maneuver, can influence the patient's outcome. It has been shown that a head-up position with a 25° inclination (reverse Trendelenburg) increases the duration of apnea without arterial desaturation, increasing the window for tracheal intubation. Another useful technique is the "ramped" position, aiming at the horizontal alignment of the sternal notch with the external auditory meatus using folded blankets or commercially available pillows (Oxford or Troop pillow) under the upper body, shoulders, and head - Head Elevated Laryngoscopy Position [HELP] [27, 28]. This would facilitate DL [29] (Fig. 26.4). Pre-oxygenation or "de-nitrogenization" is not simply

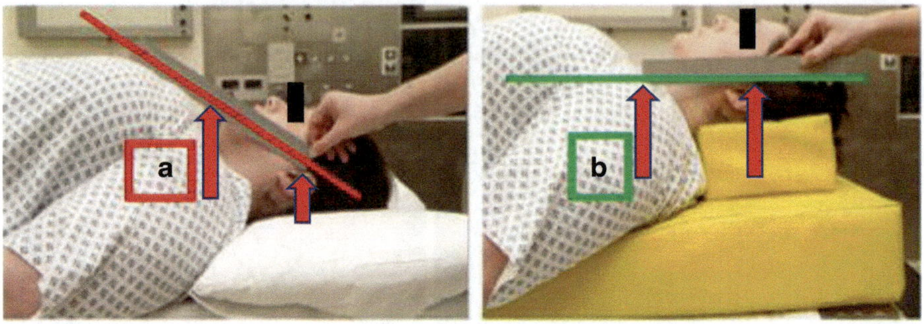

Fig. 26.4 (a) Normal pillow. (b) Oxford pillow

providing "extra oxygen" to the patient, but is a crucial step, especially in patients with suspected DI, that will allow enough time (3–5 minutes) needed to introduce the tracheal tube (Safety Apnea Rescue Time). It must be conducted correctly to ensure maximum benefit. In the absence of respiratory failure, preoxygenation using a tight-fitting face-mask, with 10 to 15 L per minute of 100% oxygen for 3 min would be sufficient. Adequate preoxygenation is preferably measured using end-tidal oxygen concentration (>85%) [30]. Obese patients, especially if suffering from OSA, benefit of positive airway pressure, supplemental nasopharyngeal oxygen insufflation, and noninvasive ventilation (NIV) before anesthesia induction. High-flow oxygenation by nasal cannula (HFNC) has been studied in intensive care units (ICUs) and in the operating room as a pre-oxygenation device and has shown the ability to extend safe apnea time during DI, and to be held during fiberoptic bronchoscopic intubation (FOI) to provide sort of "relaxed atmosphere" to the anesthetist to conduct FOI. This device can deliver up to 80 L/min with an inspired fraction of oxygen of up to 100% and generate a moderate positive supraglottic end-expiratory pressure. Moreover, in toothless or bearded patients, significant leaks around the mask can alter oxygenation, which is not a problem for HFNC. HFNC allows inserting the fiberscope in the patient's nostril to perform intubation while continuing the oxygenation and may be better tolerated [31]. However, HFNC cannot be used in all patients. Contraindications include nasal surgery, nasal bleeding, complete nasal obstruction, nasal infection, severe facial trauma, or suspected skull base fractures [32].

26.3.2 Airway Management Plans: Risk Assessment and Patient Categorization

Some experts argue that there is really no difficult airway but rather unplanned conduct of anesthesia. Evaluation and planning of anesthesia during preoperative assessment, with a strategy that includes multiple exit routes if needed, for patients with OSA, ensures a safe anesthesia with minimum unnecessary risks. El-Ganzouri et al. [33] developed a multivariate risk index, El-Ganzouri Risk Index (EGRI), that

Table 26.1 El-Ganzouri Risk Index (EGRI). Interpretation: ≥ 4 - high risk of difficult airway (93.8% specificity), < 4 - low risk of difficult airway

Variable	Points
Mouth opening	
≥ 4 cm	0
< 4 cm	1
Thyromental distance	
> 6.5 cm	0
6.0–6.5 cm	1
< 6.0 cm	2
Modified Mallampati classification	
I (soft palate, fauces, uvula, and pillars seen)	0
II (soft palate, fauces, and uvula seen)	1
III (soft palate and base of uvula seen)	2
IV (soft palate not visible)	2
Neck movement	
>90°	0
80–90°	1
<80°	2
Ability to prognath (advance lower jaw forward)	
Yes	0
No	1
Weight	
< 90 kg (198.4 lbs)	0
90–110 kg (198.4–242.5 lbs)	1
> 110 kg (242.5 lbs)	2
History of difficult intubation	
None	0
Questionable	1
Definite	2

involves the analysis of six parameters commonly performed during the preoperative evaluation. Each variable is assigned a score (0 or 1). A score ≥ 4 has a high sensitivity for predicting DI (Table 26.1). In a study by Corso et al. [34], EGRI has proven to predict DI and DMV. This would enable the operator to identify difficult cases with a single bedside test to formulate a tailored airway management plan that mitigates the potential risks. Cortellazzi et al. [35] showed that predicted difficult airway by EGRI; using video laryngoscopy (VL) had better outcomes compared to those who were managed with DL. A protocol for patients undergoing general anesthesia and scored 7 in EGRI was developed by Cortellazzi et al., and they advocated routine intubation with GlideScope® video laryngoscope (Verathon Inc., WA, USA). For patients scoring eight or more, awake FOI (AFOI) is advised with a backup Supraglottic Airway Device (SAD). In case of a score, less than seven but more than four, both DL and VL, can be implemented based on operator preference and experience, with a backup SAD. Awake intubation is frequently described in the literature as the preferred method for securing the airway in adult patients with epiglottitis, whereas children are usually intubated following an inhalational induction.

However, if topicalization is difficult due to the presence of an abscess or an uncooperative patient, an inhalational induction may still be a reasonable approach in the adult patient. In a review of the literature, only one recent case report had been found describing an inhalational induction with VL. However, this attempt was unsuccessful, mandating the need for a surgical airway [36].

26.3.3 Direct Laryngoscope (DL) Versus Video Laryngoscope (VL)

The debate of whether VL should be implemented initially in difficult cases or to give DL a chance is seen on a daily basis among experts. Some argue that a well-positioned patient with enough time to pre-oxygenate and having adjuncts, like a gum elastic bougie (GEB) or an intubating malleable stylet, can guarantee the success of the first attempt for DL, and although VL improves glottis visualization, this is usually at the expense of prolonged tracheal intubation times and does not necessarily translate into easier intubation. However, VL has definitely earned its place in modern practice. Avoiding the need to align oral and pharyngeal axes, VLs convert a difficult view into a relatively easy procedure. Several studies have shown that VLs improve intubation conditions in morbidly obese patients [37]. Using a screen to view, the intubation procedure turns it into a task performed and guided by a team. The team approach may optimize intubation attempts, limit unnecessary manipulations and trauma, and can help prevent errors such as esophageal intubations. It is also possible to record the intubation process for teaching purposes and legal documentation [38]. VLs can also be effectively used in awake techniques. It is useful to highlight that not all VLs are equal. Unfortunately, no single VL technique has shown superiority to others, with each having its pros and cons that should be weighted upon use. Operator experience must be taken into consideration also, and one should always use whatever technique he/she masters to ensure the best outcome. Among the available designs of VLs, hyper-angulated videoscopes carry some favorable features that translate into higher success rates of intubation. It is important to understand that there is a learning curve for all VLs, and particularly for hyper-angulated devices [38]. The hyper-angulation makes it easier to maneuver around obstacles like a large base of the tongue and will eliminate the need for excessive force to get a good view. This does not mean it will make the intubation easier, especially if conducted by an inexperienced operator. Successful intubation with a hyper-angulated VL mandates a stylet (or another semi-rigid introducer) with an angulation resembling the angle of the blade [38]. Of the commercially available designs of hyper-angulated VLs, the D-Blade of C-Mac® VL (KARL STORZ SE & Co. KG, Tuttlingen, Germany) has unique angulation [39] which exposes the glottis more clearly than other designs. Combined with its smaller mass, it does not occupy much of a space in the oral cavity allowing good room for manipulation and maneuvering. However, both GlideScope® and D-Blade® were tested in different clinical scenarios and different patient populations (patients with a known difficult airway, patients with cervical spine instability, patients undergoing thoracic surgeries, etc.) and showed comparable results [40, 41].

26.3.4 Fiberscopic-Assisted Video-Laryngoscope Intubation (FAVI) or Combined Technique

Although very handy and powerful tool, the fiberoptic bronchoscope alone has its restrictions and limitations. It offers a narrow frontal view of airway structures. This might be very dangerous while introducing the tube as trauma to the structures not shown can occur. Trauma to different laryngeal cartilages is a well-documented complication of difficult and even in uneventful intubation, namely, arytenoids [42–44]. In cases of epiglottis anomalies where advancing the tube can be opposed by its abnormal position (e.g., downfolding epiglottis) or morphology, this technique helps navigate the airway safely [45, 46].

In FOB, the primary operator has full control over the procedure, and the assistant is restricted to providing only limited help. Furthermore, skill and time management place restrictions on the use of the fiberoptic intubation due to rapid oxygen desaturation in patients with hemodynamic and respiratory-related comorbidities, airway masses, or redundant mucosa in some cases of OSA, which increase morbidity and mortality [47]. In an attempt to overcome these challenges, a combined intubation technique using fiberoptic bronchoscopic intubation assisted via video laryngoscope (Fibroscopic Assisted Video-laryngoscopic Intubation; FAVI) for difficult airways was described in 2004 by Doyle [48]. This combination increases the visualization of the airway and provides a more holistic view of the airway. This definitely translates into lower morbidity and mortality if conducted properly and by an experienced operator. The technique is performed by a team: an operator and an assistant. The VL is introduced by the assistant for a broad inspection of the area and appropriately identifying key landmarks (epiglottis, arytenoids, false vocal cords, and true vocal cords), followed by the introduction of the fiberoptic bronchoscope with a loaded endotracheal tube. The operator then introduces the fiberscope and advances it toward the vocal cords. After confirmation of entering the trachea, the tube is pushed gently through the cords, and with the help of the wider view provided by VL, trauma to airway structures is avoided [49].

26.3.5 Use of Supraglottic Airway Devices (SADs) as Intubating Adjuncts

Despite the great maneuverability of fiberoptic devices, they can be difficult to manipulate in an anesthetized patient because the collapse of airway muscles will close the space required to navigate the scope easily or the redundant mucosa of the upper airway in OSA patient will jostle the scope. Even with the use of fiberscope-specific oropharyngeal airways (e.g., Ovassapian plastic oropharyngeal airway), it might still be difficult, especially in the case of redundant mucosa. In this regard, SADs can provide a good conduit to fiberscopes to maintain the patency of the airway, in addition to maintaining oxygenation and ventilation throughout the procedure. This is particularly useful in critical patients and difficult airways, where procedure time might be stretched due to technical challenges. An endotracheal tube may be railroaded over a bronchoscope through the SAD, or an Aintree Intubating Catheter (Cook Critical Care, Bloomington, IN, USA) may be advanced over the bronchoscope into the trachea through the SAD, then both the fiberscope and SAD are removed leaving the intubating catheter in situ, acting as a "railroading" device for endotracheal tube, or can also be used as a ventilating device buying more time to the anesthetist.

26.3.6 Awake Fiberoptic Intubation (AFOI)

AFOI stands as the best technique for a predicted difficult airway. The safety net provided by the patient himself being awake and controlling his airway until it is secured using an endotracheal tube gives the operator a relatively relaxed working condition. Difficult Airway Society (DAS) has recently published a set of guidelines for awake tracheal intubation in adults, which outlines the best practices to conduct a safe AFOI [50]. It is of paramount importance to provide adequate topical anesthesia to the airway to avoid patient discomfort, coughing, and physiological responses associated with stimulation of the upper airway. The practice is now shifted from invasive airway blocks to the "spray-as-you-go" approach, which gives similar outcomes with fewer risks. The maximum dose of lidocaine should not exceed 9 mg/kg of body weight. Operators should be alert to the great ability of mucous membranes to absorb large amounts of drugs that are sprayed on, and it is fairly easy to hit toxicity if the operator is not cautious enough [50]. Mild to moderate sedation also facilitates the procedure. Among drugs used for sedation, remifentanil target-controlled infusion (TCI) appears to provide better conditions for AFOI when compared with propofol TCI in normal-weight patients. Dexmedetomidine is another option, providing favorable intubation conditions during AFOI, without respiratory depression and airway obstruction. However, evidence about the best sedation technique for AFOI in obese, especially those suffering from OSA, is still lacking. Sedation should ideally be administered by an independent practitioner, and it should not be used as a substitute for inadequate airway topicalization [50]. Supplemental oxygen should always be administered during awake tracheal intubation. There should be no more than three attempts, with one further attempt by a more experienced operator (3 + 1 rule) [50].

26.3.7 The Role of Tracheostomy

Despite all the different techniques that can safely secure the airway, it is important to keep Front of Neck Access or Airway (FONA) also ready, as it might come to the point that FONA would be life-saving. In some selected cases, the only way to secure the airway properly and safely is a temporary tracheostomy. This can be done under local anesthesia in an awake patient. Percutaneous Dilatational Tracheostomy (PDT) has been compared extensively to surgical tracheostomy (ST), with a favorable profile characterized by fewer wound infections, lower rates of clinically significant bleeding, and significant cost savings [51]. This procedure, however, is done with endotracheal tube inserted and entails the bronchoscopic-guided insertion of a needle into the trachea, followed by insertion of a guidewire into the lumen, and then serial dilation via the Seldinger technique. Thus, and despite having a favorable safety profile, it cannot replace awake ST in the case of non-intubated patients where placing a tube is expected to be extremely challenging or nearly impossible. Relative contraindications for PDT include but are not limited to uncorrectable coagulopathy, inability to extend the neck, cervical spine instability, aberrant neck vasculature, distortion of the anterior tracheal anatomy, overlying cellulitis or the most important which is unavailability of surgeon who can perform revision/open tracheostomy. Although safe and effective, PDT is not without risk. Of complications known to be associated with PDT, trachea-innominate artery fistulas and posterior tracheal injury tend to be the most feared.

26.4 Intraoperative Management

Unless indicated by patients' comorbidities, invasive monitoring beyond the ASA standard is not recommended for patients with OSA. The level of monitoring should also be established according to the nature of the scheduled surgical procedure. All anesthetic induction agents are known to decrease the tone of pharyngeal musculature that acts to maintain airway patency. Choosing one agent over another is based on the nature and the length of the procedure. It is prudent to use shorter acting-agents, avoid large doses of opioids that will continue exerting their action into the postoperative period, causing excessive sedation and hypoventilation, and avoid use of neuromuscular blocking agents (NMBA) as long as feasible, or use rocuronium as it has a specific reversal agent (sugammadex) that will ensure complete recovery (if used with appropriate dosage and backed by neuromuscular monitoring) [52]. This strategy will allow patients to return quickly to their baseline physiology and decrease the potential risks.

26.4.1 Mechanical Ventilation

The perfect mechanical ventilation strategy for obese patients undergoing general anesthesia is a question asked by many clinical studies. In a recent meta-analysis by Wang et al. [53], it was found that a combination of volume-controlled ventilation, associated with high positive end expiratory pressure (PEEP) value and lung recruitment maneuvers (collectively known as Protective Lung Ventilation Strategies; PLVS), is superior to other strategies of reducing the risk of atelectasis and hypoxemia and to improve oxygenation and intraoperative pulmonary compliance. Obese patients would benefit of PLVS that can be effectively applied during general anesthesia [54].

26.4.2 Special, Possibly Life-Threatening, Situations

There is always a risk of bleeding in OSA surgery, which can be serious and life-threatening. LASER is used for a more precise cut and better hemostasis. This, however, increases the risk of airway fires, in addition to other risks of using LASER in the operating theatre. Aside from OSA surgery, and generally speaking, there is always a risk of accidental intraoperative extubation, especially in the head and neck area. Taking into consideration difficulties in managing OSA patients' airways, such an event might be catastrophic under anesthesia and during surgery, and it cannot be stressed more how securing the endotracheal tube in position in this category of patients is of paramount importance and life-saving.

26.4.3 Transoral Robotic Surgery (TORS) and LASER for Epiglottoplasty

Numerous studies have shown that transoral robotic surgery (TORS) for oropharyngeal cancers is safe and yields satisfactory functional and oncological outcomes. It is increasingly considered a standard surgical approach with eligible patients. It is increasingly being used and described in the context of laryngeal cancer surgery as an alternative to open approaches, which may yield inconsistent functional results and significant rates of postoperative complications. It may also be an alternative to definitive radiotherapy, which entails significant early and late toxicities. TORS has been explored as an alternative to endoscopic LASER surgery in patients with difficult exposure, even though there is still a lack of evidence about which procedure provides better visualization of the vocal cords [55, 56]. However, several studies have tested TORS in cases of the enlarged base of tongue and epiglottis as a cause of OSA with promising outcomes that invite more research [57, 58]. In the case of LASER surgery, airway fire should be prevented and monitored closely during the surgery, and the anesthesia team should be ready for management at any time. During TORS surgery, the endotracheal tube should be resistant to compression from the robotic arms, thus requiring a wire-reinforced tube. These tubes resist compression well, but if compressed above their resistance threshold, they will buckle and then remain compressed [59].

26.5 Safe Extubation

The critical moments in airway management are intubation, time during the transfer, and extubation, with extubation ranking high in terms of risk of significant morbidity and mortality to the patients. Difficult Airway Society (DAS) developed guidelines [60] to standardize the process of tracheal extubation, minimizing patients' risk, in a stepwise approach. It starts with risk stratification of patients as high or low risk of complication during extubation.

High-risk patients include patients with:

- Severe cardiopulmonary disease.
- Congenital or acquired airway pathology.
- Morbid obesity.
- OSA.
- Severe gastroesophageal reflux.
- Patients who needed multiple attempts at intubation.

Contributing surgical factors include:

- Recurrent laryngeal nerve damage (10.6% in malignant thyroids).
- Hematoma (0.1–1.1% post-laryngeal/thyroid surgery).
- Edema and distortion of anatomy after head and neck surgery.
- Posterior fossa surgery.
- Inter-maxillary fixation.
- Drainage of the deep neck and dental abscesses.

Morbidly obese and OSA patients are regarded as high-risk, and a set of specific recommendations are suggested focused on awake tracheal extubation, managing logistics and equipment, the importance of skilled assistance, and choosing the location of extubation (operating room vs. ICU). The DAS guidelines also underline the importance of extubation over airway exchange catheters in patients for whom tracheal re-intubation is likely to be difficult. There are two schools of extubation: "Deep" and "Fully Awake." When it comes to patients with OSA, deep extubation is not an option, as the risk of airway collapse and obstruction, up to developing negative pressure pulmonary edema, is significant, and this becomes more essential if it is an airway surgery. The rationale behind extubating in a fully awake state is to ensure that all protective airway reflexes are back, and the patient can take deep breathes which will prevent atelectasis and reduce the rate of postoperative pulmonary complications. This will also enable the anesthetist to apply CPAP with full cooperation from the patient's side. Some anesthetists practice deep extubation to avoid the pressor response associated with fully awake ones, and this might be true in patients with ischemic heart disease, but the risk of airway collapse might outweigh the risk of having a sympathetic surge and straining the cardiovascular system. However, fully awake extubation does not and should not mean a struggling patient. Patient comfort should be maintained throughout the process. To achieve this, there is number of prerequisites that must be met (pre-extubation criteria):

- Arterial blood gases: Homeostasis and acid-base balance should be restored if they were disturbed for any reason intraoperatively. A large proportion of OSA patients tolerates high levels of CO_2, so "normal" CO_2 might not be a good target. The patient's baseline should be checked, and the aim is to return back to it.
- Adequate reversal of muscle blockade and confirming it with neuromuscular monitoring.
- Ensure that no residual sedatives are in circulation. Last doses of opioids should be distanced from extubation time, and opioid infusion and "context-sensitive

half-life" should be taken into consideration. If an inhalational agent is to be used, there's no conclusive evidence of the superiority of desflurane to other agents, despite having faster wash-in and wash-out times. The results of the studies conducted comparing desflurane to sevoflurane failed to demonstrate a consistent profile, and if carefully titrated to effect with the help of bispectral index (BIS), sevoflurane can give a favorable quick recovery much similar to desflurane [61–67].

- Performing a "cuff-leak test" might be advised.
- Nasopharyngeal airway might be a good option, as it is better tolerated by patients.
- Upper airway examination by fiberscope or video-scope to assess suitability for extubation: in some cases, especially with longstanding pathology or in airway surgeries, edema can render extubation risky. Therefore, a fiberscopic examination would identify potential risks and help decrease associated morbidity and mortality, and decrease the rate of reintubations, that would be an emergency ill-planned intubation should the airway become obstructed later due to edema, secretions, bleeding, or other causes.
- Patient at a head-up position, or head-up and lateral position for recovery: in sedated children examined by MRI, the area of the upper airway (the oropharynx, nasopharynx, and larynx) increased in the lateral position compared to the supine position, which translates into less chance of obstruction if extubation was performed in this position [68, 69]. However, this technique has not been studied in adults, although some experts would argue for a comparable outcome if applied to the adult population, given that in paralyzed adults under GA in lateral position, the same effect on the total cross-section is observed, as a note by Isono et al. [70]. The mechanism of this phenomenon is unknown but thought to be due to gravitational effects [68]. Since anesthesia induction and intubation are generally performed in the supine position, the supine position is familiar and comfortable for anesthetists, but lateral position technique should be considered in selected patients, nonetheless. One of the reasons anesthetists may refrain from recovery and extubation in lateral position is the inability to re-intubate easily, despite the evidence pointing to the contrary [71, 72]. This is, of course, a skill that needs training and is not orthodox in anesthesia training worldwide [73].

In case of expected difficult extubation, a number of strategies can be implemented to reduce the risk of failed extubation or losing the airway, in addition to fulfilling the pre-extubation aforementioned checklist:

- Use of steroids to decrease airway edema.
- Staged extubation over the wire (Fig. 26.5).
- Use of Tritube® (Ventinova Medical B.V., Eindhoven, The Netherlands) as the airway management technique and keep it inside the airway during recovery; it is a small-caliber tube (4.4 mm outer diameter) and would be tolerated by the patient allowing smooth recovery and backup ventilation should the weaning and extubation protract or fails (Fig. 26.6).

- Airway exchange catheters (Fig. 26.7).
- Bailey maneuver (exchange to SAD).
- Abandon extubation altogether and delay it for 24 h, To be performed in the ICU after some time and after airway rest.
- Tracheostomy, as a temporary measure, should always be an option on the table, and some patients would have no other safe alternative.

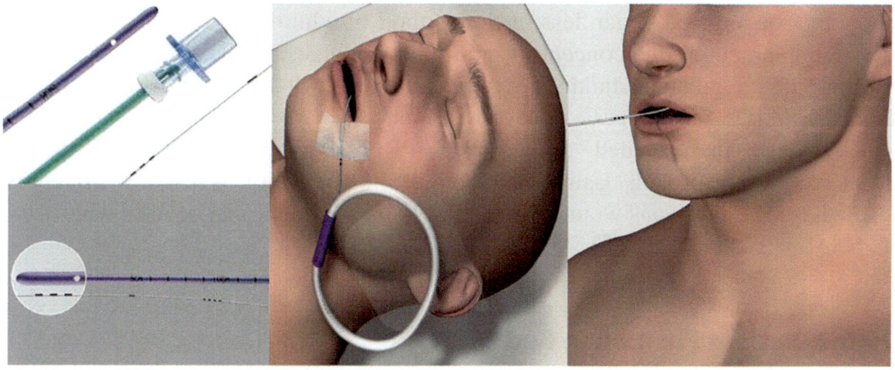

Fig. 26.5 Staged extubation set with wire

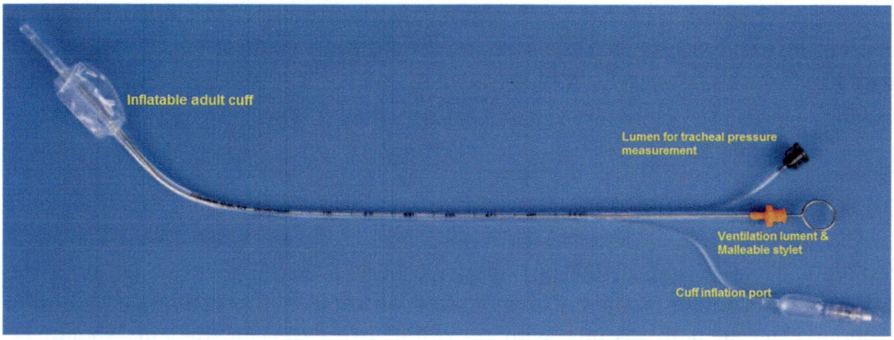

Fig. 26.6 Tritube

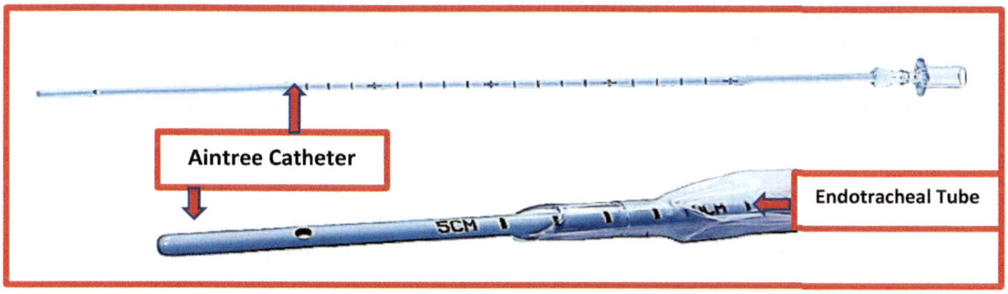

Fig. 26.7 Airway exchange catheter

26.6 Postoperative Care Management

26.6.1 Postoperative Analgesia

Managing postoperative analgesia for patients with OSA is a challenging task for any anesthetist, as a fine balance between patient comfort and potential side effects of opioids (hypoventilation and apnea) should be maintained. That is why the use of strong opioids (e.g., morphine, buprenorphine, and oxycodone) should be avoided altogether or reduced, regardless of the method of administration. This is an area where implementing the concept of multimodal analgesia makes great difference, by combining regional techniques (if applicable), Non-Steroidal Anti-Inflammatory Drugs (NSAIDs), an analgesic dose of ketamine, and paracetamol at pre-established times rather than as needed "pro re neta," (PRN) schedule, to reduce the needed doses of systemic opioids. Using weak opioids, like tramadol, as rescue treatment is also advised. Continuous wound infusion of local anesthetic can be used with comparable analgesic effects [74, 75].

26.6.2 Patient Position in Bed

As it is important during anesthesia induction, a 25–30° head-up position during the patient's stay in the post-anesthesia care unit (PACU) and in the ward increases upper airway stability [76]. This should be clearly mentioned in the postoperative nursing instructions. Again, as it was advised during extubation, lateral position with head-up can be used for postoperative nursing as it would decrease the chance of obstruction.

26.6.3 Oxygenation, Lung Recruitment, and CPAP

Supplementary oxygen in the postoperative period should be provided until the patient can maintain preoperative saturation on room air (i.e., return to baseline without external help). Along with providing extra oxygen, patients should be instructed to do "breathing exercise" or incentive spirometry, which recruits collapsed alveoli, decreasing the rate of atelectasis [77]. Significant atelectasis can cause ventilation/perfusion mismatch and consequent hypoxemia. Unresolved or neglected collapse can lead to pneumonia [78]. Moreover, CPAP application pre- and post-operatively can significantly reduce the rate of respiratory complications, especially if the patient was using CPAP at home [77]. In such patients, CPAP should be instituted in the same settings as their home settings. However, CPAP may not be useful in opioid-induced airway collapse, and prevention (by reducing the use of opioids) is always advised. It is worth mentioning that the team should be open to all possibilities, including the need to invasively ventilate a patient should he fail to respond to such non-invasive measures.

26.6.4 Ward Versus Intensive Care Unit (ICU)?

Patients disposition either to their normal beds, high dependency unit (HDU) (level I care), or ICU (level II care) is a multifactorial decision. Patients with OSA usually need adequate monitoring (SpO_2, ECG, heart rate, blood pressure, and transcutaneous CO_2 if available) and surveillance during the first 24 h post-operatively, but the level of this monitoring can be a ward nurse in simple cases with mild to moderate OSA, up to ICU with one-to-one care in cases with severe OSA and OSA-related complications. It is, of course, a preoperative decision, but it can also be revisited in the PACU, as the preoperative estimations may be under- or overdoing it. In most cases, patients who have complications in the immediate postoperative period (i.e., in PACU) will have recurring adverse events and should therefore be monitored in a higher level of care [79]. The American Society of Anesthesiology recommends a median of 3 h longer postoperative monitoring in patients with OSA after ambulatory surgery and 7 h of post-operative monitoring after the last episode of airway obstruction or hypoxemia while breathing room air in an unstimulated environment prior to discharge [80]. The organizational factors and readiness to handle such patients should also be taken into account. For more details, you can visit the algorithm of the Italian Society of Anesthesia, Analgesia, Resuscitation, and Intensive Care (SIAARTI)/Italian Association of Sleep Medicine (AIMS) Recommendations [81].

26.6.5 Criteria for Discharge Home

The literature is insufficient to offer guidance regarding the appropriate time for discharge of OSA patients at increased perioperative risk from the surgical facility to an unmonitored setting (i.e., home). Patients at increased perioperative risk from OSA should not be discharged from the hospital until they are no longer at risk of postoperative respiratory depression, which can be established by observing patients if they are able to maintain adequate oxygen saturation level on room air, in an unstimulated environment, preferably while asleep [82]. Prior to discharge, patients with known OSA on Continuous Positive Airway Pressure/Bilevel Positive Airway Pressure (CPAP/BiPAP) therapy and their caregivers should be educated to use their CPAP/BiPAP therapy whenever sleeping. If the patient has a history of non-compliance, education should be provided regarding the risks of untreated OSA, and barriers that resulted in non-compliance should be identified and addressed [83]. Before discharge, an OSA treatment plan should be in place for timely follow-up care. This plan should inform the patient of the next steps for effective treatment and compliance with CPAP/BiPAP therapy [83].

26.7 Obstructive Sleep Apnea (OSA) and Postoperative Complications

According to a recent meta-analysis, patients having OSA who are undergoing non-cardiac surgery are more prone to cardiorespiratory complications compared to non-OSA patients. These complications include, but are not limited to, desaturation in the postoperative phase, respiratory failure, cardiac events, and unplanned transferals to ICUs [84]. It is the effect of the hypnotic sedative agents used in general anesthesia or sedation that causes these patients to have such complications. The pharyngeal muscles are prone to collapse, closing the airway, which might be augmented by the sedative effect of anesthesia, leading to respiratory complications. This periodic collapse/reopening of the airway causes hypoventilation and acidosis, sympathetic activation, and hypoxia, which eventually leads to the various cardiovascular complications associated with OSA [82–84]. The risk of OSA may not normalize for several nights postoperatively, with the greatest risk on postoperative night three. Later, the disturbance and rebound in Rapid Eye Movement (REM) sleep, caused by administration of high doses of opioids in the postoperative period, which suppress REM, causes sleep deprivation and related consequences [85].

26.8 Conclusion

OSA is associated with a number of upper airway anatomical and physiological changes that pose a significant challenge to perioperative care. The effects of sedatives, analgesics, and anesthetics can worsen OSA airway and ventilation. OSA has a three-to-four-fold higher risk of DI when compared to non-OSA patients. Acute and chronic pathologies of the epiglottis that cause OSA, despite being uncommon, mandate attention from both anesthetist and surgeon, as they impose certain challenges to both diagnosis and management. The golden rule in an OSA patient is the maintenance of airway control either by the patient or by the anesthetist. Extubation is a critical time in the management of OSA patients and should be well planned ahead with multiple layers of safety.

References

1. Yang CC, Lee KW, Watanabe K, Kawakami N. The association between shift work and possible obstructive sleep apnea: a systematic review and meta-analysis. Int Arch Occup Environ Health. 2021;94(8):1763–72. https://doi.org/10.1007/s00420-021-01675-1.
2. Paul EP, Young T, Jodi HB, Mari P, Erika WH, Khin MH. Increased prevalence of sleep-disordered breathing in adults. Am J Epidemiol. 2013;177(9):1006–14. https://doi.org/10.1093/aje/kws342.
3. Ahlin S, Manco M, Panunzi S, et al. A new sensitive and accurate model to predict moderate to severe obstructive sleep apnea in patients with obesity. Medicine (Baltimore). 2019;98(32):e16687. https://doi.org/10.1097/MD.0000000000016687.

4. Peppard PE, Young T, Palta M, Dempsey J, Skatrud J. Longitudinal study of moderate weight change and sleep-disordered breathing. JAMA. 2000;284(23):3015–21. https://doi.org/10.1001/jama.284.23.3015.
5. Redline S, Tishler PV, Tosteson TD, Williamson J, Kump K, Browner I, Ferrette V, Krejci P. The familial aggregation of obstructive sleep apnea. Am J Respir Crit Care Med. 1995;151(3 I):682–7. https://doi.org/10.1164/ajrccm.151.3.7881656.
6. Calais CJ, Robertson BD, Beakes DE. Association of allergy/immunology and obstructive sleep apnea. Allergy Asthma Proc. 2016;37(6):443–9. https://doi.org/10.2500/aap.2016.37.4001. PMID: 27931299.
7. Jiang RS, Liang KL, Hsin CH, Su MC. The impact of chronic rhinosinusitis on sleep-disordered breathing. Rhinology. 2016;54(1):75–9.
8. Nakata A, Takahashi M, Ikeda T, Haratani T, Hojou M, Araki S. Perceived job stress and sleep-related breathing disturbance in Japanese male workers. Soc Sci Med. 2007;64(12):2520–32.
9. Jiang T, Tao N, Shi L, Ning L, Liu J. Associations between occupational stress and demographic characteristics in petroleum workers in the Xinjiang arid desert. Medicine (Baltimore). 2018;97(31):e11543. https://doi.org/10.1097/MD.0000000000011543. PMID: 30075521; PMCID: PMC6081070.
10. Amos JM, Durr ML, Nardone HC, Baldassari CM, Duggins A, Ishman SL. Systematic review of drug-induced sleep endoscopy scoring systems. Otolaryngol Head Neck Surg. 2018;158(2):240–8. https://doi.org/10.1177/0194599817737966.
11. Catalfumo FJ, Golz A, Westerman ST, Gilbert LM, Joachims HZ, Goldenberg D. The epiglottis and obstructive sleep apnoea syndrome. J Laryngol Otol. 1998;112(10):940–3. https://doi.org/10.1017/s0022215100142136. PMID: 10211216
12. Dedhia RC, Rosen CA, Soose RJ. What is the role of the larynx in adult obstructive sleep apnea? Laryngoscope. 2014;124(4):1029–34. https://doi.org/10.1002/lary.24494).
13. Kim HY, Sung CM, Jang HB, Kim HC, Lim SC, Yang HC. Patients with epiglottic collapse showed less severe obstructive sleep apnea and good response to treatment other than continuous positive airway pressure: a case-control study of 224 patients. J Clin Sleep Med. 2021;17:413–9. https://doi.org/10.5664/jcsm.8904.
14. Kuo IC, Hsin LJ, Lee LA, Fang TJ, Tsai MS, Lee YC, Shen SC, Li HY. Prediction of Epiglottic collapse in obstructive sleep apnea patients: epiglottic length. Nature Sci Sleep. 2021;13:1985–92. https://doi.org/10.2147/NSS.S336019.
15. Saita V, Azzolina A, Galia A, Fraggetta F. Schwannoma of the epiglottis: case report focusing on clinico-pathological aspects. Acta Otorhinolaryngol Ital. 2005;25(6):378–80.
16. Rahbar R, Litrovnik BG, Vargas SO, et al. The biology and management of laryngeal neurofibroma. Arch Otolaryngol Head Neck Surg. 2004;130(12):1400–6. https://doi.org/10.1001/archotol.130.12.1400.
17. Abdallah C. Acute epiglottitis: trends, diagnosis and management. Saudi J Anaesth. 2012;6(3):279–81. https://doi.org/10.4103/1658-354X.101222. PMID: 23162404; PMCID: PMC3498669.
18. Ahmad I, Keane O, Muldoon S. Enhancing airway assessment of patients with head and neck pathology using virtual endoscopy. Indian J Anaesth. 2017;61:782–6. https://doi.org/10.4103/ija.IJA_588_17.
19. Shallik N, Zaghw A, Dogan Z, Rahman W. The use of virtual endoscopy for diagnosis of traumatic supra-glottic airway stenosis. J Clin Anesthesiol. 2017;2:1–3.
20. Das KM, Lababidi H, Al Dandan S, Raja S, Sakkijha H, Al Zoum M, et al. Computed tomography virtual bronchoscopy: Normal variants, pitfalls, and spectrum of common and rare pathology. Can Assoc Radiol J. 2015;66:58–70. https://doi.org/10.1016/j.carj.2013.10.002.
21. Prokakis C, Koletsis EN, Dedeilias P, Fligou F, Filos K, Dougenis D. Airway trauma: a review on epidemiology, mechanisms of injury, diagnosis and treatment. J Cardiothorac Surg. 2014;9:1–8. https://doi.org/10.1186/1749-8090-9-117.
22. Xiong H, Huang X, Li Y, Li J, Xian J, Huang Y. A method for accurate reconstructions of the upper airway using magnetic resonance images. PLoS One. 2015;10:1–14. https://doi.org/10.1371/journal.pone.0130186.

23. Shallik NA, Moustafa AH, Marcus MAE, (Eds.). Virtual endoscopy and 3D reconstruction in the airways. 1st ed. Cham: Springer; 2019. https://doi.org/10.1007/978-3-030-23253-5.
24. Corso RM, Petrini F, Buccioli M, et al. Clinical utility of preoperative screening with STOP-Bang questionnaire in elective surgery. Minerva Anestesiol. 2014;80(8):877–84.
25. Cattano D, Killoran PV, Cai C, Katsiampoura AD, Corso RM, Hagberg CA. Difficult mask ventilation in general surgical population: observation of risk factors and predictors. F1000Res. 2014;27(3):204.
26. Apfelbaum JL, Hagberg CA, et al. 2022 American Society of Anesthesiologists Practice Guidelines for Management of the Difficult Airway. Anesthesiology. 2022;136:31–81. https://doi.org/10.1097/ALN.0000000000004002.
27. Levitan R, Rescuing intubation. Simple techniques to improve airway visualization. JEMS. 2001;26(3):36–42, 44–6, 48–9 passim. PMID: 11263129.
28. Schmitt HJ, Mang H. Head and neck elevation beyond the sniffing position improves laryngeal view in cases of difficult direct laryngoscopy. J Clin Anesth. 2002;14(5):335–8. https://doi.org/10.1016/s0952-8180(02)00368-9. PMID: 12208436.
29. Cattano D, Melnikov V, Khalil Y, Sridhar S, Hagberg CA. An evaluation of the rapid airway management positioner in obese patients undergoing gastric bypass or laparoscopic gastric banding surgery. Obes Surg. 2010;20(10):1436–41.
30. Higgs A, BA MG, Goddard C, Rangasami J, Suntharalingam G, Gale R, Cook TM, Difficult Airway Society, Intensive Care Society, Faculty of Intensive Care Medicine; Royal College of Anaesthetists. Guidelines for the management of tracheal intubation in critically ill adults. Br J Anaesth. 2018;120(2):323–52. https://doi.org/10.1016/j.bja.2017.10.021. Epub 2017 Nov 26. PMID: 29406182.
31. Vourc'h M, Huard D, Feuillet F, et al. Preoxygenation in difficult airway management: high-flow oxygenation by nasal cannula versus face mask (the PREOPTIDAM study). Protocol for a single-Centre randomised study. BMJ Open. 2019;9:e025909. https://doi.org/10.1136/bmjopen-2018-025909.
32. Patel A, Nouraei SAR. Transnasal humidified rapid insufflation ventilatory exchange (THRIVE): a physiological method of increasing apnoea time in patients with difficult airways. Anaesthesia. 2015;70:323e9.
33. El-Ganzouri AR, McCarthy RJ, Tuman KJ, et al. Preoperative airway assessment: predictive value of a multivariate risk index. Anesth Analg. 1996;82:1197–204.
34. Corso RM, Cattano D, Buccioli M, Carretta E, Maitan S. Post analysis simulated correlation of the El-Ganzouri airway difficulty score with difficult airway. Braz J Anesthesiol. 2016;66(3):298–303. https://doi.org/10.1016/j.bjane.2014.09.003. Epub 2014 Nov 27. PMID: 27108828.
35. Cortellazzi P, Minati L, Falcone C, Lamperti M, Caldiroli D. Predictive value of the El-Ganzouri multivariate risk index for difficult tracheal intubation: a comparison of Glidescope videolaryngoscopy and conventional Macintosh laryngoscopy. Br J Anaesth. 2007;99(6):906–11.
36. Manatpon P, Weyh AM, Gray C, Shah S, Dasika J. Airway management for an adult epiglottic abscess. Cureus. 2020;12(1):e6771. https://doi.org/10.7759/cureus.6771. PMID: 32140338; PMCID: PMC7039351.
37. Cattano D, Corso RM, Altamirano AV, Patel CB, Meese MM, Seitan C, Hagberg CA. Clinical evaluation of the C-MAC D-blade videolaryngoscope in severely obese patients: a pilot study. Br J Anaesth. 2012;109(4):647–8.
38. Brozek T, Bruthans J, Porizka M, Blaha J, Ulrichova J, Michalek P. A Randomized Comparison of Non-Channeled GlidescopeTM Titanium Versus Channeled KingVisionTM Videolaryngoscope for Orotracheal Intubation in Obese Patients with BMI> 35 kg· m− 2. Diagnostics. 2020;10(12):1024.
39. Kumar D, Gombar S, Ahuja V, Malhotra A, Gupta S. GlideScope versus D-blade for tracheal intubation in cervical spine patients: a randomised controlled trial. Indian J Anaesth. 2019;63(7):544–50. https://doi.org/10.4103/ija.IJA_3_19.
40. Huang P, Zhou R, Lu Z, et al. GlideScope® versus C-MAC®(D) videolaryngoscope versus Macintosh laryngoscope for double lumen endotracheal intubation in patients with predicted

normal airways: a randomized, controlled, prospective trial. BMC Anesthesiol. 2020;20:119. https://doi.org/10.1186/s12871-020-01012-y.
41. Serocki G, Neumann T, Scharf E, Dörges V, Cavus E. Indirect videolaryngoscopy with C-MAC D-blade and GlideScope: a randomized, controlled comparison in patients with suspected difficult airways. Minerva Anestesiol. 2013;79(2):121–9. Epub 2012 Oct 2. PMID: 23032922.
42. Rieger A, Hass I, Gross M, Gramm HJ, Eyrich K. Intubationstraumen des Larynx--eine Literaturübersicht unter besonderer Berücksichtigung der Aryknorpelluxation [Intubation trauma of the larynx--a literature review with special reference to arytenoid cartilage dislocation]. Anasthesiol Intensivmed Notfallmed Schmerzther. 1996;31(5):281–7. https://doi.org/10.1055/s-2007-995921.
43. Oh TK, Yun JY, Ryu CH, Park YN, Kim NW. Arytenoid dislocation after uneventful endotracheal intubation: a case report. Korean J Anesthesiol. 2016;69(1):93–6. https://doi.org/10.4097/kjae.2016.69.1.93.
44. Pacheco-Lopez PC, Berkow LC, Hillel AT, Akst LM. Complications of airway management. Respir Care. 2014;59(6):1006–21. https://doi.org/10.4187/respcare.02884.
45. Van Zundert A, Van Zundert T, Brimacombe J. Downfolding of the epiglottis during intubation. Anesth Analg. 2010;110(4):1246–7. https://doi.org/10.1213/ANE.0b013e3181ce716f.
46. Aoyama K, Takenaka I, Nagaoka E, et al. Potential damage to the larynx associated with light-guided intubation: a case and series of Fiberoptic examinations. Anesthesiology. 2001;94:165–7. https://doi.org/10.1097/00000542-200101000-00030.
47. Rainer L, Burkhart MT, Brock GN, et al. Is video laryngoscope-assisted flexible tracheoscope intubation feasible for patients with predicted difficult airway? A prospective, randomized clinical trial. Anesth Analg. 2014;118(6):1259–65. https://doi.org/10.1213/ANE.0000000000000220.
48. Doyle DJ. GlideScope-assisted Fiberoptic intubation: a new airway teaching method. Anesthesiology. 2004;101(5):1252.
49. Francisco OV, Cecil BR, Aaron S, Shannan CC. Videolaryngoscope assisted fiberoptic bronchoscopy for difficult intubation in upper airway cancer. Glob J Oto. 2018;14(3):555888. https://doi.org/10.19080/GJO.2018.14.555888.
50. Ahmad I, El-Boghdadly K, Bhagrath R, Hodzovic I, et al. Difficult airway society guidelines for awake tracheal intubation (ATI) in adults. Anaesthesia. 2020;75(4):509–28. https://doi.org/10.1111/anae.14904.
51. Putensen C, Theuerkauf N, Guenther U, Vargas M, Pelosi P. Percutaneous and surgical tracheostomy in critically ill adult patients: a meta-analysis. Crit Care. 2014;18(6):544.
52. Ankichetty S, Wong J, Chung F. A systematic review of the effects of sedatives and anesthetics in patients with obstructive sleep apnea. J Anaesthesiol Clin Pharmacol. 2011;27(4):447–58.
53. Wang C, Zhao N, Wang W, Guo L, Guo L, Chi C, Wang X, Pi X, Cui Y, Li E. Intraoperative mechanical ventilation strategies for obese patients: a systematic review and network meta-analysis. Obes Rev. 2015;16(6):508–17.
54. Young CC, Harris EM, Vacchiano C, Bodnar S, Bukowy B, Elliott RRD, Migliarese J, Ragains C, Trethewey B, Woodward A, Gama de Abreu M, Girard M, Futier E, Mulier JP, Pelosi P, Sprung J. Lung-protective ventilation for the surgical patient: international expert panel-based consensus recommendations. Br J Anaesth. 2019;123(6):898–913. https://doi.org/10.1016/j.bja.2019.08.017. Epub 2019 Oct 3. PMID: 31587835.
55. Gorphe P. A contemporary review of evidence for Transoral robotic surgery in laryngeal cancer. Front Oncol. 2018;8:121. https://doi.org/10.3389/fonc.2018.00121.
56. Arora A, Chaidas K, Garas G, et al. Outcome of TORS to tongue base and epiglottis in patients with OSA intolerant of conventional treatment. Sleep Breath. 2016;20(2):739–47.
57. Corso RM, Cattano D, Shallik NA. Transoral robotic surgery for obstructive sleep apnea syndrome: an Anesthetist's point of view. In: Vicini C, Hoff P, Montevecchi F, editors. Trans Oral robotic surgery for obstructive sleep apnea. Cham: Springer; 2016. https://doi.org/10.1007/978-3-319-34040-1_13.

58. Vauterin T, Garas G, Arora A. Transoral robotic surgery for obstructive sleep Apnoea-hypopnoea syndrome. ORL J Otorhinolaryngol Relat Spec. 2018;80(3–4):134–47. https://doi.org/10.1159/000489465. Epub 2018 Jun 22. PMID: 29936512.
59. Lee JA, Byun YJ, Nguyen SA, Lentsch EJ, Gillespie MB. Transoral robotic surgery versus plasma ablation for Tongue Base reduction in obstructive sleep apnea: meta-analysis. Otolaryngol Head Neck Surg. 2020;162(6):839–52. https://doi.org/10.1177/0194599820913533. Epub 2020 Mar 24. PMID: 32204654.
60. Popat M, Mitchell V, Dravid R, Patel A, Schampillai C, Higgs A. Difficult airway society guidelines for the management of tracheal extubation. Anaesthesia. 2012;67:318–40.
61. Vallejo AC, Sah N, Phelps AL, O'Donnell J, Romeo RC. Desflurane versus sevoflurane for laparoscopic gastroplasty in morbidly obese patients. J Clin Anesth. 2007;19(1):3–8. https://doi.org/10.1016/j.jclinane.2006.04.003.De.
62. De Baerdemaeker LEC, Jacobs S, Den Blauwen NMM, et al. Postoperative results after Desflurane or sevoflurane combined with remifentanil in morbidly obese patients. Obes Surg. 2006;16:728–33. https://doi.org/10.1381/096089206777346691.
63. De Baerdemaeker LEC, Struys MMRF, Jacobs S, et al. Optimization of desflurane administration in morbidly obese patients: a comparison with sevoflurane using an 'inhalation bolus' technique, BJA. Br J Anaesth. 2003;91(5):638–50. https://doi.org/10.1093/bja/aeg236.
64. Kaur A, Jain AK, Sehgal R, Sood J. Hemodynamics and early recovery characteristics of desflurane versus sevoflurane in bariatric surgery. J Anaesthesiol Clin Pharmacol. 2013;29(1):36–40. https://doi.org/10.4103/0970-9185.105792.
65. Arain SR, Barth CD, Shankar H, Ebert TJ. Choice of volatile anesthetic for the morbidly obese patient: sevoflurane or desflurane. J Clin Anesth. 2005;17(6):413–9. https://doi.org/10.1016/j.jclinane.2004.12.015. PMID: 16171660
66. Bansal T, Garg K, Katyal S, Sood D, Grewal A, Kumar A. A comparative study of desflurane versus sevoflurane in obese patients: effect on recovery profile. J Anaesthesiol Clin Pharmacol. 2020;36(4):541–5. https://doi.org/10.4103/joacp.JOACP_307_19.
67. La Colla A, La Albertin G, Colla MA. Faster wash-out and recovery for desflurane vs sevoflurane in morbidly obese patients when no premedication is used. Br J Anaesth. 2007;99(3):353–8. https://doi.org/10.1093/bja/aem197.
68. Litman RS, Wake N, Chan LM, et al. Effect of lateral positioning on upper airway size and morphology in sedated children. Anesthesiology. 2005;103:484–8.
69. Arai Y-CP, Fukunaga K, Hirota S, et al. The effects of chin lift and jaw thrustwhile in the lateral position on stridor score in anesthetized children with adenotonsillar hypertrophy. Anesth Analg. 2004;99:1638–41.
70. Isono S, Tanaka A, Nishino T. Lateral position decreases collapsibility of the passive pharynx in patients with obstructive sleep apnea. Anesthesiology. 2002;97:780–5.
71. Adachi YU, Satomoto M, Higuchi H. Tracheal intubation in the lateral position. Anesth Analg. 2004;99(3):952. https://doi.org/10.1213/01.ANE.0000131696.44401.0F.
72. Komatsu R, Nagata O, Sessler DI, Ozaki M. The intubating laryngeal mask airway facilitates tracheal intubation in the lateral position. Anesth Analg. 2004;98(3):858–61. https://doi.org/10.1213/01.ane.0000100741.46539.6b.
73. Bell D. Avoiding adverse outcomes when faced with 'difficulty with ventilation'. Anaesthesia. 2003;58(10):945–8. https://doi.org/10.1046/j.1365-2044.2003.03450.x. PMID: 12969034.
74. Paladini G, Di Carlo S, Musella G, et al. Continuous wound infiltration of local anesthetics in postoperative pain management: safety, efficacy and current perspectives. J Pain Res. 2020;13:285–94. https://doi.org/10.2147/JPR.S211234.
75. Rahman S, Zaghw A, Elazzouny O, Almenshid D, Rezk M, Imran MA, Alali M. Management of acute pain in obese patients with sleep apnea. In: Shallik NA, editor. Pain management in special circumstances [internet]. London: IntechOpen; 2018. https://doi.org/10.5772/intechopen.80350. [cited 2022 Feb 15]. https://www.intechopen.com/chapters/63061.
76. Neill AM, Angus SM, Sajkov D, McEvoy RD. Effects of sleep posture on upper airway stability in patients with obstructive sleep apnea. Am J Respir Crit Care Med. 1997;155:199–204.

77. Kelkar KV. Post-operative pulmonary complications after non-cardiothoracic surgery. Indian J Anaesth. 2015;59(9):599–605. https://doi.org/10.4103/0019-5049.165857.
78. Brodsky JB. Anesthesia for thoracic surgery. In: Healy EJ, PRT K, editors. Wylie and Churchill-Davidson's a practice of anesthesia. 7th ed. London: Arnold Publishers; 2003. p. 789–810.
79. Gali B, Whalen FX, Schroeder DR, Gay PC, Plevak DJ. Identification of patients at risk for postoperative respiratory complications using a preoperative obstructive sleep apnea screening tool and post-anesthesia care assessment. Anesthesiology. 2009;110(4):869–77.
80. Vasu TS, Grewal R, Doghramji K. Obstructive sleep apnea syndrome and perioperative complications: a systematic review of the literature. J Clin Sleep Med. 2012;8(2):199–20.
81. Piccioni F, Droghetti A, Bertani A, et al. Recommendations from the Italian intersociety consensus on perioperative anesthesia care in thoracic surgery (PACTS) part 1: preadmission and preoperative care. Perioper Med (Lond). 2020;9(1):37. https://doi.org/10.1186/s13741-020-00168-y.
82. American Society of Anesthesiologists Task Force on perioperative Management of Patients with Obstructive Sleep Apnea. Practice guidelines for the perioperative Management of Patients with obstructive sleep apnea: an updated report by the American Society of Anesthesiologists Task Force on perioperative Management of Patients with obstructive sleep apnea. Anesthesiology. 2014;120:268–86. https://doi.org/10.1097/ALN.0000000000000053).
83. Pre-and post-operative monitoring of the OSA patient, the American Association of Sleep Technologists (AAST) Technical Guideline, January 2020; https://www.aastweb.org/hubfs/Complete%20OSA%20Technical%20Guideline%20for%20Pre-%20and%20Post-Operative%20Monitorin_FINAL_UPDATED%20Post%20Board%20Call_1.28.2020.pdf
84. Kaw R, Chung F, Pasupuleti V, Mehta J, Gay PC, Hernandez AV. Meta-analysis of the association between obstructive sleep apnoea and postoperative outcome. Br J Anaesth. 2012;109(6):897–906.
85. Ramachandran SK, Haider N, Saran KA, Mathis M, Kim J, Morris M, O'Reilly M. Life threatening critical respiratory events: a retrospective study of postoperative patients found unresponsive during analgesic therapy. J Clin Anesth. 2011;23(3):207–13.

Future Directions

27

Mohamed Abdelwahab, Rakha Abdelwahab, and Robson Capasso

27.1 Introduction

27.1.1 The Problem

Obstructive sleep apnea (OSA) is a prevalent yet treatable chronic condition affecting over a billion subjects globally [1]. Subjects with OSA are reported to be up to 38% of the US population [2]. However, when we evaluated subjects with insurance coverage, this percentage was only 4.34% of all enrolled subjects, indicating that over 80% of the population likely remain undiagnosed [3]. Beyond debilitating quality of life daytime symptoms and possible partner sleep issues, associated oxygen desaturations seem to lead to worsened cardiovascular outcomes, including systemic hypertension, increased incidence of stroke, heart failure, atrial fibrillation, and coronary heart disease [4–8].

Managing OSA can be difficult, as phenotyping respiratory drive and airway collapsibility remains a challenge [5, 6]. Anatomical (including the craniofacial

Supplementary Information The online version contains supplementary material available at https://doi.org/10.1007/978-3-031-34992-8_27. The videos can be accessed individually by clicking the DOI link in the accompanying figure caption or by scanning this link with the SN More Media App.

M. Abdelwahab
Sleep Surgery Division, Department of Otolaryngology Head and Neck Surgery, Medical University of South Carolina, Charleston, SC, USA

R. Abdelwahab
Department of Otolaryngology, Head and Neck Surgery, School of Medicine, Mansoura University, Mansoura, Egypt

R. Capasso (✉)
Division of Sleep Surgery, Department of Otolaryngology-Head & Neck Surgery, Stanford University Medical Center, Stanford, CA, USA
e-mail: rcapasso@stanford.edu

M. Delakorda, N. de Vries (eds.), *The Role of Epiglottis in Obstructive Sleep Apnea*, https://doi.org/10.1007/978-3-031-34992-8_27

skeleton, neck dimensions, and airway soft tissue anatomy) [9, 10] and physiological (including the loop gain, arousal threshold, and transmural pressure) [11] phenotypes of OSA have been extensively studied. [12, 13] While our group has defined and continued to improve the comprehensive approach to OSA management since 1986 [14–16], an important step is to define the pattern, level, and triggers of airway collapse. This collapse occurs most commonly at the level of the Velum, but may involve the Oropharynx (lateral pharyngeal wall), tongue base and less commonly the Epiglottis (therefore the acronym VOTE), or a combination of any of the above [17–19]. The VOTE classification based on drug-induced sleep endoscopy (DISE), describing the dynamic airway obstruction, has guided and warranted reproducibility of our understanding of airway collapse during sleep.

Laryngeal obstruction in OSA results from collapse of the laryngeal inlet, formed by the epiglottis, aryepiglottic folds, the arytenoids, and the overlying mucosa. This may be primary (also known as "floppy epiglottis") (Fig. 27.1) or secondary, when the epiglottis is retro-displaced by the tongue base (Fig. 27.2). Epiglottic collapse may be difficult to treat with conservative therapies, such as oral appliances [20]

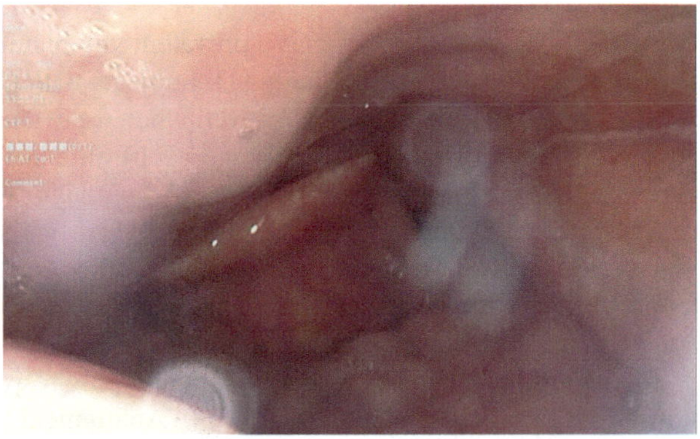

Fig. 27.1 An example of a floppy epiglottis on sleep endoscopy

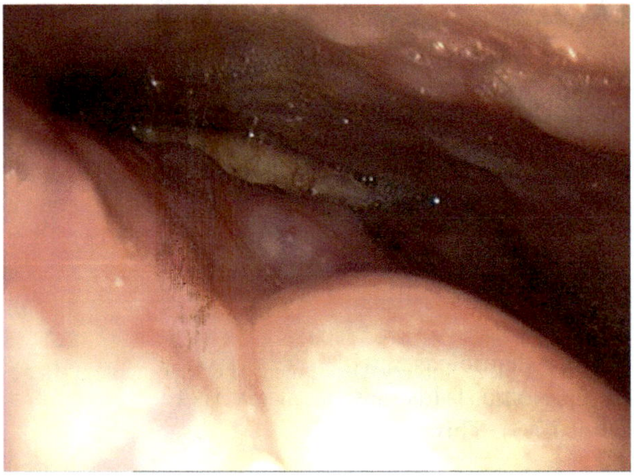

Fig. 27.2 An example of a retrodisplaced epiglottis on sleep endoscopy

and CPAP, [21] and has shown to be a predictor of OSA persistence after surgical treatments [22].

However, prior to considering a surgical intervention, it is important to investigate the following: when does the epiglottic collapse (based on DISE) requires treatment beyond positional measures, and the type of intervention required that could minimize risks of immediate and long-term swallowing dysfunction and aspiration due to a modified supraglottic anatomy.

27.1.2 Relevant Anatomy

The epiglottis is a leaf-like sheet of elastic fibrocartilage that is curled-out and laterally attached to the aryepiglottic folds. The laryngeal inlet is usually wide to avoid its collapse with inspiration according to the Bernoulli's phenomenon. The lower narrow part, the petiole, is attached to the posterior surface of the thyroid alae at their junction just above the anterior commissure. The anterior surface is separated from the hyoid and thyrohyoid membrane by pre-epiglottic space. It projects upwards and backwards behind the tongue and the hyoid bone, separated from the tongue by the vallecula. The aryepiglottic ligaments and overlying mucosa (folds) form the sides of the laryngeal inlet between the apex of arytenoid & the upper free edge of epiglottis on both sides [23, 24].

The shape can be classified into: (1) omega-shaped (sharply curved if the angle between its lateral parts was less than 90° at the central portion) epiglottis; (2) normally curved epiglottis shape; and (3) flat epiglottis. An epiglottis was classified as flat if its medial part lacked the characteristic anterior convexity [25]. In most cases of obstruction at epiglottis and/or tongue base, the epiglottis was flat (type 3), where it was lacking the typical anterior convexity in its upper part. The hypothesis was that the change of its shape is a result of degeneration of the suspensory apparatus that maintains the convexity of the epiglottis and maintains it in position. This may help identify patients with narrowing at this level [25]. Another finding was that subjects with isolated epiglottic collapse have lower mandibular plane to hyoid distance and tend to have a bigger angle of their epiglotic curvature [26]. For full details on anatomy, please review Chap. 5. Epiglottic collapse can vary based on the phenotype from a floppy epiglottis (primary) to a retro-displaced epiglottis by the tongue base (secondary) and from partial to complete collapse. The epiglottis can also collapse into two different patterns: one where it is retro-displaced in an antero-posterior (AP) direction, thereby obstructing the laryngeal inlet. This is also known as the trapdoor phenomenon. Alternatively, it can collapse in a lateral direction (omega-shaped pattern), thereby resulting in obstructing at the level of the hypopharynx or laryngeal inlet [17–19].

In pediatric cases with laryngomalacia, the epiglottis is omega-shaped, and the aryepiglottic folds are medially posed resulting in a narrow laryngeal inlet (Fig. 27.3). This narrow inlet results in collapse with inspiration presenting with

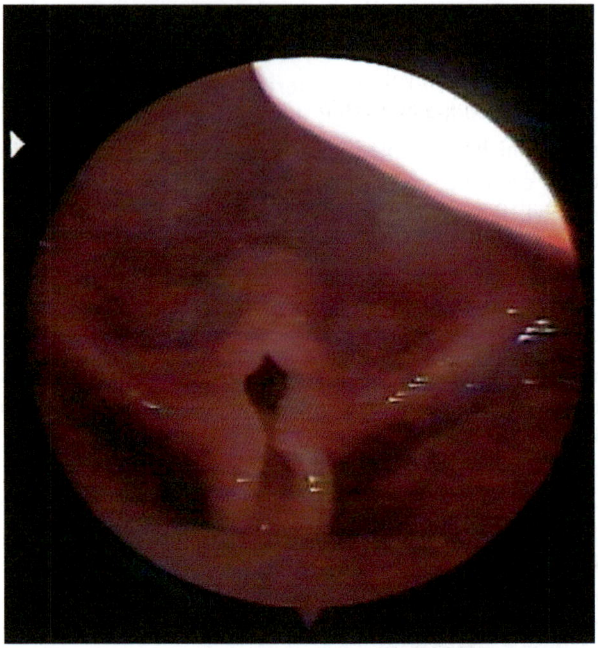

Fig. 27.3 An example of an endoscopic view of an omega shaped epiglottis in a 2-day old newborn with laryngomalacia

stridor and/or OSA. The former being the main symptom due to increasing negative pressure according to Bernoulli's effect [23, 24, 27, 28].

27.1.3 Diagnosis

Non-invasive imaging techniques such as magnetic resonance imaging (MRI) and computed tomography (CT) scan have been described to detect anatomic and functional impairments of the upper airway in OSA patients during wakefulness [29]. However, these techniques are not suitable for clinical practice due to cost and the challenge of having adequate imaging during natural sleep. While it has some limitations, DISE is the most commonly used tool for detecting the level(s), severity, and patterns of airway collapse [25]. This can guide the surgical intervention, towards either the palate, the pharynx, or the larynx.

In our practice at Stanford, we rely on manual-controlled propofol infusions. Preoperatively, the patient is given nasal decongestant (oxymetazoline). As sedation is started and before the patient is sleepy, the surgeon places the distal chip-on-tip flexible scope into the nares on the side with least obstruction. The scope is preferably passed through the middle meatus, on top of the inferior turbinate, and inferior to the middle turbinate, and advanced posteriorly until the posterior wall of the nasopharynx is reached. At this point, the scope is positioned in a rostral view (facing toward the larynx) to best visualize the airway as sedation is infused. After observing at the level of the velum that is complete and the pattern of obstruction is scored, the scope is passed distally to analyze the collapse at the level of the oropharynx. Subsequently, the scope is passed distally to observe the tongue base and epiglottis.

We also document the following in all DISE reports:

(a) Lowest O_2 saturation;
(b) Improvement of desaturation with jaw thrust.
(c) Improvement of desaturation with mouth closure.
(d) Comment on epiglottis collapse, if any, either primary or secondary to tongue base collapse.
(e) If lateral head movement improves or eliminate epiglottic collapse [30–32]·

Moreover, we report other potential structures of interest, such as mass lesions of the enlarged adenoids, posterior pharyngeal pathologies, or laryngeal pathologies of the inlet or the glottis. For full details on DISE, please review Chap. 8.

27.2 Surgical Indication (What to Know)

Surgical approach to epiglottic collapse is not without controversies and has been suggested for primary or isolated epiglottic collapse, epiglottis collapse as part of the multilevel OSA especially with tongue base collapse [21, 26, 33–35]. While epiglottic collapse is likely to fail conservative options as CPAP, positional therapy may play a role in opening the retrolingual and retro-epiglottic airway [36]. It was reported that tongue base and epiglottis collapse caused obstruction twice as frequent in positional OSA when contrasted with non-positional OSA groups [37].

When there is an association between tongue base and epiglottic collapse, it is considered that there is an additional value on simultaneous tongue base and epiglottic surgeries [34, 38–41]. There is insufficient data regarding the effect of epiglottis interventions alone, as most of the available literature describes the result of epiglottic surgery as a part of multilevel surgery for OSA patients [33]. Different shapes of the epiglottis have also been used as predictors of OSA severity [42]. In the pediatric age group, there is a more conclusive body of evidence suggesting that minimally invasive approaches in experienced hands have more substantive results. Laryngomalacia is the leading cause of congenital stridor in infants, accounting for 60%–70% of cases [28, 43]. The congenital form manifests within 2 weeks during infancy. On the other hand, non-congenital laryngomalacia presents after the age of 2 years old. Occult or state-dependent laryngomalacia presents with stridor in children, limited to sleep or exercise. Indications for surgical interventions include dyspnea, cor pulmonale, failure to thrive, cyanosis, and OSA [27, 44–49]. Supraglottoplasty has shown to improve both congenital and non-congenital laryngomalacia achieving surgical success [50].

27.3 Surgical Techniques

While the first line of treatment for OSA continues to be CPAP [51–53], former studies suggest that CPAP may be ineffective in the treatment of OSA resulting from a floppy epiglottis as it may lead to the trapdoor phenomenon described above [18]. That being said, most of the evidence available regards how CPAP may exacerbate this problem is based on case reports [21, 54–57]. Some procedures can address multiple levels of airway obstruction simultaneously, and epiglottis surgery can also be done separately or as a part of a multilevel approach for OSA. [58–62] Partial epiglottectomy is one of the procedures that provides predictable solutions for the floppy epiglottis collapses that obstructs the laryngeal inlet during sleep [34, 41, 63–68]. However, the risks of aspiration and dysphagia are present and can be of concern, and can pose a challenging decision-making situation in non-severe cases, or older patients [69, 70]. Studies have shown that combining partial epiglottectomy with other sleep surgery procedures can raise the cure rate from 50% to around 65% [63]. Commonly described procedures reported include additional midline glossectomy [34], UPPP with or without glossectomy, and hyoepiglottoplasty [41, 68, 71].

If a decision to proceed with surgery after a detailed discussion and evaluation is opted, the approaches and the surgical tools reported in this book and in the literature are variable. These include the use of diathermy [65, 66], cold instruments, CO_2 laser [65–67], coblation [72], and TORS-assisted partial epiglottectomy [41]. From a technical standpoint, there has been a change from aggressive resection to more preservative methodologies. Examples of more preservative approaches include V-shaped epiglottectomy of the upper-central part, leaving the inferior half intact to protect against aspiration [64]. CO_2 laser has been described for resection as well as for reshaping the epiglottis configuration by irradiating the superficial layers of the cartilage, resulting in warping of the epiglottis towards the radiation, in other words, anteriorly away from the airway [73]. Epiglottis stiffening procedures have also been described, after exposition of the epiglottis with direct micro-laryngoscopy, the lower half of the lingual epiglottis is cauterized in between the lateral glosso-epiglottic folds reaching the perichondrium while avoiding reaching the free margin of the epiglottis itself [35]. Hyoid suspension represents another extra-pharyngeal surgical option for epiglottic collapse with promising results [17–19, 22]. Additionally, after the introduction of upper airway stimulation surgery, studies have reported that the impact of this extrapharyngeal procedure can relieve collapse at the level of the epiglottis along with the tongue base collapse (Video 27.1) [74]. In children with congenital or non-congenital laryngomalacia and OSA, supraglottoplasty can be tailored accordingly and has been shown to be both effective and safe [49, 75]. It can be performed using cold knife [76–78], microdebrider [78], or laser techniques [79], depending on surgeon's training and preference (Fig. 27.4).

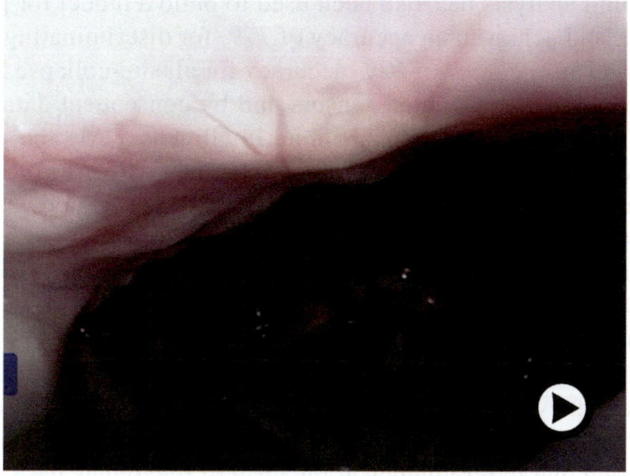

Fig. 27.4 (Video 27.1) The effect of hypoglossal nerve stimulation on velum, lateral pharyngeal wall, tongue base, and epiglottis (► https://doi.org/10.1007/000-bfw)

27.4 Future Research

The use of novel tools and mobile technology has the potential to revolutionize the way that health services are delivered, increasing access to health care at a lower cost in both developing and developed countries [80]. Future projects should focus on finding non-invasive alternatives to determine upper airway level of collapse beyond the time observed in a DISE, and correlate epiglottic collapse with airway reduction and clinically relevant daytime symptoms or other health issues. Moreover, intrapharyngeal versus extrapharyngeal procedures is another trajectory that requires careful investigations [81]. There have been recent efforts to screen for OSA with emerging technologies. For example, the SleepMinder™ (SM) is a novel non-contact device that employs radiofrequency wave technology to assess the breathing pattern, and thereby estimate OSA severity. The median SM measured AHI at home (SM-HOME) correlated significantly with polysomnography (PSG) AHI. The median SM-HOME performance against PSG in the sleep clinic cohort showed a sensitivity and specificity of 72% and 94% for AHI $\geq$ 15 [82].

Innovative, non-invasive techniques have been recently studied as additional tools or even as replacements for DISE. The shape of nasal pressure transducer flow waveforms has been suggested to identify the site-of-airway collapse with variable degrees of accuracy [83]. Pneumotachograph flow has been used to differentiate epiglottic from non-epiglottic collapse [84]. Epiglottic collapse produces particular quantifiable flow features that can be distinguished from the features produced by nonepiglottic-related obstructions and can be reliably estimated from high-fidelity (unfiltered amplification) nasal pressure signals collected during clinical sleep studies. The main predictors of epiglottic collapse were abrupt discontinuity and jaggedness [84].

Snoring sound analysis has also been used to build a model for predicting the site of collapse and achieved an accuracy of 77% for discriminating hypopharyngeal collapse and an accuracy of 62% accuracy for all site-collapse [85]. With the increased number of sleep-related sensors and by consequent data volume, and utilization of waveform and audio Artificial Intelligence (AI) analysis, it is possible to foresee an adequate airway anatomic collapse description in the not so distant future in addition to the traditional metrics generated in a sleep test. Moreover, it was proposed that acoustic energy produced at the level of the hypopharynx, particularly tongue base and epiglottis, experience low frequency absorption. The effect would be to diminish the high amplitude transients by increased damping and to reduce the asymmetry extent [86]. It was also reported that after sound frequency analysis of different snoring sites, epiglottis snoring has a peak frequency of 490 hertz (Hz), while the vibrations at the tonsils and lateral pharyngeal wall have a peak frequency of 170 Hz [87]. Similarly, other studies supported that the frequency at the level of the tongue base and epiglottis tend to have an increase in pitch frequency in tongue base and epiglottis compared with soft palate [88].

Based on a recent metanalysis, bed/mattress-based and contact-free devices were shown to have a promising role for screening and monitoring OSA. While not selective for the level of collapse, bed/mattress-based devices showed a high sensitivity overall, as well as the best sensitivity in detecting moderate and severe cases [89]. With the use of real world data, sleep medicine physicians and surgeons are able to answer questions using artificial intelligence and machine learning [3]. Machine learning and deep learning approaches have gained traction in recent years for different tasks [90]. Some were used for classifying sleep–wake cycle [91].

Ultrasound imaging as a radiation-free tool has also been used to evaluate OSA severity and pathogenesis [92]. Tongue area measurements were significantly different between patients with varying severities of OSA during normal breathing and during Müller manoeuvre, and also differed in normal breathing and during the Müller manoeuvre. Patients with moderate or severe OSA exhibited minimal movement of the tongue, while subjects with mild OSA demonstrated bidirectional tongue motions during a transition from normal breathing to the Müller manoeuvre in wakefulness [92].

Snoring is a key symptom of OSA caused by upper airway collapse resulting in vibration of different tissues and turbulence in the airflow. Multiple trials have used snoring to characterize the site of obstruction, particularly in distinguishing tongue base from non-tongue base collapse [85, 87, 93]. Using simultaneous nasal flow and pharyngeal pressure recordings during natural sleep, Genta et al. classified the flow shape according to the degree of negative effort dependence (NED), defined as the reduction percentage in inspiratory flow from peak to midinspiratory flow with increasing respiratory effort. Epiglottic collapse showed to have a severe NED with abrupt termination of the inspiratory flow [83].

27.5 Conclusion

While DISE, and the use of the VOTE classification, have helped identify and phenotype airway collapse, the field of OSA is in need for non-invasive tools for diagnosis, monitoring, and long-term follow-up of our patients. Epiglottis collapse may contribute to failure of both non-surgical and surgical treatments, therefore identifying cases when it is a clinically relevant phenomenon and balance against the short- and long-term risks of treatment should be the goal to improve treatment outcomes. Future studies are directed towards the validation of new ways to monitor and identify characteristics of different levels of collapse.

References

1. Benjafield A Eastwood PR, Heinzer RC, Ip MS. Global prevalence of obstructive sleep apnea in adults: estimation using currently available data. In. San Diego, CA 2018.
2. Senaratna CV, Perret JL, Lodge CJ, et al. Prevalence of obstructive sleep apnea in the general population: a systematic review. Sleep Med Rev. 2017;34:70–81.
3. Abdelwahab M, Marques S, Previdelli I, Capasso R. Peri-operative antibiotic use in sleep surgery: clinical relevance. Otolaryngol Head Neck Surg. 2021;166:993.
4. Lyons OD, Bradley TD. Heart failure and sleep apnea. Can J Cardiol. 2015;31(7):898–908.
5. Ibrahim B, de Freitas Mendonca MI, Gombar S, Callahan A, Jung K, Capasso R. Association of Systemic Diseases with Surgical Treatment for obstructive sleep apnea compared with continuous positive airway pressure. JAMA Otolaryngol Head Neck Surg. 2021;147(4):329–35.
6. Sapina E, Torres G, Barbe F, Sanchez-de-la-Torre M. The use of precision medicine to manage obstructive sleep apnea treatment in patients with resistant hypertension: current evidence and future directions. Curr Hypertens Rep. 2018;20(7):60.
7. Gami AS, Howard DE, Olson EJ, Somers VK. Day-night pattern of sudden death in obstructive sleep apnea. N Engl J Med. 2005;352(12):1206–14.
8. Punjabi NM, Caffo BS, Goodwin JL, et al. Sleep-disordered breathing and mortality: a prospective cohort study. PLoS Med. 2009;6(8):e1000132.
9. Lee RW, Chan AS, Grunstein RR, Cistulli PA. Craniofacial phenotyping in obstructive sleep apnea--a novel quantitative photographic approach. Sleep. 2009;32(1):37–45.
10. Liu KH, Chu WC, To KW, et al. Sonographic measurement of lateral parapharyngeal wall thickness in patients with obstructive sleep apnea. Sleep. 2007;30(11):1503–8.
11. Owens RL, Edwards BA, Eckert DJ, et al. An integrative model of physiological traits can be used to predict obstructive sleep apnea and response to non positive airway pressure therapy. Sleep. 2015;38(6):961–70.
12. Efficacy of Maxillomandibular Advancement Examined with Drug-Induced Sleep Endoscopy and Computational Fluid Dynamics Airflow Modeling 2016.
13. Liu SYC, Huon LK, Powell NB, et al. Lateral Pharyngeal Wall tension after Maxillomandibular advancement for obstructive sleep apnea is a marker for surgical success: observations from drug-induced sleep endoscopy. J Oral Maxillofac Surg. 2015;73(8):1575–82.
14. Riley RW, Powell NB, Guilleminault C. Obstructive sleep apnea syndrome: a review of 306 consecutively treated surgical patients. Otolaryngol Head Neck Surg. 1993;108(2):117–25.
15. Riley RW, Powell NB, Guilleminault C, Nino-Murcia G. Maxillary, mandibular, and hyoid advancement: an alternative to tracheostomy in obstructive sleep apnea syndrome. Otolaryngol Head Neck Surg. 1986;94(5):584–8.
16. Liu SY, Awad M, Riley R, Capasso R. The role of the revised Stanford protocol in Today's precision medicine. Sleep Med Clin. 2019;14(1):99–107.

17. Altintas A, Yegin Y, Celik M, Kaya KH, Koc AK, Kayhan FT. Interobserver consistency of drug-induced sleep endoscopy in diagnosing obstructive sleep apnea using a VOTE classification system. J Craniofac Surg. 2018;29(2):e140–3.
18. Kezirian EJ, Hohenhorst W, de Vries N. Drug-induced sleep endoscopy: the VOTE classification. Eur Arch Otorhinolaryngol. 2011;268(8):1233–6.
19. Yegin Y, Celik M, Kaya KH, Koc AK, Kayhan FT. Comparison of drug-induced sleep endoscopy and Muller's maneuver in diagnosing obstructive sleep apnea using the VOTE classification system. Braz J Otorhinolaryngol. 2017;83(4):445–50.
20. Kent DT, Rogers R, Soose RJ. Drug-induced sedation endoscopy in the evaluation of OSA patients with incomplete Oral appliance therapy response. Otolaryngol Head Neck Surg. 2015;153(2):302–7.
21. Verse T, Pirsig W. Age-related changes in the epiglottis causing failure of nasal continuous positive airway pressure therapy. J Laryngol Otol. 1999;113(11):1022–5.
22. Kezirian EJ. Nonresponders to pharyngeal surgery for obstructive sleep apnea: insights from drug-induced sleep endoscopy. Laryngoscope. 2011;121(6):1320–6.
23. Holzki J, Brown KA, Carroll RG, Cote CJ. The anatomy of the pediatric airway: has our knowledge changed in 120 years? A review of historic and recent investigations of the anatomy of the pediatric larynx. Paediatr Anaesth. 2018;28(1):13–22.
24. Noordzij JP, Ossoff RH. Anatomy and physiology of the larynx. Otolaryngol Clin N Am. 2006;39(1):1–10.
25. Delakorda M, Ovsenik N. Epiglottis shape as a predictor of obstruction level in patients with sleep apnea. Sleep Breath. 2019;23(1):311–7.
26. Sung CM, Kim HC, Yang HC. The clinical characteristics of patients with an isolate epiglottic collapse. Auris Nasus Larynx. 2020;47(3):450–7.
27. Solomons NB, Prescott CA. Laryngomalacia. A review and the surgical management for severe cases. Int J Pediatr Otorhinolaryngol. 1987;13(1):31–9.
28. Thorne MC, Garetz SL. Laryngomalacia: review and summary of current clinical practice in 2015. Paediatr Respir Rev. 2016;17:3–8.
29. Sutherland K, Deane SA, Chan AS, et al. Comparative effects of two oral appliances on upper airway structure in obstructive sleep apnea. Sleep. 2011;34(4):469–77.
30. Safiruddin F, Koutsourelakis I, de Vries N. Analysis of the influence of head rotation during drug-induced sleep endoscopy in obstructive sleep apnea. Laryngoscope. 2014;124(9):2195–9.
31. Beelen A, Vonk PE, de Vries N. Drug-induced sleep endoscopy: the effect of different passive maneuvers on the distribution of collapse patterns of the upper airway in obstructive sleep apnea patients. Sleep Breath. 2018;22(4):909–17.
32. Vonk PE, Ravesloot MJL, Kasius KM, van Maanen JP, de Vries N. Floppy epiglottis during drug-induced sleep endoscopy: an almost complete resolution by adopting the lateral posture. Sleep Breath. 2020;24(1):103–9.
33. Kwon OE, Jung SY, Al-Dilaijan K, Min JY, Lee KH, Kim SW. Is epiglottis surgery necessary for obstructive sleep apnea patients with epiglottis obstruction? Laryngoscope. 2019;129(11):2658–62.
34. Mickelson SA, Rosenthal L. Midline glossectomy and epiglottidectomy for obstructive sleep apnea syndrome. Laryngoscope. 1997;107(5):614–9.
35. Salamanca F, Leone F, Bianchi A, Bellotto RGS, Costantini F, Salvatori P. Surgical treatment of epiglottis collapse in obstructive sleep apnoea syndrome: epiglottis stiffening operation. Acta Otorhinolaryngol Ital. 2019;39(6):404–8.
36. Safiruddin F, Koutsourelakis I, de Vries N. Upper airway collapse during drug induced sleep endoscopy: head rotation in supine position compared with lateral head and trunk position. Eur Arch Otorhinolaryngol. 2015;272(2):485–8.
37. Victores AJ, Hamblin J, Gilbert J, Switzer C, Takashima M. Usefulness of sleep endoscopy in predicting positional obstructive sleep apnea. Otolaryngol Head Neck Surg. 2014;150(3):487–93.

38. Hybaskova J, Jor O, Novak V, Zelenik K, Matousek P, Kominek P. Drug-induced sleep endoscopy changes the treatment concept in patients with obstructive sleep Apnoea. Biomed Res Int. 2016;2016:6583216.
39. Arora A, Chaidas K, Garas G, et al. Outcome of TORS to tongue base and epiglottis in patients with OSA intolerant of conventional treatment. Sleep Breath. 2016;20(2):739–47.
40. Huang GJ, Luo MS, Chen MZ, Chen GP, Fu MY. Exploration of transoral robotic surgery in the treatment of pediatric obstructive sleep apnea-hypopnea syndrome. Lin Chung Er Bi Yan Hou Tou Jing Wai Ke Za Zhi. 2017;31(22):1782–4.
41. Lin HS, Rowley JA, Badr MS, et al. Transoral robotic surgery for treatment of obstructive sleep apnea-hypopnea syndrome. Laryngoscope. 2013;123(7):1811–6.
42. Gazayerli M, Bleibel W, Elhorr A, Maxwell D, Seifeldin R. A correlation between the shape of the epiglottis and obstructive sleep apnea. Surg Endosc. 2006;20(5):836–7.
43. Cotton RT, Richardson MA. Congenital laryngeal anomalies. Otolaryngol Clin N Am. 1981;14(1):203–18.
44. Faria J, Behar P. Medical and surgical management of congenital laryngomalacia: a case-control study. Otolaryngol Head Neck Surg. 2014;151(5):845–51.
45. Holinger LD, Konior RJ. Surgical management of severe laryngomalacia. Laryngoscope. 1989;99(2):136–42.
46. Kavanagh KT, Babin RW. Endoscopic surgical management for laryngomalacia. Case report and review of the literature. Ann Otol Rhinol Laryngol. 1987;96(6):650–3.
47. Lv Y, Huang Q, Lv J, Wu H. Surgical management for severe congenital laryngomalacia: 16 consecutive cases. Lin Chung Er Bi Yan Hou Tou Jing Wai Ke Za Zhi. 2013;27(9):475–8.
48. Richter GT, Thompson DM. The surgical management of laryngomalacia. Otolaryngol Clin N Am. 2008;41(5):837–64. vii
49. Toynton SC, Saunders MW, Bailey CM. Aryepiglottoplasty for laryngomalacia: 100 consecutive cases. J Laryngol Otol. 2001;115(1):35–8.
50. Lee CF, Hsu WC, Lee CH, Lin MT, Kang KT. Treatment outcomes of supraglottoplasty for pediatric obstructive sleep apnea: a meta-analysis. Int J Pediatr Otorhinolaryngol. 2016;87:18–27.
51. Martinez-Garcia MA, Capote F, Campos-Rodriguez F, et al. Effect of CPAP on blood pressure in patients with obstructive sleep apnea and resistant hypertension: the HIPARCO randomized clinical trial. JAMA. 2013;310(22):2407–15.
52. Penzel T, Riedl M, Gapelyuk A, et al. Effect of CPAP therapy on daytime cardiovascular regulations in patients with obstructive sleep apnea. Comput Biol Med. 2012;42(3):328–34.
53. Vlachantoni IT, Dikaiakou E, Antonopoulos CN, Stefanadis C, Daskalopoulou SS, Petridou ET. Effects of continuous positive airway pressure (CPAP) treatment for obstructive sleep apnea in arterial stiffness: a meta-analysis. Sleep Med Rev. 2013;17(1):19–28.
54. Dedhia RC, Rosen CA, Soose RJ. What is the role of the larynx in adult obstructive sleep apnea? Laryngoscope. 2014;124(4):1029–34.
55. Shimohata T, Shinoda H, Nakayama H, et al. Daytime hypoxemia, sleep-disordered breathing, and laryngopharyngeal findings in multiple system atrophy. Arch Neurol. 2007;64(6):856–61.
56. Chetty KG, Kadifa F, Berry RB, Mahutte CK. Acquired laryngomalacia as a cause of obstructive sleep apnea. Chest. 1994;106(6):1898–9.
57. Andersen AP, Alving J, Lildholdt T, Wulff CH. Obstructive sleep apnea initiated by a lax epiglottis. A contraindication for continuous positive airway pressure. Chest. 1987;91(4):621–3.
58. Lin HC, Friedman M, Chang HW, Gurpinar B. The efficacy of multilevel surgery of the upper airway in adults with obstructive sleep apnea/hypopnea syndrome. Laryngoscope. 2008;118(5):902–8.
59. Richard W, Kox D, den Herder C, van Tinteren H, de Vries N. One stage multilevel surgery (uvulopalatopharyngoplasty, hyoid suspension, radiofrequent ablation of the tongue base with/without genioglossus advancement), in obstructive sleep apnea syndrome. Eur Arch Otorhinolaryngol. 2007;264(4):439–44.
60. Verse T, Baisch A, Maurer JT, Stuck BA, Hormann K. Multilevel surgery for obstructive sleep apnea: short-term results. Otolaryngol Head Neck Surg. 2006;134(4):571–7.

61. Kotecha BT, Hannan SA, Khalil HM, Georgalas C, Bailey P. Sleep nasendoscopy: a 10-year retrospective audit study. Eur Arch Otorhinolaryngol. 2007;264(11):1361–7.
62. Schwab RJ, Gefter WB, Hoffman EA, Gupta KB, Pack AI. Dynamic upper airway imaging during awake respiration in normal subjects and patients with sleep disordered breathing. Am Rev Respir Dis. 1993;148(5):1385–400.
63. Catalfumo FJ, Golz A, Westerman ST, Gilbert LM, Joachims HZ, Goldenberg D. The epiglottis and obstructive sleep apnoea syndrome. J Laryngol Otol. 1998;112(10):940–3.
64. Kanemaru S, Kojima H, Fukushima H, et al. A case of floppy epiglottis in adult: a simple surgical remedy. Auris Nasus Larynx. 2007;34(3):409–11.
65. Harries PG, Randall CJ. Adult floppy epiglottis: a simple surgical remedy. J Laryngol Otol. 1995;109(9):871–2.
66. Oluwasanmi AF, Mal RK. Diathermy epiglottectomy: endoscopic technique. J Laryngol Otol. 2001;115(4):289–92.
67. Golz A, Goldenberg D, Westerman ST, et al. Laser partial epiglottidectomy as a treatment for obstructive sleep apnea and laryngomalacia. Ann Otol Rhinol Laryngol. 2000;109(12 Pt 1):1140–5.
68. Toh ST, Han HJ, Tay HN, Kiong KL. Transoral robotic surgery for obstructive sleep apnea in Asian patients: a Singapore sleep Centre experience. JAMA Otolaryngol Head Neck Surg. 2014;140(7):624–9.
69. Rastatter JC, Schroeder JW, Hoff SR, Holinger LD. Aspiration before and after Supraglottoplasty regardless of technique. Int J Otolaryngol. 2010;2010:1.
70. Schroeder JW Jr, Thakkar KH, Poznanovic SA, Holinger LD. Aspiration following CO(2) laser-assisted supraglottoplasty. Int J Pediatr Otorhinolaryngol. 2008;72(7):985–90.
71. Sorrenti G, Piccin O, Mondini S, Ceroni AR. One-phase management of severe obstructive sleep apnea: tongue base reduction with hyoepiglottoplasty plus uvulopalatopharyngoplasty. Otolaryngol Head Neck Surg. 2006;135(6):906–10.
72. Bahgat A, Bahgat Y. Robo-cob technique; transoral endoscopic coblation tongue base resection in obstructive sleep apnea patients. Sleep Breath. 2021;25(1):411–5.
73. Bourolias C, Hajiioannou J, Sobol E, Velegrakis G, Helidonis E. Epiglottis reshaping using CO2 laser: a minimally invasive technique and its potent applications. Head Face Med. 2008;4:15.
74. Heiser C, Edenharter G, Bas M, Wirth M, Hofauer B. Palatoglossus coupling in selective upper airway stimulation. Laryngoscope. 2017;127(10):E378–83.
75. Roger G, Denoyelle F, Triglia JM, Garabedian EN. Severe laryngomalacia: surgical indications and results in 115 patients. Laryngoscope. 1995;105(10):1111–7.
76. Zalzal GH, Anon JB, Cotton RT. Epiglottoplasty for the treatment of laryngomalacia. Ann Otol Rhinol Laryngol. 1987;96(1 Pt 1):72–6.
77. Groblewski JC, Shah RK, Zalzal GH. Microdebrider-assisted supraglottoplasty for laryngomalacia. Ann Otol Rhinol Laryngol. 2009;118(8):592–7.
78. Zalzal GH, Collins WO. Microdebrider-assisted supraglottoplasty. Int J Pediatr Otorhinolaryngol. 2005;69(3):305–9.
79. Seid AB, Park SM, Kearns MJ, Gugenheim S. Laser division of the aryepiglottic folds for severe laryngomalacia. Int J Pediatr Otorhinolaryngol. 1985;10(2):153–8.
80. Free C, Phillips G, Felix L, Galli L, Patel V, Edwards P. The effectiveness of M-health technologies for improving health and health services: a systematic review protocol. BMC Res Notes. 2010;3:250.
81. Yu MS, Ibrahim B, Riley RW, Liu SY. Maxillomandibular advancement and upper airway stimulation: Extrapharyngeal surgery for obstructive sleep apnea. Clin Exp Otorhinolaryngol. 2020;13(3):225–33.
82. Crinion SJ, Tiron R, Lyon G, et al. Ambulatory detection of sleep apnea using a non-contact biomotion sensor. J Sleep Res. 2020;29(1):e12889.
83. Genta PR, Sands SA, Butler JP, et al. Airflow shape is associated with the pharyngeal structure causing OSA. Chest. 2017;152(3):537–46.

84. Azarbarzin A, Marques M, Sands SA, et al. Predicting epiglottic collapse in patients with obstructive sleep apnoea. Eur Respir J. 2017;50(3):1700345.
85. Sebastian A, Cistulli PA, Cohen G, de Chazal P. Automated identification of the predominant site of upper airway collapse in obstructive sleep apnoea patients using snore signal. Physiol Meas. 2020;41(9):095005.
86. Beeton RJ, Wells I, Ebden P, Whittet HB, Clarke J. Snore site discrimination using statistical moments of free field snoring sounds recorded during sleep nasendoscopy. Physiol Meas. 2007;28(10):1225–36.
87. Agrawal S, Stone P, McGuinness K, Morris J, Camilleri AE. Sound frequency analysis and the site of snoring in natural and induced sleep. Clin Otolaryngol Allied Sci. 2002;27(3):162–6.
88. Won TB, Kim SY, Lee WH, et al. Acoustic characteristics of snoring according to obstruction site determined by sleep videofluoroscopy. Acta Otolaryngol. 2012;132(Suppl 1):S13–20.
89. Rosa T, Bellardi K, Viana A Jr, Ma Y, Capasso R. Digital health and sleep-disordered breathing: a systematic review and meta-analysis. J Clin Sleep Med. 2018;14(9):1605–20.
90. Perez-Pozuelo I, Zhai B, Palotti J, et al. The future of sleep health: a data-driven revolution in sleep science and medicine. NPJ Digit Med. 2020;3:42.
91. Binder S, Baier PC, Molle M, Inostroza M, Born J, Marshall L. Sleep enhances memory consolidation in the hippocampus-dependent object-place recognition task in rats. Neurobiol Learn Mem. 2012;97(2):213–9.
92. Manlises CO, Chen JW, Huang CC. Dynamic tongue area measurements in ultrasound images for adults with obstructive sleep apnea. J Sleep Res. 2020;29(4):e13032.
93. Qian K, Janott C, Pandit V, et al. Classification of the excitation location of snore sounds in the upper airway by acoustic multifeature analysis. IEEE Trans Biomed Eng. 2017;64(8):1731–41.

GPSR Compliance

The European Union's (EU) General Product Safety Regulation (GPSR) is a set of rules that requires consumer products to be safe and our obligations to ensure this.

If you have any concerns about our products, you can contact us on ProductSafety@springernature.com

In case Publisher is established outside the EU, the EU authorized representative is:

Springer Nature Customer Service Center GmbH
Europaplatz 3
69115 Heidelberg, Germany

Batch number: 10732031

Printed by Printforce, the Netherlands